T0336530

Investment Framework for Nutrition 2024

Scan the QR code to see all titles in this series.

HUMAN DEVELOPMENT PERSPECTIVES

Investment Framework for Nutrition 2024

Meera Shekar
Kyoko Shibata Okamura
Mireya Vilar-Compte
Chiara Dell'Aira

Editors

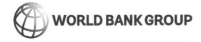 **WORLD BANK GROUP**

© 2024 International Bank for Reconstruction and Development / The World Bank
1818 H Street NW, Washington, DC 20433
Telephone: 202-473-1000; Internet: www.worldbank.org

Some rights reserved

1 2 3 4   27 26 25 24

This work is a product of the staff of The World Bank with external contributions. The findings, interpretations, and conclusions expressed in this work do not necessarily reflect the views of The World Bank, its Board of Executive Directors, or the governments they represent.

The World Bank does not guarantee the accuracy, completeness, or currency of the data included in this work and does not assume responsibility for any errors, omissions, or discrepancies in the information, or liability with respect to the use of or failure to use the information, methods, processes, or conclusions set forth. The boundaries, colors, denominations, links/footnotes, and other information shown in this work do not imply any judgment on the part of The World Bank concerning the legal status of any territory or the endorsement or acceptance of such boundaries. The citation of works authored by others does not mean The World Bank endorses the views expressed by those authors or the content of their works.

Nothing herein shall constitute or be construed or considered to be a limitation upon or waiver of the privileges and immunities of The World Bank, all of which are specifically reserved.

Rights and Permissions

This work is available under the Creative Commons Attribution 3.0 IGO license (CC BY 3.0 IGO) http://creativecommons.org/licenses/by/3.0/igo. Under the Creative Commons Attribution license, you are free to copy, distribute, transmit, and adapt this work, including for commercial purposes, under the following conditions:

Attribution—Please cite the work as follows: Shekar, Meera, Kyoko Shibata Okamura, Mireya Vilar-Compte, and Chiara Dell'Aira, eds. 2024. *Investment Framework for Nutrition 2024*. Human Development Perspectives. Washington, DC: World Bank. doi:10.1596/978-1-2162-2. License: Creative Commons Attribution CC BY 3.0 IGO

Translations—If you create a translation of this work, please add the following disclaimer along with the attribution: *This translation was not created by The World Bank and should not be considered an official World Bank translation. The World Bank shall not be liable for any content or error in this translation.*

Adaptations—If you create an adaptation of this work, please add the following disclaimer along with the attribution: *This is an adaptation of an original work by The World Bank. Views and opinions expressed in the adaptation are the sole responsibility of the author or authors of the adaptation and are not endorsed by The World Bank.*

Third-party content—The World Bank does not necessarily own each component of the content contained within the work. The World Bank therefore does not warrant that the use of any third-party-owned individual component or part contained in the work will not infringe on the rights of those third parties. The risk of claims resulting from such infringement rests solely with you. If you wish to re-use a component of the work, it is your responsibility to determine whether permission is needed for that re-use and to obtain permission from the copyright owner. Examples of components can include, but are not limited to, tables, figures, or images.

All queries on rights and licenses should be addressed to World Bank Publications, The World Bank, 1818 H Street NW, Washington, DC 20433, USA; e-mail: pubrights@worldbank.org.

ISBN (paper): 978-1-4648-2162-2
ISBN (electronic): 978-1-4648-2163-9
SKU: 212162
DOI: 10.1596/978-1-4648-2162-2

Cover photo: © Lucian Coman / Shutterstock. Used with the permission of Lucian Coman / Shutterstock. Further permission required for reuse.

Cover and interior design: Bill Pragluski, Critical Stages, Inc.

Library of Congress Control Number: 2024919325.

Human Development Perspectives

The books in this series address main and emerging development issues of a global/regional nature through original research and findings in the areas of education, gender, health, nutrition, population, and social protection and jobs. The series is aimed at policy makers and area experts and is overseen by the Human Development Practice Group chief economist.

Previous titles in this series

Feng Zhao, Rialda Kovacevic, David Bishai, and Jeff Weintraub, eds. *Strategic Investment for Health System Resilience: A Three-Layer Framework* (2024).

Magdalena Bendini and Amanda E. Devercelli (eds.), *Quality Early Learning: Nurturing Children's Potential* (2022).

Margaret Grosh, Phillippe Leite, Matthew Wai-Poi, and Emil Tesliuc (eds.), *Revisiting Targeting in Social Assistance: A New Look at Old Dilemmas* (2022).

Feng Zhao, Clemens Benedikt, and David Wilson (eds.), *Tackling the World's Fastest-Growing HIV Epidemic: More Efficient HIV Responses in Eastern Europe and Central Asia* (2020).

Meera Shekar and Barry Popkin (eds.), *Obesity: Health and Economic Consequences of an Impending Global Challenge* (2020).

Truman Packard, Ugo Gentilini, Margaret Grosh, Philip O'Keefe, Robert Palacios, David Robalino, and Indhira Santos, *Protecting All: Risk Sharing for a Diverse and Diversifying World of Work* (2019).

Damien de Walque (ed.), *Risking Your Health: Causes, Consequences, and Interventions to Prevent Risky Behaviors* (2014).

Rita Almeida, Jere Behrman, and David Robalino (eds.), *The Right Skills for the Job? Rethinking Training Policies for Workers* (2012).

Barbara Bruns, Deon Filmer, and Harry Anthony Patrinos, *Making Schools Work: New Evidence on Accountability Reforms* (2011).

Harold Alderman (ed.), *No Small Matter: The Impact of Poverty, Shocks, and Human Capital Investments in Early Childhood Development* (2011).

All books in the Human Development Perspectives series are available at https://openknowledge.worldbank.org/handle/10986/2161.

Contents

Boxes

Figures

Maps

Tables

Foreword

With only six years remaining until the Sustainable Development Goals (SDGs) end line of 2030, the world stands at a critical juncture. Central to the World Bank Group's commitment to eliminate extreme poverty on a livable planet is the recognition of the vital role nutrition plays in fostering sustainable development and building human capital. Despite significant progress on SDG 2.2 over the past decades, recent crises, compounded by climate change and conflicts, have exacerbated food insecurity, malnutrition, and poverty.

Child stunting, wasting, anemia, obesity, low birthweight, and maternal anemia persist at alarming rates, especially in lower- and middle-income countries in which more than 148 million children are still stunted and 1 in 3 women is anemic. These trends jeopardize future human capital and economic productivity and significantly increase the risk of poor learning outcomes, illness, death, and rising health care cost burdens.

Nutrition serves as both a maker and a marker of human capital, with both undernutrition and obesity significantly affecting it. The Human Capital Index paints a bleak picture of future economic productivity in the developing world, with scores below 0.40 in most African nations and hovering around 0.48 in South Asia, which means that children in Africa and South Asia will grow up to be only 40 or 48 percent as productive as they could be, respectively.

Unlike many other development investments, investments in nutrition are durable, inalienable, and portable. They are durable because investments made during the critical first 1,000 days of a child's life last a lifetime. They are inalienable and portable because they belong to the child regardless of their location or circumstances. They are among the most effective tools for sustainable development, offering a return of $23 for every $1 invested.

Building on the 2017 Investment Framework for Nutrition, this report updates the latest evidence and serves as a comprehensive guide to the most effective interventions and policy measures to improve nutrition outcomes. It emphasizes the importance of multisectoral approaches and brings in interactions with gender and climate. Additionally, it complements previous financing estimates with important new approaches to innovative financing, such as repurposing agrifood subsidies for healthier and more sustainable options, thereby enhancing nutrition and climate co-benefits. The report serves as a key guide for domestic and official development assistance commitments in the lead-up to the global Nutrition for Growth summit to be hosted by the government of France in March 2025. It also informs the implementation of the World Bank Group's new Food and Nutrition Security (FNS) Global Challenge Program, laying a robust foundation for addressing three interconnected issues: enhancing FNS crisis prevention, preparedness, and response mechanisms; promoting innovative, high-impact cross-sectoral solutions to improve nutrition outcomes; and scaling low-emissions, climate-resilient food systems. These action areas provide powerful, scalable solutions that can be implemented across countries, leveraging the World Bank Group's unique capacity to mobilize public, private, and philanthropic financing for development.

Mamta Murthi
Vice President, Human Development

Acknowledgments

This publication was led by Meera Shekar, Kyoko Shibata Okamura, Mireya Vilar-Compte, and Chiara Dell'Aira. The report benefited from substantial inputs and support from the American Institutes for Research (AIR), Burnet Institute in Australia, Research Center for Equitable Development (EQUDE) at Universidad Iberoamericana, Results for Development (R4D) Institute, Stronger Foundations for Nutrition, Alive & Thrive, and Northwestern University. Financial support for this work was provided by the Bill and Melinda Gates Foundation (BMGF) and the government of Japan through the World Bank Nutrition Multi-Donor Trust Fund for Scaling Up Nutrition.

Hoa Thi Mai Nguyen (World Bank), Nick Scott (Burnet Institute), and Michelle Mehta (World Bank) were lead authors on chapters 2, 7, and 8, respectively, and Jonathan Kweku Akuoku, Mia Blakstad, Lisa Shireen Saldanha, Kate Mandeville, Libby Hattersley, Felipe Dizon, Ali Winoto Subandoro, and Mary D'Alimonte (R4D) coauthored one or more of the chapters, laying the groundwork for this work's broad scope and depth.

The following colleagues contributed to relevant chapters: Stephen Geoffrey Dorey, Loreta Rufo, and the Climate and Health team, as well as Anne Marie Provo, Chris Jackson, and Francis Addeah Darko of the World Bank (chapter 4); Claire Chase of the World Bank, Thomas de Hoop and the team at AIR, Sonia Hernandez-Cordero, Pablo Gaitán-Rossi and the EQUDE team at Universidad Iberoamericana, Sera Young of Northwestern University, and Roger Mathisen of the Alive & Thrive team (chapter 5); Reem Alsukait, Christopher Herbst, Ceren Ozer, Danielle Bloom, Norman Maldonado, Roberto Iunes, Yu Shibui, and Kajali Paintal Goswami of the World Bank, as well as Elisa Cadena at the Research Center on Health Economics and Social Protection, Universidad Icesi (chapter 6); Camila Corvalán and Marcela Reyes of the University of Chile, Fernando Mediano of the

Catholic University of Chile, and Cristián Cofre of the Chilean Ministry of Health (chapter 7); Anne Marie Provo and Rogers Ayiko of the World Bank (chapter 8); and Abbe McCarter and Caroline Andridge from R4D, as well as Emily Custer at the Stronger Foundations for Nutrition (chapter 9).

The report greatly benefited from thoughtful comments provided by peer reviewers: Afshan Khan, coordinator of the Scaling Up Nutrition Movement; Rahul Rawat (BMGF); Abigail Perry (World Food Program); Saul Guerrero Oteyza (United Nations Children's Fund [UNICEF]); and Jed Friedman (World Bank). Kathryn Dewey (University of California, Davis), Emanuela Galasso (World Bank), Helena Guarin (European Commission [EC]), Heather McBride (Canada), Lynette Neufeld (Food and Agriculture Organization of the United Nations [FAO]), and Purnima Menon (International Food Policy Research Institute [IFPRI]) provided additional valuable comments. The authors extend their deepest gratitude to the members of the Technical Advisory Group (TAG) and Policy Advisory Group (PAG) for their invaluable contributions to guiding this work. PAG members were Afshan Khan (Scaling Up Nutrition [SUN]), Helena Guarin (EC), Heather McBride (Global Affairs Canada); TAG members were Anna Hakobyan (Children's Investment Fund Foundation [CIFF]), Augustin Flory (consultant), Avani Kapur (Center for Policy Research, India), Emanuela Galasso (World Bank), Felipe Dizon (World Bank), George Ouma (African Development Bank), Jed Friedman (World Bank), Kathryn Dewey (University of California, Davis), Lynnette Neufeld (FAO), Paddy Wilmott (Foreign, Commonwealth and Development Office), Purnima Menon (IFPRI), Rahul Rawat (BMGF), and Victor Aguayo (UNICEF). Emanuela Galasso, Kathryn Dewey, and Rahul Rawat went beyond the call of duty to support the team with a careful review of the evidence base.

Many thanks are due to Juan Pablo Uribe (director, Health, Nutrition and Population/Global Financing Facility, World Bank) for chairing the TAG/PAG meetings and the decision meeting and to Norbert Schady (chief economist, Human Development, World Bank) for his careful review and advice in finalizing the report.

The team thanks Michael R. Fisher for his incredibly skilled editing and David Lloyd for preparing the excellent graphics. Kathie Porta Baker was the copy editor. Jewel McFadden served as the acquisitions officer, Mary Fisk managed the production process, and Orlando Mota handled the printing and electronic file preparation.

Last, the team expresses their sincere appreciation to all those who have contributed to this report. Their insights and expertise have been crucial in enriching the content and depth of this report, and each of them is a co-owner of this report.

About the Editors and Contributors

About the Editors

Chiara Dell'Aira is a nutrition specialist (Young Professional) in the Health, Nutrition, and Population Global Practice at the World Bank. She provides technical and analytical support to large-scale nutrition projects through research and global engagement activities and works with multidisciplinary teams on the intersections of nutrition with climate, agriculture, gender, and food security. Before working with the World Bank, she worked with the Pan American Health Organization, academia, and nongovernmental organizations. She holds an MSc in global health from the University of Copenhagen.

Kyoko Shibata Okamura is a senior nutrition specialist in the Health, Nutrition, and Population Global Practice at the World Bank. Building on her extensive experience in managing large-scale nutrition programs in countries such as Ethiopia and Nepal, she has more recently been working on nutrition financing, healthy diet, and food systems. She has a master's degree in health sciences in human nutrition from the Johns Hopkins Bloomberg School of Public Health.

Meera Shekar is global lead for nutrition in the Health, Nutrition, and Population Global Practice at the World Bank. She has lived and worked across the globe and has extensive operational experience in Africa, East Asia, Latin America, the Middle East, and South Asia. Before joining the World Bank, she worked with UNICEF in Ethiopia, the Philippines, and Tanzania. She has a PhD in international nutrition, epidemiology, and population studies from Cornell University.

Mireya Vilar-Compte is a senior nutrition consultant in the Health, Nutrition, and Population Global Practice at the World Bank and an associate professor in public health (on leave) at Montclair State University. She specializes in global public health with an emphasis on maternal and child health and nutrition. She has led research grants and consultancies across the globe with national, international, and not-for-profit organizations. She has a PhD in health policy from New York University.

About the Chapter Authors

Jonathan Kweku Akuoku is a nutrition specialist in the Health, Nutrition, and Population Global Practice at the World Bank.

Mia Blakstad is a social protection specialist in the Social Protection and Jobs Global Practice at the World Bank.

Mary D'Alimonte is a program director at the Results for Development Institute.

Felipe Dizon is a senior economist in the Agriculture and Food Global Practice at the World Bank.

Libby Hattersley is a consultant in the Health, Nutrition, and Population Global Practice at the World Bank.

Kate Mandeville is a senior health specialist in the Health, Nutrition, and Population Global Practice at the World Bank.

Michelle Mehta is a nutrition specialist in the Health, Nutrition, and Population Global Practice at the World Bank.

Hoa Thi Mai Nguyen is a nutrition specialist consultant in the Health, Nutrition, and Population Global Practice at the World Bank.

Lisa Shareen Saldanha is a senior nutrition specialist in the Health, Nutrition, and Population Global Practice at the World Bank.

Nick Scott is the head of modeling and biostatistics at the Burnet Institute.

Ali Winoto Subandoro is a senior nutrition specialist in the Health, Nutrition, and Population Global Practice at the World Bank.

Glossary

Adult overweight and obesity refers to an individual age 18 years or older with a body mass index (BMI) of 25 kilograms per square meter (kg/m²) or higher. Within this range, a BMI of 25 to less than 30 kg/m² is classified as overweight, and a BMI of 30 kg/m² or higher is considered obesity. Obesity severity is categorized into three classes: class 1 for a BMI of 30 to less than 35 kg/m², class 2 for a BMI of 35 to less than 40 kg/m², and class 3 for a BMI of 40 kg/m² or higher.

Anemia in pregnant women and children younger than age five years is defined as a hemoglobin concentration less than 110 grams per liter (g/L) at sea level, and anemia in nonpregnant women is defined as a hemoglobin concentration less than 120 g/L. The current WHO thresholds for mild, moderate, and severe anemia are 110–119, 80–109, and less than 80 g/L, respectively, for nonpregnant women and 100–109, 70–99, and less than 70 g/L, respectively, for pregnant women. The hemoglobin concentration cutoff points may differ by age, gender, physiological status, smoking habits, and altitude at which the population being assessed lives.

A **benefit–cost ratio** summarizes the overall value of a project or proposal. It is the ratio of the benefits of a project or proposal, expressed in monetary terms, relative to its costs, also expressed in monetary terms. The benefit–cost ratio takes into account the amount of monetary gain realized by implementing a project versus the amount it costs to execute the project. The higher the ratio, the better the investment. A general rule is that if the benefit from a project is greater than its cost, the project is a good investment.

Child overweight and obesity refers to a child who is too heavy for their height. Child overweight and obesity is measured as a percentage of children ages 0 to 59 months who are above 2 standard deviations from median weight for height according to the WHO Child Growth Standards.

Child stunting refers to a child who is too short for their age and is the result of chronic or recurrent malnutrition. Stunting is measured as a percentage of children ages 0 to 59 months who are below –2 standard deviations from median height for age according to the World Health Organization (WHO) Child Growth Standards.

Child wasting refers to a child who is too thin for their height. Wasting is the result of recent rapid weight loss or the failure to gain weight. Wasting is measured as a percentage of children ages 0 to 59 months who are below –2 standard deviations from median weight for height of the WHO Child Growth Standards.

Complementary feeding refers to the process of introducing solid and semisolid foods to an infant's diet in addition to breast milk to meet the nutritional requirements of the infant, typically starting around age six months.

Cost–benefit analysis is an approach to economic analysis that weighs the cost of an intervention against its benefits. The approach involves assigning a monetary value to the benefits of an intervention and estimating the expected present value of the net benefits, known as the net present value. Net benefits are the difference between the cost and monetary value of benefits of the intervention. The net present value is defined mathematically as

$$Net\ present\ value = \sum_{t=1}^{T} \frac{C_t}{(1+r)^t} - C_0$$

where C_t is net cash inflows, C_0 is the initial investment, the index t is the time period, and r is the discount rate. A positive net present value, when discounted at appropriate rates, indicates that the present value of cash inflows (benefits) exceeds the present value of cash outflows (cost of financing). Interventions with net present values that are at least as high as alternative interventions provide greater benefits than interventions with net present values equal to or lower than alternatives. The results of cost–benefit analysis can also be expressed in terms of the benefit–cost ratio.

Double burden of malnutrition refers to the coexistence of undernutrition (wasting, stunting, and micronutrient deficiencies) along with overweight and obesity and diet-related noncommunicable diseases within individuals, households, and populations throughout life.

Exclusive breastfeeding refers to when an infant receives only breast milk for the first six months of life and no other foods or liquids are provided, including water.

Low birthweight refers to a weight at birth of less than 2,500 grams or 5.5 pounds regardless of gestational age.

Maternal short stature refers to a mother with height less than 145 centimeters (cm).

Syndemic refers to two or more diseases that co-occur, interacting synergistically, with common societal drivers. In the context of this book, *syndemic* is used to refer to the coexisting and interacting pandemics of obesity, undernutrition, and climate change, referred to as the *global syndemic* by the Lancet Commission.

Executive Summary

Introduction

With only six years remaining until the Sustainable Development Goals (SDGs) end date of 2030, the world is at a pivotal moment. Despite a commendable 44 percent decrease in child stunting rates between 1990 and 2022, a staggering 148 million children worldwide are still stunted. Wasting and low birthweight (LBW) remain stubbornly high; 45 million children suffered from wasting in 2022, and 1 in 7 children were born with LBW in 2020. The rate of anemia is increasing, affecting 3 in 10 women globally. Concurrently, obesity rates are also increasing across the globe. In 2022, approximately 45 percent of adults were overweight or obese, with more than 70 percent of those individuals living in low- and middle-income countries (LMICs).

Nutrition is a marker of human capital, and both undernutrition and obesity are key contributors to the Human Capital Index. This index paints a bleak picture of future economic productivity in low-income countries (LICs) and middle-income countries (MICs); most African nations score below 0.40 and South Asia hovers around 0.48, which means that children in Africa and South Asia will grow up to be only 40 percent or 48 percent, respectively, as productive as they could be.

In 2017, *An Investment Framework for Nutrition* (Shekar et al. 2017) focused on the global SDG target 2.2, addressing child stunting and wasting among children younger than age five and breastfeeding and anemia among women. By aligning financing needs with potential for impact, the framework provided the foundation for transformative investments and donor and country commitments at the 2021 Tokyo Nutrition for Growth (N4G) summit. This report builds on this foundation, expanding its scope to include LBW and obesity and integrating critical policy guidance with gender and climate change. It serves as a compendium of cost-effective, evidence-based investments and policy measures for countries to draw on and as a key resource for the commitments forthcoming at the 2025 N4G summit in France.

In its pursuit of a world free of poverty and a livable planet, the World Bank has identified food and nutrition security as one of six priority global challenges. This report aligns with the new Global Challenge Program on Food and Nutrition Security (FNS) and provides a powerful evidence base for three interconnected action areas: scaling up (1) FNS crisis prevention, preparedness, and response; (2) innovative, high-impact cross-sectoral nutrition solutions; and (3) low-emissions and climate-resilient food systems with an eye toward mobilizing private sector resources for this agenda.

The Evidence

Prenatal Interventions

Iron and iron–folic acid (I/IFA) supplementation during pregnancy is linked to significant reductions (49 percent) in maternal anemia. Multiple micronutrient supplements (MMS) outperform I/IFA by reducing LBW by 12–15 percent and small-for-gestational age births by 7–12 percent. MMS significantly decrease stillbirths by 9 percent. Calcium supplementation in LMICs during pregnancy has a pronounced effect on the risk of preeclampsia (reducing it by 48 percent) and on birth outcomes, including a reduction in LBW and preterm births (by 16 percent and 47 percent, respectively). Intermittent preventive treatment of malaria in pregnancy using sulfadoxine–pyrimethamine (IPTp-SP) remains effective and has positive impacts, including a 10 percent reduction in maternal anemia and a 21 percent reduction in risk of LBW. Maternity leave is associated with increased breastfeeding duration and increased probability of exclusive breastfeeding.

Interventions Targeting Children

Delayed cord clamping at birth is associated with increased total hemoglobin after birth (from 1.6 to 2.4 g/dL higher) among infants and significant reductions in anemia (by 8 percent among children ages 6–12 months), but more research is needed to understand its long-term protection and implementation in LMICs. Kangaroo mother care (KMC) significantly reduces neonatal mortality (by 32 percent), all-cause mortality (by 35 percent by 2 months and 25 percent by 6 months), and severe infection and sepsis (by 15 percent). It improves early breastfeeding initiation (2.6 days earlier), exclusive breastfeeding (by 52 percent at discharge or at 28 days), and growth. Vitamin A supplementation in children ages 6–59 months reduces all-cause mortality and diarrhea incidence (by 12 percent and 15 percent, respectively). Prophylactic zinc reduces the incidence of diarrhea among children ages 1–59 months by 9 percent. Small-quantity lipid-based nutrient supplements (SQ-LNS) are strongly associated with reductions in stunting (by 12 percent), severe stunting (by 17 percent), wasting (by 14 percent), severe wasting (by 31 percent), anemia (by 16–34 percent), and all-cause mortality (by 27 percent) among children ages 6–24 months. Interventions focused on breastfeeding counseling and education significantly increase reported rates of early initiation by 20 percent and are linked to a 100 percent improvement in reported exclusive breastfeeding rates, with corresponding reductions in projected diarrhea incidence rates. School nutrition interventions, including deworming, can reduce anemia prevalence among displaced, rural, or low-income schoolchildren when iron-fortified products or supplements are provided.

Interventions Targeting the General Population

Cash-plus-nutrition interventions (that is, cash transfers accompanied by nutrition education, behavior change communications, and supplements) can reduce the incidence of child stunting by 15–20 percent. Evidence of the effects of cash transfers on wasting is inconclusive, and further research is needed. Agriculture programs (for example, vegetable gardens and homestead food production) and livestock interventions may have positive effects on dietary diversity and anemia but not on stunting. Further studies are needed on these issues, especially considering their importance in climate change adaptation and mitigation. Water, sanitation, and hygiene (WASH) interventions that include nutrition services can improve height for age (standardized mean difference of 0.13–0.15) and can also reduce the risk of diarrhea among children and all-cause child mortality by 30–50 percent and about 30 percent, respectively. Iron-fortified foods, with or without other micronutrients, effectively reduce the overall prevalence of anemia; wheat flour, soy sauce, condiments, and double-fortified salt show significant impacts. Biofortification of agricultural produce has the potential to improve micronutrient deficiencies.

These interventions can be delivered through the appropriate sectors— health, agriculture, social protection, water, and education—as well as the private sector, thereby maximizing multiple delivery platforms and allowing for much greater scale-up (refer to figure ES.1). To implement many of these interventions at scale, however, significant technical and implementation support are needed with respect to national guidelines, protocols, product supply chains, capacity development, and so forth.

Figure ES.1 Nutrition Services Can Be Delivered through Several Sectors

Policies and regulations

- Antenatal care and nutritional supplements during pregnancy
- Interventions in the perinatal period
- Infancy and childhood preventive care, nutritional supplements, and growth monitoring
- Nutrition education and counseling

- Food fortification
- Nutrition commodities

Health

Social protection

Private sector

Institutions and commodities delivered

Institutions and governance

- Cash transfers (conditional, unconditional)
- Food transfers and vouchers
- Other social protection schemes

Outcomes aligned with SDG 2.2
Stunting | Wasting | Anemia | Low birthweight and birth outcomes | Overweight and obesity | Breastfeeding

Morbidity | Mortality | Other nutrition indicators

- Integrated agriculture and nutrition
- Agriculture and livelihoods
- Homestead food production and vegetable garden
- Agriculture and livestock
- Agriculture and gender
- Biofortification

Education

Water and sanitation

Agriculture

- Early childhood development and nurturing care
- School health, nutrition, and hygiene

- Multiple or single WASH components
- WASH interventions with nutrition interventions

Food systems and climate

Source: Original figure for this publication.
Note: SDG = Sustainable Development Goal; WASH = water, sanitation, and hygiene.

A strategically designed package of policy instruments is essential to complement these interventions and influence consumer preferences by modifying social environments, food environments, and commercial determinants of health and dietary behaviors, as highlighted in figure ES.2. Such policies include Infant and Young Child Nutrition, the Baby Friendly Hospital Initiative, and the International Code of Marketing of Breast-Milk Substitutes. Fiscal policy measures such as nutrition-targeted health taxes affect prices and consumption of unhealthy products and simultaneously increase domestic revenues. To date, these measures have focused primarily on sugar-sweetened beverages (SSBs), which are now covered by such taxes across 57 percent of the world's population, but some countries have extended these taxes to ultraprocessed and other unhealthy foods. To be

Figure ES.2 Effective and Coherent Policy Actions to Support Nutrition Investments

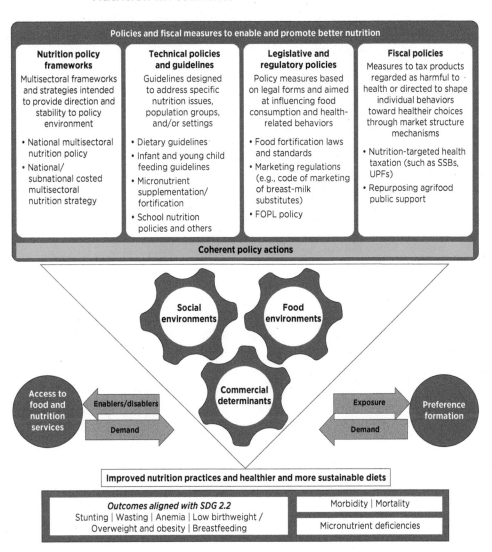

Source: Original figure for this publication.
Note: FOPL = front-of-package labeling; SDG = Sustainable Development Goal; SSB = sugar-sweetened beverage; UPFs = ultraprocessed foods.

effective, these nutrition-targeted health taxes must be designed in the context of the broader policy environment—including production incentives, consumer subsidies, and price controls throughout food supply chains—as well as complementary actions that can help shift social norms to healthier dietary choices and practices, such as front-of-package labeling, marketing regulations, and mass media and digital communication campaigns. Furthermore, repurposing of public support for agrifood, such as producer subsidies and trade policies, which currently amounts to

$638–$851 billion per year globally, is key to shifting food systems to healthier and more sustainable diets. Policy coherence is vital—for example, although the health sector discourages consumption of sugar, sugar is one of the most highly subsidized crops in the agrifood sector. Countries that develop and implement a coherent package of regulatory and fiscal policies and policy frameworks—accompanied by strong social communication strategies that are carefully calibrated to national contexts, the economic and political landscape, institutional capacities, and the epidemiology of malnutrition—and that hold each sector accountable can maximize economic and health benefits and minimize negative externalities, including climate impacts.

The Climate–Nutrition Nexus and Key Gender Considerations

Climate change, undernutrition, and obesity form a complex nexus that undermines health and development, disproportionately affecting the most vulnerable communities and countries globally. There is a significant relationship between climate change proxies (droughts, floods, and climate variability) and malnutrition. Drought conditions raise the likelihood of both wasting and underweight by almost 50 percent; in a high climate-change scenario, a relative rise of 23 percent in severe stunting in Sub-Saharan Africa and 62 percent in South Asia is expected by the 2050s. Climate change also exacerbates obesity through the reduced availability and accessibility of fresh food products and a dietary shift to less expensive ultraprocessed foods (UPFs). Women are particularly vulnerable to climate change because of their physiological differences from men, such as reduced heat dissipation through sweating, higher working metabolic rates, and thicker subcutaneous fat that impedes radiative cooling. Women are also more exposed to climate hazards through their role in agriculture and water collection, wherein they are forced to walk longer distances, often in extreme temperatures. During climate-related disasters, women face higher mortality rates and decreased life expectancy, as well as increased risks of physical, sexual, and domestic violence.

Globally, fresh, minimally processed foods and their culinary preparation are increasingly being displaced by UPFs. Brazil has experienced a 21 percent increase in diet-related greenhouse gas (GHG) emissions, largely attributed to the growing consumption of UPFs. These hyperpalatable, cheap, ready-to-consume food products—often energy-dense and rich in sodium, sugar, and unhealthy fats—raise serious concerns for planetary and human health. As dietary patterns around the world continue to shift, the negative effects of UPF consumption are also expected to increase. Concurrently, global demand for protein from livestock-based foods is projected to rise by 14 percent per person and by 38 percent overall between 2020 and 2050, with the fastest growth in demand anticipated in South Asia and Sub-Saharan Africa.

Overall, nutrition and climate decision-makers need to carefully scrutinize both nutritional needs and environmental sustainability to achieve balanced and effective solutions for people and the planet. Investing in climate adaptation and mitigation presents a dual opportunity to address climate challenges while improving nutrition outcomes. Women, whose health and livelihood tend to be most susceptible to climate change, play a crucial role in food systems and should be key beneficiaries of nutrition-smart adaptation interventions. Countries are showing the way forward. For example, Indonesia has established an integrated and climate-responsive monitoring and evaluation system to better understand the links between nutrition and climate, and Madagascar has integrated several climate mitigation and adaptation activities into phase two of its Improving Nutrition Outcomes Using the Multiphase Programmatic Approach, with support from the World Bank.

Despite the significant contribution of the agrifood sector to GHG emissions and a recent surge in climate financing, only 4.3 percent of climate funds currently target the agrifood sector, and only 2.4 percent of the key multilateral climate fund investments are child-responsive. It is critical to allocate financing more efficiently and leverage opportunities to advance nutrition-sensitive investments through the agriculture, social protection, and WASH sectors. Examples of climate–nutrition win–wins include imposing taxes on unhealthy foods with a significant carbon footprint such as UPFs and commercial milk formulas.

Financing Needs to Scale Up Evidence-Based Nutrition Actions

Scaling up a discrete set of evidence-based nutrition interventions to 90 percent coverage will require an additional $128 billion (discounted) for the 10-year period 2025–34 (approximately an additional $13 billion per year), which amounts to $13 per pregnant woman and $17 per child younger than age five per annum. This amount is in addition to the estimated $6.3 billion per annum that is already being spent to maintain status quo coverage.

Of the additional financing needs, $52 billion (40 percent) is required for the first five-year period (2025–29), and $76 billion (60 percent) is required for the subsequent five years (2030–34). Of the total $128 billion needed, $98 billion (77 percent) of that amount is for low- and lower-middle-income countries. On a regional basis, $43 billion is required for South Asia, $34 billion for Sub-Saharan Africa, $19 billion for East Asia and Pacific, and $16 billion for the Middle East and North Africa, reflecting the disproportionate burden of poor nutrition outcomes in these regions (refer to figure ES.3).

**Figure ES.3 Additional Financing Needs by Region
(Billion US$, Discounted)**

$6 (5%)

$16 (12%)

$43 (34%)

$19 (15%)

$34 (26%)

$9 (7%)

■ South Asia

□ Sub-Saharan Africa

□ Latin America and the Caribbean

■ East Asia and Pacific

□ Middle East and North Africa

□ Europe and Central Asia

Source: Original figure for this publication.

These investments could avert 6.2 million deaths among children younger than age five and 980,000 stillbirths in 2025–34. They could have positive impacts on several nutrition outcomes, for example, averting the following:

• 27 million stunting cases among children turning age five (over and above the current World Health Organization projections of 17.5 million fewer stunted children in 2034)

• 47 million episodes of wasting

• 77 million cases of anemia among children younger than age five

• Nearly 7 million cases of LBW

• 144 million cases of maternal anemia.

In addition, 85 million additional children could be exclusively breastfed.

Although these investments are critical, it is also possible to improve nutrition outcomes by optimizing current spending.

For example, if only 25 percent or 50 percent of the financing needs could be met in low-resource contexts, countries could maximize their impact by investing in the most cost-effective combination of interventions for their specific context. Depending on country-specific epidemiological indicators and policy and implementation contexts, a cost-effective package of interventions could be some combination of cash transfers to poor families accompanied by nutrition education, vitamin A supplementation, SQ-LNS for children, micronutrient powders and preventive zinc supplementation for children (although there are currently no feasible platforms for scaling up preventive zinc), intermittent preventive treatment of malaria in pregnancy (IPTp) and MMS for pregnant women, delayed cord clamping during childbirth, and KMC. Once these interventions are scaled up, and as budgets allow, other interventions can be added (refer to figure ES.4). Each country will, however, need to tailor the most cost-effective combination of these interventions through the health or social protection sectors, including potential delivery platforms, and complement them with investments such as biofortification through the agriculture sector, WASH investments through the water sector, and nutrition education and deworming through education platforms.

Figure ES.4 Optimized Annual Spending Allocations: Potential Scenarios If 0 Percent, 25 Percent, or 50 Percent of Additional Financing Needs Are Met

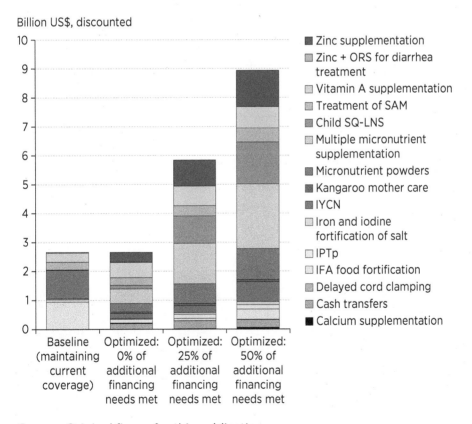

Billion US$, discounted

Legend:
- Zinc supplementation
- Zinc + ORS for diarrhea treatment
- Vitamin A supplementation
- Treatment of SAM
- Child SQ-LNS
- Multiple micronutrient supplementation
- Micronutrient powders
- Kangaroo mother care
- IYCN
- Iron and iodine fortification of salt
- IPTp
- IFA food fortification
- Delayed cord clamping
- Cash transfers
- Calcium supplementation

X-axis categories:
- Baseline (maintaining current coverage)
- Optimized: 0% of additional financing needs met
- Optimized: 25% of additional financing needs met
- Optimized: 50% of additional financing needs met

Source: Original figure for this publication.
Note: IFA = iron–folic acid; IPTp = intermittent preventive treatment of malaria in pregnancy; IYCN = infant and young child nutrition; ORS = oral rehydration solution; SAM = severe acute malnutrition; SQ-LNS = small-quantity lipid-based nutrient supplements.

Financing needs for obesity prevention policies are significantly lower, albeit harder to quantify with the evidence available. Case studies in Bulgaria, Mexico, and South Africa estimate the costs of food labeling, mass media campaigns, mobile apps, and regulation of advertisements at approximately $3.4–$3.6 purchasing power parity (PPP) per capita annually. The case studies estimate that for each $1 PPP invested, approximately $4–$5 PPP, on average, will be returned in economic benefits each year for 2020–50, with large positive impacts on labor market productivity. Furthermore, some of the fiscal policies to address obesity, such as taxes on unhealthy foods, have the potential to raise tax revenues, thereby increasing fiscal space in these countries. In Colombia, for example, such taxes are expected to raise up to $700 million annually in taxes that could then potentially be invested in improving nutrition.

The full scale-up of interventions to address undernutrition is estimated to generate $2.4 trillion in economic benefits, with a benefit–cost ratio of 23. For every $1 invested in addressing undernutrition, a return of $23 is expected.

The economic benefits associated with the investments in child and maternal nutrition alone far outweigh the costs of inaction, which run around $41 trillion over 10 years, with $21 trillion in economic productivity losses resulting from undernutrition and micronutrient deficiencies and an estimated $20 trillion in economic and social costs from overweight and obesity. While we need additional financing for nutrition, we must also improve the efficiency of spending to get more nutrition from the money available (figure ES.5).

Figure ES.5 More Money for Nutrition and More Nutrition for the Money

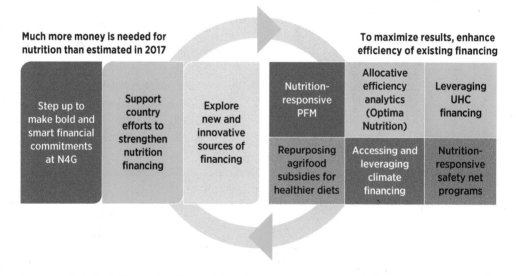

Source: Original figure for this publication.
Note: N4G = Nutrition for Growth; PFM = public financial management; UHC = universal health coverage.

The Way Forward

Overall, traditional financing sources from both development assistance and domestic sources are projected to be constrained and are unlikely to meet financing needs. Given this scenario, it is imperative for the nutrition community to support countries' efforts to step up and renew financial commitments at the Paris N4G Summit and at the same time explore new and innovative sources of financing by including nutrition in universal health coverage and adaptive safety net programs, repurposing agrifood subsidies for healthy diets, and leveraging climate funds. Nontraditional and innovative sources—including sovereign wealth funds and environmental, social, and governance (ESG) investments in the private sector—offer yet another new opportunity. Yet nutrition lags behind other sectors in catalyzing these sources, even though food systems hold some of the most powerful opportunities to improve human and planetary health while increasing productivity, and the private sector has a key role to play in this process.

The new Global Challenge Program on FNS launched by the World Bank is designed with an eye toward private capital mobilization, as well as toward innovative sources, recognizing that domestic resources and other development financing will not suffice to address the scale of global challenges.

In mobilizing private capital, the nutrition sector has much to learn from the climate movement, which benefited from public capital investing in new technologies to the point at which renewable energy can now be generated more cheaply than fossil fuel energy. To catalyze significant ESG investing for food and nutrition security from the private sector, the community needs to bring together metrics, advocacy, catalytic capital (leveraging the balance sheets of development finance institutions and multilateral development bank communities), and strategic capital by incentivizing and encouraging companies and investors to invest in the food systems of tomorrow. With this in place, private sector investment groups will pivot to nutrition-positive investments, as they did with climate investment initiatives. The key here is to educate investors on the return potential of investing in nutrition, not simply to address an investment returns perspective but also to increase labor productivity in the private and public sectors.

Further work is needed in the following five key domains:

- **Development assistance and domestic resources:** Ensure that development assistance resources catalyze converging actions across donors and national governments and that they balance the current focus on humanitarian aid to reduce child wasting with forward-looking preventive actions that will build resilience and reduce future needs for such aid. Support countries to enhance domestic resource allocations for preventive nutrition actions.

- **Innovative financing approaches:** Explore additional innovative financing sources, including using climate financing, repurposing agrifood subsidies, and mobilizing private sector sources, such as ESG investing. Further enhance mechanisms and tools to integrate preventive nutrition interventions and policies as well as fiscal policies, such as taxation and regulation of marketing of unhealthy foods, into national universal health coverage plans and packages.

- **Empirical research:** Encourage additional empirical research on climate, gender, WASH, and nutrition. Their biological underpinnings are known, but evidence on the size of their impact on nutrition outcomes is insufficient. Develop empirical estimates of the costs, opportunities, and challenges of implementing obesity-reduction policies. Once estimates and costs are available, they could be included in future iterations of impact models, such as the Optima Nutrition allocative efficiency analysis tool.

- **Maximization of delivery platforms for scaling up:** Continue to explore how adaptive safety net programs can be designed to deliver high-impact nutrition interventions and how synergies with the WASH, education, and agriculture sectors could be maximized. Identify setting-specific approaches that might influence the scale and effectiveness of interventions.

- **Technical and implementation support to countries to scale up:** Provide technical and implementation support to countries to scale up nutrition programming and policies across all relevant sectors, and work with countries to understand how resources can be optimized, public financial management enhanced, and nutrition budgets better tracked in ways that align with their strategic plans.

Call to Action

Increased investments in reducing undernutrition and obesity are crucial to meeting nutrition financing needs. These investments have unparalleled potential to build human capital; drive economic growth and prosperity; and, when carefully designed, provide additional climate co-benefits. For every $1 invested in addressing undernutrition, $23 are returned, and an estimated $2.4 trillion is generated in economic benefits. The economic benefits associated with these investments far outweigh the costs of inaction, which run around $41 trillion over 10 years, including $21 trillion in economic productivity losses due to undernutrition and micronutrient deficiencies and $20 trillion in economic and social costs from overweight and obesity.

The costs of inaction are far too high—trillions of dollars worth of lost human capital that will impinge on future economic productivity, 6.2 million more child deaths, 27 million more stunted children, 47 million more episodes of child wasting, and 144 million more cases of maternal anemia. The urgency cannot be overstated. Each day without action to improve nutrition outcomes diminishes the growth and prosperity of countries around the world and the ability to shape a more prosperous and equitable world on a livable planet for all.

Reference

Shekar, Meera, Jakub Kakietek, Julia Dayton Eberwein, and Dylan Walters. 2017. *An Investment Framework for Nutrition: Reaching the Global Targets for Stunting, Anemia, Breastfeeding, and Wasting.* Directions in Development. Washington, DC: World Bank. https://doi.org/10.1596/978-1-4648-1010-7.

Abbreviations

ACF	Action contre la Faim
AGA	appropriate for gestational age
AIR	American Institutes for Research
ANC	antenatal care
ASR	adult survival rate
AWWs	Anganwadi workers
BCC	behavior change communication
BEP	balanced energy supplementation
BF	breastfeeding
BFHI	Baby Friendly Hospital Initiative
BMGF	Bill & Melinda Gates Foundation
BMI	body mass index
CGIAR	Consortium of International Agricultural Research Centers
CHOICE	Choosing Interventions that are Cost-Effective
CI	confidence interval
CIAT	International Center for Tropical Agriculture
CLM	Cellule de Lutte Contre la Malnutrition
cm	centimeters
cm/week	centimeters per week
CMF	commercial milk formula
CNAP	Climate and Nutrition Adaptation Plan
CO_2	carbon dioxide
CRS	Creditor Reporting System
DALYs	disability-adjusted life years
DCC	delayed cord clamping
DDS	dietary diversity score
DHS	Demographic and Health Surveys
DID	difference in differences

EBF	exclusive breastfeeding
EC	European Commission
ECD	early childhood development
ECF	Eleanor Crook Foundation
EQUDE	Research Center for Equitable Development
ESG	environmental, social, and governance
ESG-Nutrition	ESG investing and nutrition and health in the food sector
FAO	Food and Agriculture Organization (of the United Nations)
FNS	Food and Nutrition Security
FOLU	Food and Land Use Coalition
FOP	front of package
FOPL	front-of-package labeling
FTV	food transfer and voucher
g	gram
g/day	grams per day
g/dL	grams per deciliter
g/L	grams per liter
GCA	Global Center on Adaptation
GCP	Global Challenge Program
GDP	gross domestic product
GFFN	Good Food Finance Network
GHED	Global Health Expenditure Database
GHG	greenhouse gas
GOI	Government of Indonesia
HAZ	height-for-age z-score
Hb	hemoglobin
HCI	Human Capital Index
HCR	Human Capital Review
HE	health expenditure
HFP	homestead food production
HICs	high-income countries
HIES	household income and expenditure surveys
ICDS	Integrated Child Development Services
ICDS-CAS	ICDS Common Application Software
IFA	iron–folic acid
IFAD	International Fund for Agricultural Development
IFAS	iron and folic acid supplementation
IFC	International Finance Corporation
IFMIS	Integrated Financial Management Information System
IFPRI	International Food Policy Research Institute
IFRC	International Federation of the Red Cross and Red Crescent

IHME	Institute for Health Metrics and Evaluation
I/IFA	iron/iron–folic acid
ILO	International Labour Organization
INEY	Investing in Nutrition and Early Years
IPTp	intermittent preventive treatment of malaria in pregnancy
ISO	International Organization for Standardization
IU	international units
IYCF	infant and young child feeding
IYCN	infant and young child nutrition
kcal/d	kilocalories per day
kg/m²	kilograms per square meter
KMC	kangaroo mother care
L	liter
LAZ	length-for-age z score
LBW	low birthweight
LICs	low-income countries
LiST	Lives Saved Tool
LLA	locally led adaptation
LMICs	low- and middle-income countries
LNS	lipid-based nutrient supplements
LSFF	large-scale food fortification
LY	life year
M&E	monitoring and evaluation
MAM	moderate acute malnutrition
MCT	maternity cash transfer
MD	mean difference
MDD	minimum dietary diversity
µg	micrograms
MICs	middle-income countries
ml	milliliters
MMS	multiple micronutrient supplements
MNP	micronutrient powder
MoHSP	Ministry of Health and Social Protection
MQ-LNS	medium-quantity lipid-based nutrients
MSPAN	Multi-Sectoral Nutrition Action Plan
NCD	noncommunicable disease
NCP	Nutrition Convergence Program
N4G	Nutrition-for Growth
NIN	National Institute of Nutrition
NPERs	Nutrition Public Expenditure Reviews
NSDS	Nutrition-Sensitive Direct Support
OECD	Organisation for Economic Co-operation and Development

OHCHR	Office of the United Nations High Commissioner for Human Rights
OR	odds ratio
ORS	oral rehydration solution
PAG	Policy Advisory Group
PAHO	Pan American Health Organization
PER	public expenditure review
PFM	public financial management
PHC	primary health care
pp	percentage points
PPP	purchasing power parity
PR	prevalence ratio
RCTs	randomized controlled trials
RD	risk difference
R4D	Results for Development
RisC	Risk Factor Collaboration
ROR	relative odds ratio
RR	risk ratio
RUTF	ready-to-use therapeutic food
SAM	severe acute malnutrition
SBC	social and behavior change
SDG	Sustainable Development Goal
SE	standard error
SGA	small for gestational age
SHA	System of Health Accounts
SMD	standardized mean difference
SQ-LNS	small-quantity lipid-based nutrients
SP	sulfadoxine–pyrimethamine
SPHeP-NCDs	Strategic Public Health Planning for NCDs
SSB	sugar-sweetened beverage
SUN	Scaling Up Nutrition
SWF	sovereign wealth fund
TAG	Technical Advisory Group
U5MR	under-5 mortality rate
UHC	universal health coverage
UMICs	upper-middle-income countries
UNDESA	United Nations Department of Economic and Social Affairs
UNICEF	United Nations Children's Fund
UPFs	ultraprocessed foods
USDHHS	US Department of Health and Human Services
USFB	unhealthy snack foods and beverages
VAS	vitamin A supplementation

WASH	water, sanitation and hygiene
WAZ	weight-for-age z score
WFP	World Food Program
WHA	World Health Assembly
WHO	World Health Organization
WHZ	weight-for-height z score
WISE	Water Insecurity Experience (Scales)
WRA	women of reproductive age

All dollar amounts are US dollars unless otherwise indicated.

1

Objective and Scope of the 2024 Update

Meera Shekar and Kyoko Shibata Okamura

Introduction

In response to the polycrises of climate change and geopolitical conflicts, food price increases, and an unprecedented global pandemic over the past several years, the World Bank has identified six new Global Challenge Programs (GCPs) as it fulfills its vision of working toward a world free of poverty on a livable planet, and it has established comprehensive and coordinated efforts to address them. These new GCPs are Fast-Track Water Security and Climate Adaptation; Energy Transition, Efficiency, and Access; Enhanced Health Emergency Prevention, Preparedness, and Response; Accelerating Digitalization; Food and Nutrition Security (FNS); and Forests for Development, Climate, and Biodiversity. All GCPs are expected to lay out solutions that are scalable and replicable across World Bank Group institutions. The GCP on FNS focuses on scaling up three interconnected action areas: (1) FNS crisis prevention, preparedness, and response; (2) innovative,[1] high-impact cross-sectoral nutrition solutions; and (3) low emissions and climate-resilient food systems. These cross-sectoral action areas are intended to deliver powerful solutions that can be replicated and scaled up across countries, reflecting the World Bank Group's comparative advantage to mobilize public, private, and philanthropic funding for development. This report serves as a compendium of cost-effective, evidence-based interventions and effective policy measures for countries to draw on to scale up high-impact nutrition actions.

The 2017 *An Investment Framework for Nutrition* (Shekar et al. 2017) outlined the financing needed to address four nutrition targets—child stunting, wasting, breastfeeding, and anemia among women—in support of SDG 2.2 under the Zero Hunger target. The report also for the first time linked these financing needs to their potential for impact and results and proposed a framework for mobilizing the needed resources. The framework was instrumental in providing a basis for donor and country commitments presented at the Tokyo Nutrition for Growth (N4G) summit in 2021 and in providing country clients with the best available evidence to maximize the impact of their investments.

Unlike investments in physical infrastructure, investments in nutrition generate benefits that are durable, inalienable, and portable. These investments also fuel progress toward all 17 SDGs, including education and the alleviation of poverty, and they are key to improving human capital. Ensuring optimum nutrition—particularly early in life—can permanently alter an individual's developmental trajectory and maximize their productive potential. The global food system today generates $10 trillion in market values per year. However, it also results in $12 trillion of hidden costs in health burdens, environmental impacts, and socioeconomic vulnerabilities, including $2.7 trillion from obesity-related noncommunicable diseases, $1.8 trillion from undernutrition, and $1.5 trillion from greenhouse gas emissions, reflecting significant global market failures (FOLU 2019).

This 2024 update will serve as a basis for donor and client country commitments at the next N4G in Paris in 2025 and will continue to guide country clients with the most updated evidence as they design their programs.

The update builds on the 2017 framework by doing the following:

- Expanding the outcomes of interest to include low birthweight and birth outcomes and overweight and obesity, in addition to child stunting, wasting, breastfeeding, and anemia

- Including new evidence on interventions, such as small-quantity lipid-based nutrient supplements (SQ-LNS) for children and multiple micronutrient supplements for pregnant women

- Including emerging new evidence on interventions with a multisectoral approach

- Adding key perspectives on gender and the links between nutrition and climate change

- Adding the latest landscape and evidence for effective policy measures to address the nutrition–food systems–climate nexus

- Updating the financing needs and financing framework with an added focus on innovative financing, including new potential resources, such as leveraging and repurposing existing private and public financing for better nutritional outcomes.

Although there are many relevant nutritional outcomes, this report focuses primarily on those aligned with SDG 2.2. Improving outcomes requires a combination of interventions across several sectors, coupled with enabling factors and policies such as adequate governance structures, institutional arrangements, functional norms and regulations, and adequate resources, among others. Whereas previous reports have referred to nutrition-specific and nutrition-sensitive interventions, and the latest *Lancet* series on nutrition refers to direct and indirect interventions, this change in nomenclature has not been universally accepted by all agencies and often creates confusion. To avoid the dissonance associated with both nomenclatures and to align with country-level implementation platforms, the actions proposed in this report are organized according to target groups (prenatal, perinatal, children, and general population) and delivery platforms across health, social protection, agriculture, water and sanitation, and education, including the private sector.

What Worked Well in the 2017 Investment Framework—and What Did Not Work as Well

Experience from the 2017 framework shows that it provided useful guidance for both domestic governments and development assistance partners as they formulated their financial commitments for the Tokyo N4G summit in 2021. It also provided advocates and national advisors with a target for formulating their development assistance commitments (see, for example, the 2024 report from Generation Nutrition Coalition (Generation Nutrition 2024) on commitments from the European Commission). Aid-tracking groups such as the Global Nutrition Report and the Results for Development have used the recommendations in the 2017 framework as markers for how well aid is aligned with high-impact investments (refer to chapter 9). Countries also used the technical guidance in prioritizing interventions within their country contexts, especially when resources were constrained.

The framework listed some high-priority areas for future research, including research on scalable strategies for delivering high-impact interventions through nonhealth sectors, allocative and technical efficiency for nutrition investments, and efforts to identify interventions to prevent child wasting. All of these areas have seen significant progress with the development of new interventions such as SQ-LNS and careful documentation of their impacts and costs. New tools have been developed, and country teams are being trained on tools such as Optima Nutrition to prioritize actions within limited budgets, as well as nutrition budget tracking tools and tools to strengthen public financial management, so as to maximize the impact of available resources. Progress has also been made on another key area highlighted in 2017: the links between water and sanitation and nutrition outcomes (Kremer et al. 2023), as well as the use of adaptive safety nets to improve nutrition outcomes, although more work is still needed to establish the empirical value of these links. One key area in which less progress has been made is leveraging innovative financing. These and other relevant areas for further work are summarized in chapter 9.

Nutrition sits at the heart of the current polycrises, and child and maternal malnutrition is driven by recurrent and intersecting shocks, including conflict; climate change; a global pandemic; unsustainable debt levels; and market disruptions in energy, food, and fertilizers, with compound effects on both individual and societal health. Food price inflation, for example, has dire consequences for child undernutrition in low- and middle-income nations. A recent study analyzing 1.27 million preschoolers from 44 countries (Headey and Ruel 2023) found that, on average, a 5 percent rise in food prices over a three-month period led to a 14 percent increased risk of severe wasting. Infants are particularly vulnerable, and boys and those from impoverished rural settings are most affected. Food inflation during the mother's prenatal period also predicts long-term stunting of their children at ages two to five years. The most vulnerable, particularly women and young children, experience lifelong health and cognitive development consequences, including reduced education, lost income, and a devastating intergenerational cycle of malnutrition that leads to lost productivity, ballooning health care costs, and lost human capital and reduced gross domestic product countrywide and globally.

Although the impact of these interlocking crises on nutrition is clear, the reverse is also true: investment in nutrition can be a powerful catalyst for achieving at least 12 of the 17 SDGs, including a range of global health goals, and unlocking the human capital potential of the next generation. Every $1 invested in preventing malnutrition is estimated to deliver $23 in net benefits. These benefits are inalienable because once they are locked in during a child's early years, they cannot be rescinded. Tackling malnutrition in all its forms is possible, as evidenced by improvements in child stunting over the past two decades, as shown in the 2017 *An Investment Framework for Nutrition* (Shekar et al. 2017) and in this 2024 update, although recent crises have led to some backsliding. Nutrition investments must be recognized as central and indispensable parts of addressing the most pressing global challenges—and they need to be financed accordingly.

Note

1. Sustainable Development Goal 2.2 targets include stunting, wasting, breast feeding, anemia among women, low birthweight, and obesity.

References

FOLU (Food and Land Use Coalition). 2019. *Growing Better: Ten Critical Transitions to Transform Food and Land Use.* The Global Consultation Report of the Food and Land Use Coalition. London: FOLU. https://www.foodandlandusecoalition.org /wp-content/uploads/2019/09/FOLU-GrowingBetter-GlobalReport.pdf.

Generation Nutrition. 2024. "L'Union européenne et ses États membres doivent intensifier leurs efforts pour lutter contre la sous-nutrition mondiale" [Rethinking the EU's ODA Investments in Nutrition: Catalyzing Transformative Change]. Paris: Generation Nutrition. https://www.actioncontrelafaim.org/a-la -une/lunion-europeenne-et-ses-etats-membres-doivent-intensifier-leurs-efforts -pour-lutter-contre-la-sous-nutrition-mondiale/.

Headey, Derek, and Marie Ruel. 2023. "Food Inflation and Child Undernutrition in Low- and Middle-Income Countries." *Nature Communications* 14 (1): 5761. https://doi.org/10.1038/s41467-023-41543-9.

Kremer, Michael, Stephen P. Luby, Ricardo Maartens, Brandon Tan, and Witold Więcek. 2023. "Water Treatment and Child Mortality: A Meta-Analysis and Cost-Effectiveness Analysis." Working Paper No. 30835, National Bureau of Economic Research, Cambridge, MA. https://www.nber.org/system/files /working_papers/w30835/w30835.pdf.

Shekar, Meera, Jakub Kakietek, Julia Dayton Eberwein, and Dylan Walters. 2017. *An Investment Framework for Nutrition.* Washington, DC: World Bank. https://doi .org/10.1596/978-1-4648-1010-7.

2

Maternal and Child Nutrition Trends

Hoa Thi Mai Nguyen, Mireya Vilar-Compte, and Jonathan Kweku Akuoku

KEY MESSAGES

- Although child stunting rates across the globe declined an impressive 44 percent between 1990 and 2022, malnutrition rates remain high, with 148 million children still stunted. The global progress in malnutrition reduction is slow with anemia rates increasing among women of reproductive age; child stunting, wasting, and low birthweight (LBW) rates stagnating; and rates of childhood and adult obesity increasing.

- In 2019, anemia affected 3 in 10 women of reproductive age, totaling 571 million women with anemia worldwide—an increase of 78 million since 2000. Between 2012 and 2019, progress was seen only in Latin America and the Caribbean, whereas South Asia and Sub-Saharan Africa, which carried the highest anemia burden, showed no progress, and all other regions saw an increase.

- Available data between 2003–19 revealed approximately 1.2 billion nonpregnant women globally had a deficiency in at least one of three core micronutrients (iron, zinc, and folic acid), mostly in low- and middle-income countries (LMICs).

- Over the past decade, the number of stunted children has risen in 34 countries—15 countries in Sub-Saharan Africa, 6 in East Asia and Pacific, 6 in the Middle East and North Africa, 3 in Latin America and the Caribbean, 3 in Europe and Central Asia, and 1 in North America.

- In 2022, more than 50 percent of the world's 45 million children suffering from wasting lived in South Asia (mostly in India); one-fourth in Sub-Saharan Africa (11.1 million); and slightly more than one-tenth in East Asia and Pacific (5 million).

- Despite improvements in the proportion of women breastfeeding, countries are still far from desirable outcomes. Exclusive breastfeeding rates in low-income, lower-middle-income, and upper-middle-income countries were 51.2 percent, 46.7 percent, and 37.0 percent, respectively, in 2019.

- In 2020, 1 in 7 children globally was born with LBW, a ratio virtually unchanged since 2012. Of the 19.8 million children born with LBW globally, the majority were in South Asia and Sub-Saharan Africa (8.7 million and 5.6 million, respectively), with the rest distributed across other regions.

- Two-fifths of children ages 6 months to 59 months globally were considered anemic in 2019, totaling 269 million. Between 2012 and 2019, at least 92 countries made no progress or had an increase in the prevalence of child anemia.

- An estimated 372 million children ages 6 months to 59 months were deficient in at least one of three core micronutrients (iron, zinc, and vitamin A), predominantly in LMICs.

- In 2022, approximately 45 percent of adults ages 18 and older had excess weight, with a total of nearly 2.5 billion classified as overweight or obese. Of these, more than 907 million were obese, and women exhibited a higher prevalence of obesity than men. Between 1990 and 2022, the prevalence of obesity rose consistently among both genders across all regions.

- Approximately 57 percent of countries globally are grappling with the double burden of malnutrition, predominantly in LMICs across Sub-Saharan Africa, East Asia and Pacific, and Latin America and the Caribbean. Increases in the prevalence of overweight and obesity are driving the worsening levels of this double burden. From 2016 to 2022, the prevalence of overweight and obesity among women rose in 103 countries. As of 2022, approximately 122 countries (77 percent) face a very high burden of overweight and obesity among women.

Introduction: Progress toward SDG 2

Nearly two decades since the adoption of Sustainable Development Goal 2 (SDG 2) and its target 2.2 to end all forms of malnutrition, the world is facing significant challenges. Recent crises, armed conflicts, and climate change have had a profound impact on global economic growth, food security, and health systems. Hunger and food insecurity, which increased sharply in 2019, have remained at high levels, with 735 million people undernourished and 2.4 billion food insecure in 2022 (refer to figures 2.1 and 2.2). Rates of anemia among women of reproductive age have risen; previously observed declines in child stunting rates, wasting, and LBW have stalled; and the prevalence of childhood overweight and obesity is increasing. With these challenges, the world is falling off track in many key nutrition indicators (refer to figure 2.3).

Figure 2.1 Prevalence of Undernourishment and Number of People Undernourished, 2000–22

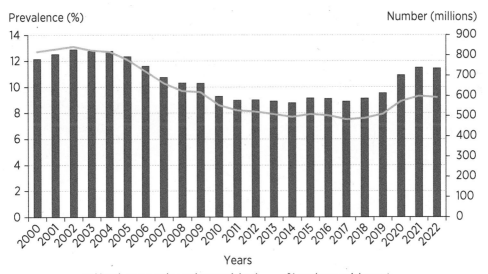

■ Number, people undernourished ——— % undernourishment

Source: Original figure for this publication based on data from FAO, IFAD, UNICEF, WFP, and WHO 2023.

Figure 2.2 Evolution of Global Moderate or Severe Food Insecurity, 2014–22

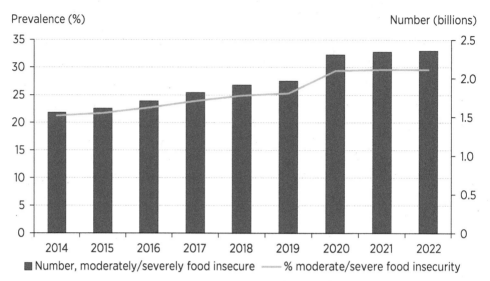

Source: Original figure for this publication based on data from FAO, IFAD, UNICEF, WFP, and WHO 2023.

Figure 2.3 Global Progress toward the SDG Nutrition Targets, 2000–22

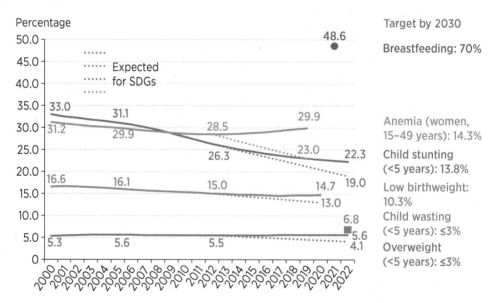

Sources: Original figure for this publication based on Neves et al. 2023 (breastfeeding); UNICEF 2023 (breastfeeding); WHO 2023a (anemia); *World Bank Open Data* 2023 (anemia); UNICEF, WHO, and World Bank 2023 (stunting, wasting, and overweight/obesity); WHO 2023b (low birthweight).
Note: The SDG Nutrition Targets are currently being revised by the WHO. SDG = Sustainable Development Goal.

Forms of Malnutrition and Target Groups

Designed to incentivize key stakeholders to work toward preventing all forms of malnutrition throughout a person's life, SDG target 2.2 places a strong emphasis on maternal and child nutrition during the first 1,000 days, from conception to a child's second birthday (refer to figure 2.4). Improving anemia among women of reproductive age (15–49 years) and micronutrient deficiencies in pregnancy is crucial during the period of conception and breastfeeding exclusively for the first six months, and reducing stunting, wasting, anemia, micronutrient deficiency, and overweight and obesity among children younger than age five years are fundamental factors that can have long-lasting impacts on human capital and productivity.

Figure 2.4 Nutrition Target Groups during the Life Course

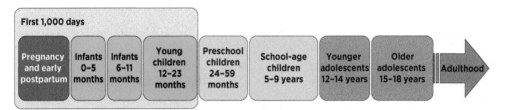

Source: Original figure for this publication.

Maternal Malnutrition

Anemia among Women of Reproductive Age

Anemia among women of reproductive age leads to severe consequences for both women and their children, including maternal and perinatal mortality, intrauterine growth restriction, LBW children, impaired cognitive function, heightened risk of infection, and reduced physical work capacity (Shekar et al. 2017). Globally, anemia among women of reproductive age has been creeping up since 2012 (refer to figure 2.5). As of 2019, 3 in 10 women of reproductive age were anemic, or a total of about 571 million women worldwide—an increase of 78 million women compared with data as of 2000 (WHO 2023a; World Bank 2023). Between 2012 and 2019, the global anemia rate has been stagnant among pregnant women (from 37.0 percent to 36.5 percent) and has slightly increased among nonpregnant women (from 28.1 percent to 29.6 percent).

Figure 2.5 Prevalence of Anemia among Women of Reproductive Age, 2000–19

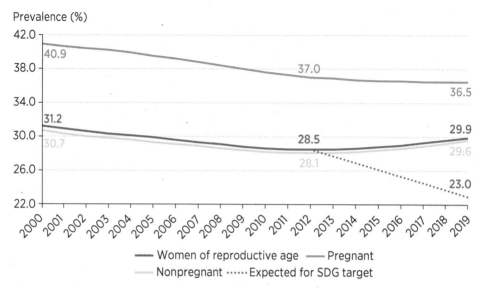

Prevalence (%)

Legend: Women of reproductive age — Pregnant — Nonpregnant ······ Expected for SDG target

Sources: WHO 2023a; World Bank 2023.
Note: SDG = Sustainable Development Goal. The SDG Nutrition Targets are currently being revised by the WHO.

Between 2012 and 2019, Latin America and the Caribbean experienced a modest reduction in anemia among women of reproductive age (from 18.2 percent to 17.3 percent). Meanwhile, South Asia and Sub-Saharan Africa, which carried the highest burden, made no progress: in South Asia, the rate decreased from 49.6 percent to 49.4 percent, and in Sub-Saharan Africa, it decreased from 41.0 percent to 40.6 percent. All other regions saw increases: in East Asia and Pacific, the rate increased from 18.0 percent to 19.4 percent; in Europe and Central Asia, from 16.0 percent to 17.4 percent; in the Middle East and North Africa, from 30.0 percent to 30.4 percent; and in North America, from 9.9 percent to 11.7 percent. Globally, 52 countries made modest progress in anemia reduction (with reductions ranging from 0.1 to 8.8 percentage points), and at least 134 countries either made no progress or experienced an increase (with increases ranging from 0 to 7.4 percentage points).

Micronutrient Deficiencies among Women

Although most cases of anemia are caused by iron deficiency, deficiencies in other micronutrients are also major concerns because they contribute to increased morbidity and mortality among women of reproductive age. Globally, more than two-thirds (69 percent) of nonpregnant women ages 15–49 are deficient in at least one of three core micronutrients (iron, zinc, and folate; Stevens et al. 2022).[1] Such deficiencies affect at least 1.2 billion nonpregnant women worldwide, most of whom reside in LMICs. Of these, nearly one-third live in East Asia and Pacific (384 million) and more than one-fourth in South Asia (307 million). In terms of prevalence, Sub-Saharan Africa has the highest prevalence of women with any micronutrient deficiency (80 percent), followed by South Asia (74 percent) and East Asia and Pacific (72 percent).

Child Malnutrition

Stunting

As a predictor of many childhood developmental constraints and future economic opportunities, stunting is at the forefront of the global nutrition and development agenda. As of 2022, approximately 1 in 5 children younger than age five years (22.3 percent) were stunted worldwide (UNICEF, WHO, and World Bank 2023; refer to figure 2.6). Two-thirds of the 148 million stunted children globally resided in Sub-Saharan Africa (59.3 million) and South Asia (53.4 million), with India having a very high prevalence rate and the largest number of stunted children (refer to box 2.1). Although stunting prevalence has been trending downward in these two regions since 2000, the decline has plateaued. Meanwhile, East Asia and Pacific as well as North America have experienced increases in recent years (refer to figure 2.6). Between 2012 and 2022, at least 34 countries showed an increase in the number of stunted children (15 countries in Sub-Saharan Africa, six in East Asia and Pacific, six in the Middle East and Central Africa, three in Latin America and the Caribbean, three in Europe and Central Asia, and one in North America). Albeit several countries such as Bangladesh, Burkina Faso, Nepal, Rwanda, and Tajikistan have experienced considerable declines in child stunting (box 2.2), India continues to carry the largest global burden of child stunting (box 2.1) as well as child wasting.

Figure 2.6 Stunting Prevalence, Global and by Region, 2000–22 (Modeled Estimates)

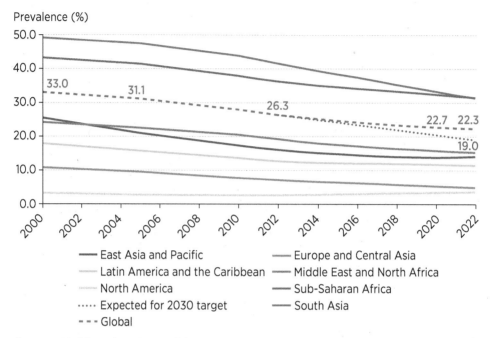

Source: UNICEF, WHO, World Bank 2023. The SDG Nutrition Targets are currently being revised by the WHO.

Box 2.1

Child Stunting in India

India carries the largest global burden of child stunting and has much higher stunting rates than other countries with similar GDP rates.

Figure B2.1.1 High Burden of Child Stunting in India

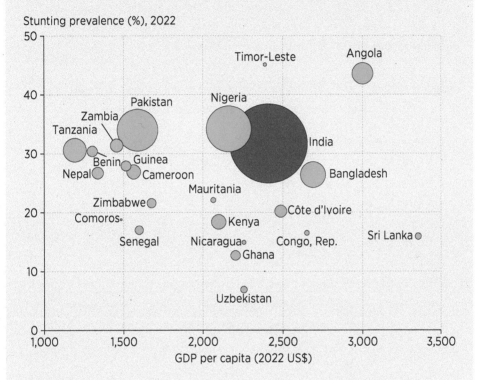

Stunting prevalence (%), 2022

GDP per capita (2022 US$)

Sources: GDP per capita (current US$) from World Bank Group, World Development Indicators. https://data.worldbank.org/indicator/NY.GDP .PCAP.CD. Accessed 6/24/2024. Stunting data from UNICEF/WHO/WB Joint Malnutrition Estimates 2023. https://data.unicef.org/topic/nutrition /malnutrition/. Accessed August 1, 2023.
Note: GDP per capita is gross domestic product divided by midyear population.

Box 2.2

Where Is the Greatest Decline in Child Stunting Seen?

Between 2012 and 2022, the 10 countries with the greatest decline in the prevalence of stunting were Nepal, the Comoros, Bangladesh, Lao People's Democratic Republic, Tajikistan, Republic of Yemen,

(continued)

Box 2.2

Where Is the Greatest Decline in Child Stunting Seen? *(continued)*

Cambodia, Burkina Faso, Rwanda, and Afghanistan (with an absolute reduction range of 11.2–13.6 percentage points; refer to figure B2.2.1). Additionally, the 10 countries with the greatest reduction in the number of stunted children were India, China, Pakistan, Bangladesh, Indonesia, Kenya, Iraq, Viet Nam, Nepal, and Myanmar (with an absolute reduction range of 0.34–16.4 million).

Figure B2.2.1 Top 10 Countries with Greatest Decline in Stunting Prevalence, 2012–22 (Modeled Estimates)

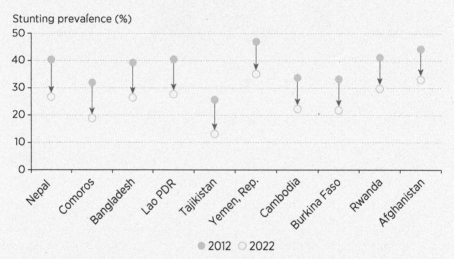

Sources: Stunting data from UNICEF/WHO/WB Joint Malnutrition Estimates 2023. https://data.unicef.org/topic/nutrition/malnutrition/. Accessed August 1, 2023.

Wasting

As of 2022, nearly 1 in 15 children younger than age five years globally (6.8 percent) were moderately or severely wasted, with a total of 45 million wasted children globally (UNICEF, WHO, and World Bank 2023; refer to figure 2.7). South Asia had the highest prevalence of wasting at 14.8 percent for moderate and severe wasting and 4.9 percent for severe wasting (refer to figure 2.7). In 2022, more than half of wasted children younger than age five years were in South Asia (25.2 million), one-fourth were in Sub-Saharan Africa (11.1 million), and more than one-tenth were in East Asia and Pacific (5 million). The number of wasted children in India alone accounted for nearly half of the world's wasted children (21.9 million).

Figure 2.7 Wasting Prevalance, Global and by Region, 2022

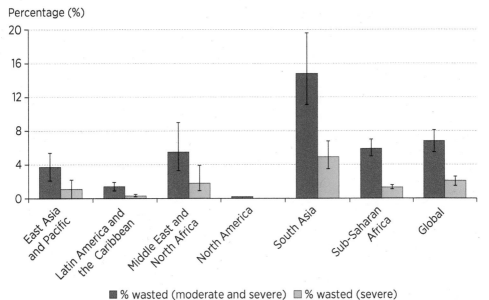

Percentage (%)

■ % wasted (moderate and severe) ■ % wasted (severe)

Source: UNICEF, WHO, and World Bank 2023.

Low Birthweight

The consequences of LBW can span a lifetime, including heightened risks of mortality in the neonatal period, stunted growth in childhood, and chronic conditions such as obesity and diabetes in adulthood (Blencowe et al. 2019). As of 2020, 1 in 7 children (19.8 million) globally were born with LBW (WHO 2023b). The global prevalence of LBW trended down between 2000 and 2012, but that reduction has since stagnated through 2020 (refer to figure 2.8). South Asia had the highest prevalence of LBW children globally (24.9 percent as of 2020), although the regional rate has declined over the past two decades. Nearly half of LBW children globally were born in South Asia (8.7 million), just more than one-fourth in Sub-Saharan Africa (5.6 million), approximately one-tenth in East Asia and Pacific (2.2 million), and the rest in other regions (ranging from 0.3 to 1.3 million).

Figure 2.8 Low Birthweight Prevalence and Number, 2000–20

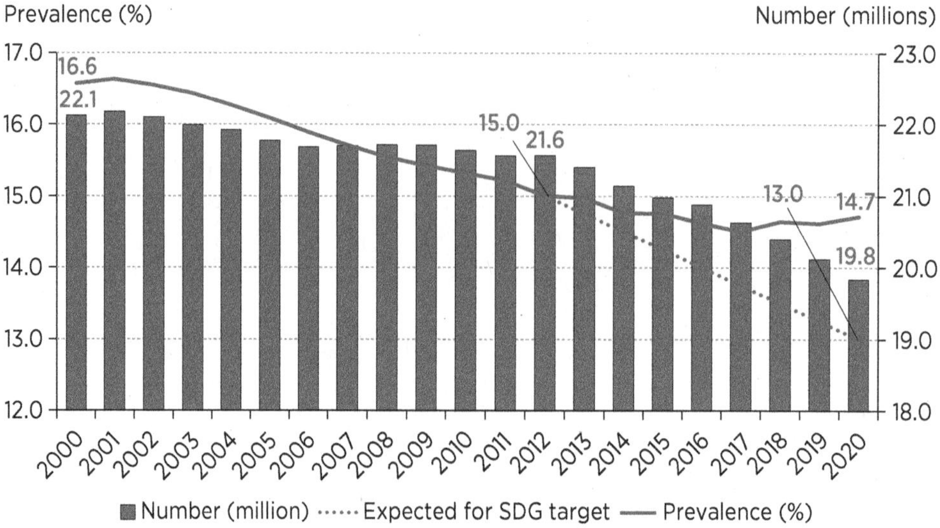

Prevalence (%)   Number (millions)

■ Number (million) ······ Expected for SDG target —— Prevalence (%)

Source: WHO 2023b.
Note: SDG = Sustainable Development Goal. The SDG Nutrition Targets are currently being revised by the WHO.

Breastfeeding

Optimal breastfeeding, including early initiation of breastfeeding, exclusively breastfeeding for the child's first six months of life, and continued breastfeeding until the child is at least two years old, provides strong disease and malnutrition prevention and overall health protection effects to mothers and children. Mothers who breastfeed benefit from prolonged birth spacing and reduced risks of breast and ovarian cancer, type 2 diabetes, and high blood pressure. Breastfed children are better protected from morbidity and mortality than nonbreastfed children, and they reap better health, nutritional, cognitive, and long-term economic benefits (Shekar et al. 2017). As of 2019, the global prevalence of exclusive breastfeeding among infants younger than age six months (the SDG target outcome) was 48.6 percent, a substantial increase from 35.4 percent in 2000 (Neves et al. 2021; UNICEF 2023; refer to figure 2.9). Despite improvements, countries are still far from reaching desirable outcomes with exclusive breastfeeding rates in low-income, lower-middle-income, and upper-middle-income countries at 51.2 percent, 46.7 percent, and

37.0 percent, respectively (refer to figure 2.9). Although all other regions showed an increase in exclusive breastfeeding rates, the Middle East and North Africa experienced a decrease, from 42.9 percent in 2000 to 30.2 percent in 2019.

Figure 2.9 Exclusive Breastfeeding Prevalence, Global and by Country Income Group, 2000 and 2019

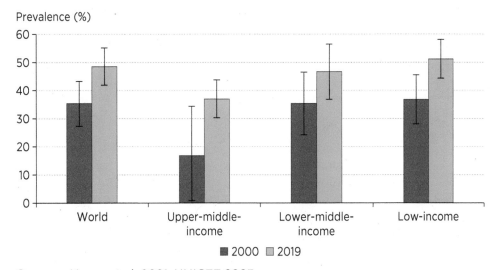

Sources: Neves et al. 2021; UNICEF 2023.
Note: No data available for high-income countries.

Anemia and Micronutrient Deficiencies among Children

Children with anemia are more likely to experience poor weight gain, frequent respiratory and intestinal infections, and impaired development (Saloojee and Pettifor 2021). As of 2019, anemia affected approximately 39.8 percent of children worldwide, which equates to 2 in 5 children ages 6 months to 59 months (or 269 million; WHO 2023a; World Bank 2023; refer to figure 2.10). Anemia among children has been trending down globally since 2000, yet the decline has stagnated since 2012. As of 2019, both Sub-Saharan Africa and South Asia had the highest prevalence of children with anemia, at 60.5 percent and 51.7 percent, respectively (refer to figure 2.10). Between 2012 and 2019, at least 92 countries either made no progress or experienced an increase in the prevalence of childhood anemia, with increases ranging from 0 to 9.9 percentage points.

Figure 2.10 Anemia Prevalence among Children Ages 6–59 Months, Global and by Region, 2000–19

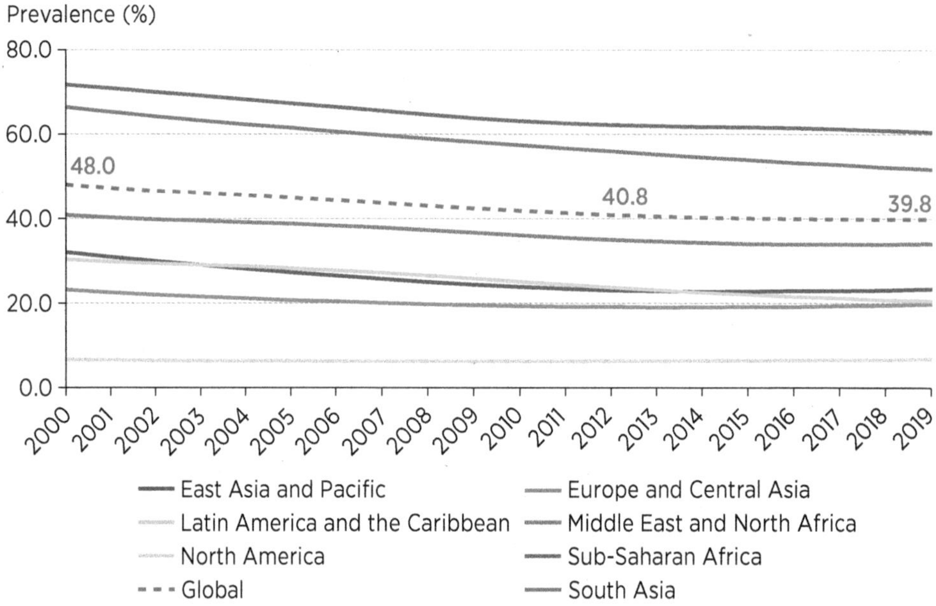

Prevalence (%)

Legend:
- East Asia and Pacific
- Europe and Central Asia
- Latin America and the Caribbean
- Middle East and North Africa
- North America
- Sub-Saharan Africa
- Global
- South Asia

Sources: WHO 2023; World Bank 2023.

Worldwide, 56 percent of children ages 6 months to 59 months (372 million) were deficient in at least one of three core micronutrients (iron, zinc, and vitamin A) (Stevens et al. 2022). Most of these children (92 percent) resided in LMICs. The three most-affected regions were Sub-Saharan Africa, East Asia and Pacific, and South Asia.

Childhood Overweight and Obesity

Given that childhood obesity greatly affects the chances of adult obesity, overweight and obesity during childhood has damaging impacts on children's health and economic potential in the long run, with long-term debilitating noncommunicable diseases (NCDs) in adulthood (Shekar and Popkin 2020; Simmonds et al. 2016; Ward et al. 2017). As of 2022, the global prevalence of overweight and obesity among children younger than age five years was 5.6 percent, totaling 37 million overweight or obese children (UNICEF, WHO, and World Bank 2023; refer to figure 2.11). Between 2012 and 2022, Europe and Central Asia was the only region to have a notable decreased prevalence of childhood obesity (from 9.3 percent to 7.1 percent). Meanwhile, its prevalence was stagnant in South Asia (changing from just 2.6 percent to 2.7 percent), Sub-Saharan Africa (changing from 3.7 percent to 3.6 percent), and the Middle East and North Africa (changing from 10.6 percent to 10.3 percent). Two regions that had a clear linear rising trend between 2000 and 2022 were East Asia and Pacific, which saw an increase from 5.1 percent to 8.2 percent, and Latin America and the Caribbean, which saw an increase from 6.8 percent to 8.6 percent (refer to figure 2.11 and box 2.3). In the decade between 2012 and 2022, rates increased most in the upper-middle-income country group (10 percent relative increase), followed by the lower-middle-income group (5 percent relative increase), and the high-income group (3 percent relative increase).

Figure 2.11 Prevalence of Overweight and Obesity among Children Younger than Age Five Years, Global and by Region, 2000–22 (Modeled Estimates)

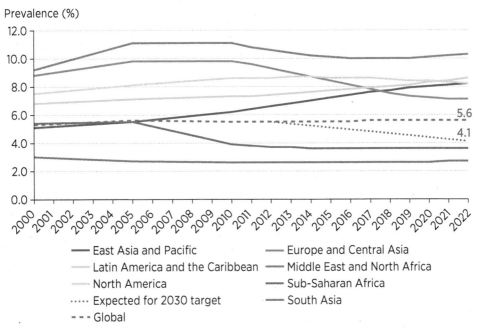

Source: UNICEF, WHO, World Bank 2023. The SDG Nutrition Targets are currently being revised by the WHO.

Box 2.3

Where Is the Greatest Increase in Child Overweight and Obesity Seen?

Between 2012 and 2022, the 10 countries experiencing the highest surge in the prevalence of child overweight and obesity were Australia, Papua New Guinea, Viet Nam, Tunisia, Oman, Jordan, Ecuador, Paraguay, Trinidad and Tobago, and Cameroon (with an absolute increase range of 3.4–8.1 percentage points;

(continued)

Box 2.3

Where Is the Greatest Increase in Child Overweight and Obesity Seen? *(continued)*

refer to figure B2.3.1). As of 2022, East Asia and Pacific had the largest number of overweight and obese children at 11 million, followed by Sub-Saharan Africa (6.8 million), the Middle East and North Africa (5 million), South Asia (4.6 million), Latin America and the Caribbean (4.2 million), Europe and Central Asia (3.7 million), and North America (1.7 million).

Figure B2.3.1 Ten Countries with Greatest Absolute Increase in Prevalence of Child Overweight and Obesity, 2012–22 (Modeled Estimates)

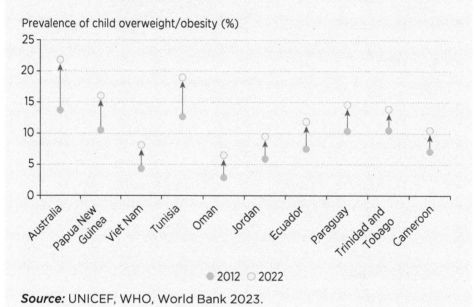

Source: UNICEF, WHO, World Bank 2023.

Nutrition among School-Age Children and Adolescents

Data collection and research on nutrition among school-age children and adolescents ages five to 19 years are scarce and underinvested (Norris et al. 2022), yet substantial gaps in their growth and nutrition status have been identified across countries (Stevens et al. 2022). In 2020, the difference in mean height between the countries with the tallest and shortest 19-year-old adolescents was at least 20 cm, and the difference in mean body mass index (BMI) between the countries with the highest and lowest adolescent BMIs was approximately 9–10 kg/m² (Norris et al. 2022; Sawyer 2020). A healthy growth trajectory in early childhood can be stalled or reversed with age if children gain too much weight but too little height as they grow older. This pattern has been observed in many countries in Sub-Saharan Africa, as well as in New Zealand and the United States among both boys and girls, in Malaysia and some Pacific Island nations among boys, and in Mexico among girls (Norris et al. 2022; Sawyer 2020).

Adult Overweight and Obesity

Along with unhealthy diets and physical inactivity, overweight and obesity is one of the top three preventable causes of NCDs; it accounts for 74 percent of global mortality each year (Shekar and Popkin 2020; WHO 2023c). As of 2022, an estimated 44.8 percent of the global adult population age 18 and older carried excess weight, with 28.5 percent classified as overweight (BMI = 25 kg/m² to <30 kg/m²) and 16.3 percent classified as obese (BMI ≥ 30 kg/m²; NCD-RisC 2024a, 2024b; UNDESA 2022). This translates to nearly 2.5 billion overweight or obese adults worldwide, of whom more than 907 million were obese. Women exhibited a higher prevalence of obesity than men at all severity levels (refer to figure 2.12).

Figure 2.12 Prevalence of Overweight and Obesity (Overall and by Class) among Adult Women and Men, 2022

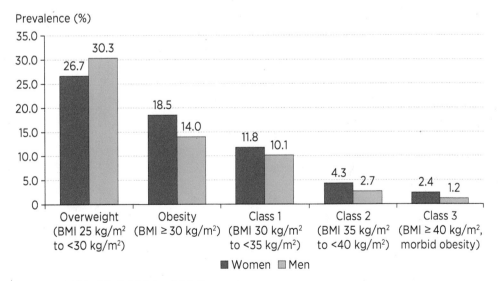

Source: NCD-RisC 2024a, 2024b.
Note: BMI = body mass index. BMI = weight (kg) / height² (m²).

From 1990 to 2022, the prevalence of obesity has risen consistently among both genders across all regions, although the rate of increase varied between women and men within the same region (NCD-RisC 2024a, 2024b; UNDESA 2022). Countries such as Pakistan, Afghanistan, Brazil, Argentina and Chile have seen the greatest absolute increase in obesity prevalence among adult women between 2012 and 2022 (box 2.4).

Box 2.4

Where Is the Greatest Increase in Adult Obesity Seen?

Between 2012 and 2022, the 10 countries experiencing the greatest increase in the prevalence of obesity among adult women were Afghanistan, Panama, Pakistan, The Bahamas, Mauritania, Jamaica, Brazil, Chile, Romania, and Argentina (with an absolute increase range of 9.4–11.9 percentage points; refer to figure B2.4.1). Meanwhile, the 10 countries with the greatest rise in the prevalence of obesity among adult men were Romania, Pakistan, Uzbekistan, Croatia, Georgia, Tonga, Argentina, Hungary, Chile, and Peru (with an absolute increase range of 8.8–15.4 percentage points).

Figure B2.4.1 Ten Countries with the Greatest Absolute Increase in Obesity Prevalence among Adult Women, 2012–22

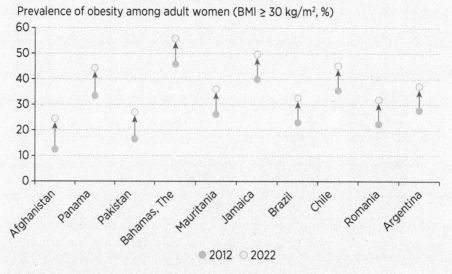

Source: NCD-RisC 2024a, 2024b.
Note: BMI = body mass index. BMI = weight (kg) / height^2 (m^2)

Double Burden of Malnutrition

The double burden of malnutrition—the coexistence of undernutrition (wasting, stunting, and micronutrient deficiencies) and overweight and obesity—imposes significant health and economic consequences on both individuals and populations, including heightened health care costs, decreased productivity, and impeded sustainable social and economic development (WHO 2017). As of 2022, 57 percent of countries worldwide were experiencing this double burden, measured by a concurrence of stunting rates at or above 10 percent among children younger than age five years and overweight and obesity rates at or above 20 percent among women (NCD-RisC 2024a, 2024b; UNICEF, WHO, and World Bank 2023; refer to annex 2A, table 2A.1).[2] Among these countries, nearly half were lower-middle-income (47 percent), more than one-fourth were low-income (26 percent), and one-fifth were upper-middle-income (21 percent). A majority of the countries with double burden were in Sub-Saharan Africa (47 percent), followed by East Asia and Pacific (17 percent), and Latin America and the Caribbean (14 percent). Other regions accounted for smaller proportions: the Middle East and North Africa (9 percent), South Asia (9 percent), and Europe and Central Asia (4 percent).

Between 2016 and 2022, the number of countries with a very high level of double burden increased from 8 to 14. However, the number of countries with high and moderate levels of double burden decreased from 53 to 33 and 47 to 43, respectively, and the number of countries with a low level of or no double burden increased from 42 to 68 (NCD-RisC 2024b; Shekar and Popkin 2020; UNICEF, WHO, and World Bank 2023; refer to figure 2.13 and annex 2A, table 2A.2). Lower levels of double burden in 2022 compared with 2016 were mainly because of a reduced level of stunting; meanwhile, higher levels of double burden were mainly because of worsening levels of overweight and obesity. In this period, the prevalence of overweight and obesity among women increased in 103 countries, with 41 countries experiencing at least a 10 percentage point increase. As of 2022, up to 122 countries worldwide (77 percent) had very high level of overweight and obesity among women, a marked increase from 95 countries (65 percent) in 2016 (refer to annex 2A, table 2A.3). Estimating the double burden as a combined prevalence of underweight and obesity among children and adults, recent research has also asserted that increases in obesity are driving rises in this double burden (NCD-RisC 2024b).

Figure 2.13 Changes in the Proportion of Countries by Burden Level of Public Health Significance

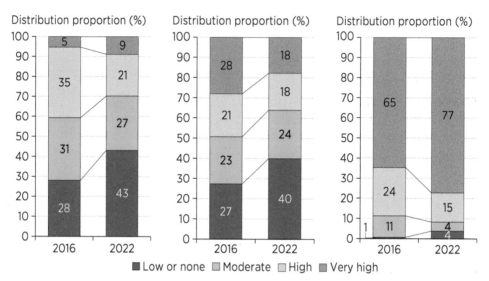

Source: Original figure for this publication based on data from NCD-RisC 2024a, 2024b; UNICEF, WHO, and World Bank 2023.

Notes

1. Estimates are based on country data between 2003 and 2019, where the median year of data collection was 2013 and the population estimates were based on the year 2013.
2. Analyses were limited to the countries with data available for both stunting among children younger than age five years and overweight and obesity among women.

References

Blencowe, Hanna, Julia Krasevec, Mercedes de Onis, Robert E. Black, Gretchen A. Stevens, Elaine Borghi, Chika Hayashi, et al. 2019. "National, Regional, and Worldwide Estimates of Low Birthweight in 2015, with Trends from 2000: A Systematic Analysis." *The Lancet Global Health* 7 (7): e849–60. https://doi.org /10.1016/S2214-109X(18)30565-5.

FAO, IFAD, UNICEF, WFP, and WHO. 2023. "The State of Food Security and Nutrition in the World 2023: Urbanization, Agrifood Systems Transformation and Healthy Diets across the Rural–Urban Continuum." https://doi.org/10.4060 /cc3017en.

NCD-RisC (NCD Risk Factor Collaboration). 2024a. "National Adult Body-Mass Index." https://www.ncdrisc.org/data-downloads-adiposity.html.

NCD-RisC (NCD Risk Factor Collaboration). 2024b. "Worldwide Trends in Underweight and Obesity from 1990 to 2022: A Pooled Analysis of 3663 Population-Representative Studies with 222 Million Children, Adolescents, and Adults." *The Lancet* 403 (10431): 1027–50. https://doi.org/10.1016/S0140-6736(23)02750-2.

Neves, Paulo A.R., Juliana S. Vaz, Fatima S. Maia, Philip Baker, Giovanna Gatica-Domíguez, Ellen Piwoz, Nigel Rollins, et al. 2021. "Rates and Time Trends in the Consumption of Breastmilk, Formula, and Animal Milk by Children Younger than 2 Years from 2000 to 2019: Analysis of 113 Countries." *The Lancet Child & Adolescent Health* 5 (9): 619–30. https://doi.org/10.1016/S2352-4642(21)00163-2.

Norris, Shane A., Edward A. Frongillo, Maureen M. Black, Yanhui Dong, Caroline Fall, Michelle Lampl, Angela D. Liese, et al. 2022. "Nutrition in Adolescent Growth and Development." *The Lancet* 399(10320): 172–84. https://doi.org/10.1016/S0140-6736(21)01590-7.

Saloojee, Haroon, and John M. Pettifor. 2001. "Iron Deficiency and Impaired Child Development." *BMJ* 323 (7326): 1377–78. https://doi.org/10.1136/bmj.323.7326.1377.

Sawyer, Susan M. 2020. "Global Growth Trends in School-Aged Children and Adolescents." *The Lancet* 396 (10261): 1465–67. https://doi.org/10.1016/S0140-6736(20)32232-7.

Shekar, Meera, Jakub Kakietek, Julia Dayton Eberwein, and Dylan Walters. 2017. *An Investment Framework for Nutrition.* Washington, DC: World Bank. https://doi.org/10.1596/978-1-4648-1010-7.

Shekar, Meera, and Barry Popkin. 2020. *Obesity: Health and Economic Consequences of an Impending Global Challenge.* Washington, DC: World Bank.

Simmonds, M., A. Llewellyn, C.G. Owen, and N. Woolacott. 2016. "Predicting Adult Obesity from Childhood Obesity: A Systematic Review and Meta-Analysis." *Obesity Reviews* 17 (2): 95–107.

Stevens, Gretchen A., Ty Beal, Mduduzi N. N. Mbuya, Hanqi Luo, and Lynnette M. Neufeld; Global Micronutrient Deficiencies Research Group. 2022. "Micronutrient Deficiencies among Preschool-Aged Children and Women of Reproductive Age Worldwide: A Pooled Analysis of Individual-Level Data from Population-Representative Surveys." *The Lancet Global Health* 10 (11): e1590–99. https://doi.org/10.1016/S2214-109X(22)00367-9.

UNDESA (United Nations Department of Economic and Social Affairs), Population Division. 2022. "World Population Prospects 2022." New York: UNDESA. Accessed November 30, 2023. https://population.un.org/wpp/Download/Standard/MostUsed/.

UNICEF (United Nations Children's Fund). 2023. "Infant and Young Child Feeding."
UNICEF data. Accessed September 4, 2023. https://data.unicef.org/topic
/nutrition/infant-and-young-child-feeding/.

UNICEF (United Nations Children's Fund), WHO (World Health Organization), and
World Bank. 2023. "Joint Child Malnutrition Estimates Database, May 2023."
Accessed September 4, 2023. https://data.unicef.org/topic/nutrition
/malnutrition.

Ward, Zachary J., Michael W. Long, Stephen C. Resch, Catherine M. Giles, Angie L.
Cradock, and Steven L. Gortmaker. 2017. "Simulation of Growth Trajectories of
Childhood Obesity into Adulthood." *New England Journal of Medicine* 377 (22):
2145–53. https://doi.org/10.1056/NEJMoa1703860.

WHO (World Health Organization). 2017. *The Double Burden of Malnutrition: Policy
Brief.* Geneva: WHO. https://www.who.int/publications-detail-redirect/WHO
-NMH-NHD-17.3.

WHO (World Health Organization). 2023a. "Anaemia in Women and Children."
Global Health Observatory database (accessed September 5, 2023). Geneva:
WHO. https://www.who.int/data/gho/data/themes/topics/anaemia_in_women
_and_children.

WHO (World Health Organization). 2023b. "Joint Low Birthweight Estimates."
Geneva: WHO. https://www.who.int/teams/nutrition-and-food-safety
/monitoring-nutritional-status-and-food-safety-and-events/joint-low
-birthweight-estimates.

WHO (World Health Organization). 2023c. "Noncommunicable Diseases." Geneva:
WHO. https://www.who.int/news-room/fact-sheets/detail/noncommunicable
-diseases.

World Bank. 2023. *World Bank Open Data.* Washington, DC: World Bank. Accessed
September 5, 2023. https://data.worldbank.org.

3

Safeguarding Human Capital amid a Global Food and Nutrition Crisis

Meera Shekar

KEY MESSAGES

- Human capital, as measured by the World Bank's Human Capital Index (HCI), is a critical marker of future economic productivity. Globally, a child born in 2020 could expect to be only 56 percent, on average, as productive as they could be.

- In Africa, most countries have an HCI performance value below 0.40; South Asia has a slightly higher average HCI value, at 0.48; and East Asia and Pacific's HCI value is 0.59. These values suggest that children in these regions will grow to become just 40 percent, 48 percent, and 59 percent, respectively, as productive as they could be.

- Nutrition is a maker and a marker of human capital. Both undernutrition and obesity are key contributors to the HCI and important markers of poor HCI performance. Improving all types of nutritional deficiencies is therefore essential to protecting future human capital, especially in the context of recent and ongoing polycrises that have wreaked havoc on developing economies.

Human Capital

Human capital can be broadly defined as the combination of knowledge, skills, and health that people invest in and accumulate throughout their lives and that enables them to realize their potential as productive members of society and their country. It is measured annually with the Human Capital Index.

Human Capital Index

The Human Capital Index (HCI) combines indicators of health and education into a single measurement of the human capital that a child born today can expect to obtain by their 18th birthday, given the risks of poor education and health that may prevail in the country where they live. The HCI is measured in units of productivity relative to a benchmark of complete education and full health, and its value ranges from 0 to 1. An HCI value of 0.3 for a country indicates, for example, that a child born today in that country can expect to be only 30 percent as productive as a future worker who enjoyed complete education and full health and nutrition. The methodology of the HCI is anchored in the extensive literature on development accounting (Kraay 2018).

The index is designed to highlight how improvements in current health and education outcomes can shape the productivity of the next generation of workers. However, because the HCI captures outcomes, it is not designed to be a checklist of potential policy actions. Instead, the nature and scale of nutritional interventions and actions designed to build human capital will necessarily be different in different countries, based on the epidemiology, institutional capacity, and cost-effectiveness of interventions and policy options in a country, as highlighted in chapters 5 and 6.

Nutrition as a Key Element of the HCI

Early childhood stunting is one of the best indicators of overall societal well-being and inequity (de Onis and Branca 2016). Early malnutrition reduces schooling attainment, decreases adult wages, and makes children less likely to escape poverty as adults (Hoddinott et al. 2008; Martorell 2017). Conversely, reductions in stunting are estimated to increase overall potential economic productivity. Decisions made by families to invest in their children and their health likely underlie the large differences observed between high- and low-income households in their ability to protect human capital from climate hazards, such as excessive heat, air pollution, and flooding, as well as their ability to adapt to climate change, as detailed in chapter 4.

Figure 3.1 lists the top-level components of the HCI. Each indicator included in the estimation of a country's HCI is closely linked to nutrition. Undernutrition contributes to more than 45 percent of child deaths in low- and middle-income countries (LMICs) (Black et al. 2008; Caulfield et al. 2004). Evidence also shows that children with stunting or anemia are more likely to drop out of school and that they learn less in school than

Figure 3.1 Nutrition Is a Key Component of the Human Capital Index

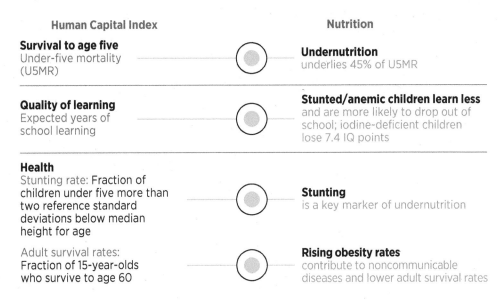

Human Capital Index	Nutrition
Survival to age five Under-five mortality (U5MR)	**Undernutrition** underlies 45% of U5MR
Quality of learning Expected years of school learning	**Stunted/anemic children learn less** and are more likely to drop out of school; iodine-deficient children lose 7.4 IQ points
Health Stunting rate: Fraction of children under five more than two reference standard deviations below median height for age	**Stunting** is a key marker of undernutrition
Adult survival rates: Fraction of 15-year-olds who survive to age 60	**Rising obesity rates** contribute to noncommunicable diseases and lower adult survival rates

Source: Original figure for this publication.

healthy children (Alderman et al. 2017; Chang et al. 2002; Samson et al. 2022). Furthermore, iodine-deficient children lose, on average, at least 7.4 IQ points (Bougma et al. 2013; Ming et al. 2005), and stunting is a key marker of poor health in childhood. Finally, new evidence shows that overweight and obesity, and associated noncommunicable diseases, affect adult survival rates. Cardiovascular disease and cancer account for the greatest mortality risk associated with obesity (Abdelaal, le Roux, and Docherty 2017).

Therefore, improving both ends of the malnutrition spectrum— undernutrition and obesity—is crucial to building and protecting human capital and future economic productivity.

In Africa, most countries have an HCI below 0.40; thus, as adults, children in these countries will be able to maximize only 40 percent of their full economic potential. Child stunting, one of the indicators that make up the HCI, is a significant contributor to low HCI in many countries, not only in Africa but also in South Asia. In about half of the countries in Sub-Saharan Africa, more than 30 percent of children are stunted. South Asia's average HCI is slightly higher than Africa's at 0.48, but five of the seven countries in the region have child stunting rates greater than 30 percent (World Bank 2023).

As cited in chapter 1, a recent study suggests that food price hikes even over a period of a few months can put young children at a much greater risk of severe wasting, which is not just a threat to their health and cognitive development but often leads to death (Headey and Ruel 2023). Infants are particularly vulnerable, and boys and those from impoverished rural settings appear to be most affected. Food inflation during the prenatal period also predicts long-term stunting of children ages two to five. Other studies have shown that food inflation leads to shifts toward consumption of less healthy foods, including ultraprocessed foods, that are associated with rising obesity, noncommunicable diseases, and decreases in adult survival rates. Global warming, too, has been shown to have an impact on nutritional health: a 1°C increase in temperature correlates with 5 percent and 2 percent increases, respectively, in body mass index among girls and women in developing countries. Exposure to extreme temperatures during pregnancy can cause significant birth defects, especially in LMICs, where health care services and resources are less available (Bustinza et al. 2013). Ending malnutrition is therefore a critical input for economic and human development, prosperity, and equity—and for improvements in human capital. This is especially relevant in the context of recent polycrises of pandemics, conflicts, and climate change that have precipitated increases in food prices and reduced access to basic health services.

References

Abdelaal, Mahmoud, Carel W. le Roux, and Neil G Docherty. 2017. "Morbidity and Mortality Associated with Obesity." *Annals of Translational Medicine* 5 (7): 161. https://doi.org/10.21037/atm.2017.03.107.

Alderman, Harold, Jere R. Behrman, Paul Glewwe, Lia Fernald, and Susan Walker. 2017. "Evidence of Impact of Interventions on Growth and Development during Early and Middle Childhood." In *Child and Adolescent Health and Development*, Vol. 8 of Disease Control Priorities, edited by Donald A. P. Bundy, Nilanthi de Silva, Susan Horton, Dean T. Jamison, and George C. Patton, 79–98. Washington, DC: International Bank for Reconstruction and Development /World Bank. https://doi.org/10.1596/978-1-4648-0423-6.

Black, Robert E., Lindsay H. Allen, Zulfiqar A. Bhutta, Mercedes de Onis, Majid Ezzati, Colin Mathers, and Juan Rivera; Maternal and Child Undernutrition Study Group. 2008. "Maternal and Child Undernutrition: Global and Regional Exposures and Health Consequences." *The Lancet* 371 (9608): 243–60.

Bougma, Karim, Francis E. Aboud, Kimberly B. Harding, and Grace S. Marquis. 2013. "Iodine and Mental Development of Children 5 Years Old and Under: A Systematic Review and Meta-Analysis." *Nutrients* 5 (4): 1384–1416. https://doi.org/10.3390/nu5041384.

Bustinza, Ray, Germain Lebel, Pierre Gosselin, Diane Bélanger, and Fateh Chebana. 2013. "Health Impacts of the July 2010 Heat Wave in Québec, Canada." *BMC Public Health* 13: 56. https://doi.org/10.1186/1471-2458-13-56.

Caulfield, Laura E., Mercedes de Onis, Monika Blössner, and Robert E. Black. 2004. "Undernutrition as an Underlying Cause of Child Deaths Associated with Diarrhea, Pneumonia, Malaria, and Measles." *American Journal of Clinical Nutrition* 80 (1): 193–98. https://doi.org/10.1093/ajcn/80.1.193.

Chang, S.M., S.P. Walker, S. Grantham-McGregor, and C.A. Powell. 2002. "Early Childhood Stunting and Later Behaviour and School Achievement." *Journal of Child Psychology and Psychiatry* 43 (6): 775–83. https://doi.org/10.1111/1469-7610.00088.

de Onis, Mercedes, and Francesco Branca. 2016. "Childhood Stunting: A Global Perspective." *Maternal & Child Nutrition* 12 (S1): 12–26. https://doi.org/10.1111/mcn.12231.

Headey, Derek, and Marie Ruel. 2023. "Food Inflation and Child Undernutrition in Low and Middle Income Countries." *Nature Communications* 14: 5761. https://doi.org/10.1038/s41467-023-41543-9.

Hoddinott, John, John A. Maluccio, Jere R. Behrman, Rafael Flores, and Reynaldo Martorell. 2008. "Effect of a Nutrition Intervention during Early Childhood on Economic Productivity in Guatemalan Adults." *The Lancet* 371 (9610): 411–16. https://doi.org/10.1016/S0140-6736(08)60205-6.

Kraay, Aart C. 2018. *Methodology for a World Bank Human Capital Index.* Policy Research Working Paper No. 8593, World Bank, Washington, DC. http://documents.worldbank.org/curated/en/300071537907028892/Methodology-for-a-World-Bank-Human-Capital-Index.

Martorell, Reynaldo. 2017. "Improved Nutrition in the First 1000 Days and Adult Human Capital and Health." *American Journal of Human Biology* 29 (2). https://doi.org/10.1002/ajhb.22952.

Ming, Qian, Dong Wang, William E. Watkins, Val Gebski, Yu Qin Yan, Mu Li, and Zu Pei Chen. 2005. "The Effects of Iodine on Intelligence in Children: A Meta Analysis of Studies Conducted in China." *Asia Pacific Journal of Clinical Nutrition* 14 (1): 32–42.

Samson, Kaitlyn L. I., Jordie A. J. Fischer, and Marion L. Roche. 2022. "Iron Status, Anemia, and Iron Interventions and Their Associations with Cognitive and Academic Performance in Adolescents: A Systematic Review." *Nutrients* 14 (1): 224. https://doi.org/10.3390/nu14010224.

World Bank. 2023. Human Capital Index (database). Washington, DC: World Bank. (Accessed March 5, 2023), https://datacatalog.worldbank.org/int/search/dataset/0038030/human-capital-index.

4

Exploring the Intersection of Nutrition, Climate Change, and Gender: Shared Burdens, Shared Benefits

Chiara Dell'Aira and Meera Shekar

KEY MESSAGES

- Climate change, undernutrition, and obesity are closely intertwined, creating a syndemic that deeply undermines health and development. Because of their low adaptive capacity, low-income countries—and communities affected by poverty in general—are uniquely affected by an increased susceptibility to climate change, aggravating their existing high burden of malnutrition.

- Climate-induced factors—from disrupted food systems, shifting diets, and diminishing nutrient concentrations in crops to increased risk of diseases—fuel global malnutrition. By 2050, more than half a million additional climate-related deaths from dietary changes are anticipated globally: a total of 1.4 billion women and children will be at risk of iron deficiency, 24 million children are projected to become undernourished, and stunting rates are forecast to rise by 23 percent in Sub-Saharan Africa and 62 percent in South Asia.

- Climate change exacerbates obesity by altering food availability and accessibility, promoting the intake of less healthy ultraprocessed foods (UPFs), and reducing physical activity.

- Women bear the brunt of climate change—for example, by virtue of their water collection duties in 70 percent of countries and enduring extreme heat while pregnant. This affects their own health and livelihood and perpetuates intergenerational impacts on nutrition. Heat exposure in pregnancy increases the risk of low birthweight by 25.3 percent. Women are the backbone of food and nutrition security, composing 40 percent of the agricultural labor force in developing countries, and they should be the priority for locally led climate–nutrition interventions. Interventions targeting women may also positively affect their children—another disproportionately vulnerable population in both climate and nutrition spaces. Women-centered investments based on locally led adaptations are anticipated to enhance resilience and mitigation capacities, improve efficiency through better returns on investments, and ensure equitable distribution of the positive impacts.

- Food systems as well as nutrition also deeply affect climate. The agrifood sector contributes more than 30 percent of total annual global greenhouse gas emissions, and food loss and waste account for 8–10 percent. UPFs contribute to one-third of all diet-related emissions in high-income countries, and the carbon footprint from commercial milk formulas is estimated at 11–14 kilograms of carbon dioxide per kilogram sold. Investments in breastfeeding need to be recognized as a carbon offset in global strategies for sustainable food, health, and economic systems. The United Nations Children's Fund's Children's Climate Risk Index is a helpful tool to identify countries in which children are most threatened by climate change, allowing protective actions to be prioritized. Climate investments that are intentional in targeting both women and children are best placed to achieve maximum returns on nutrition and health outcomes and consequently improve human capital. Overall, decision-makers must carefully assess nutritional needs along with environmental sustainability.

- Despite a surge in climate financing, only 4.3 percent of climate funds currently target the agrifood sector, and only 2.4 percent of the key multilateral climate fund investments are currently supporting child-responsive activities. Allocating financing more efficiently and leveraging opportunities to advance nutrition-sensitive investments are critical.

- Many avenues for integrated action exist, but more research is needed: very few experimental studies link climate adaptation strategies with nutrition outcomes.

Social and Economic Costs of Malnutrition and Climate Change

Climate change exacerbates the burden of malnutrition in multiple ways, all with serious implications for health and for social and economic outcomes. Building on the work of the International Food Policy Research Institute (IFPRI 2015), figure 4.1 illustrates the direct and cascading effects of climate change on nutrition outcomes, using an adapted version of the United Nations Children's Fund (UNICEF) nutrition conceptual model (UNICEF 2013) as it applies to the Investment Framework for Nutrition's outcomes of interest: stunting, wasting, anemia, low birthweight (LBW) and birth outcomes, overweight and obesity, and breastfeeding.

Increasing temperatures, along with the escalating frequency and intensity of extreme weather events, upend the enabling environment that is essential to maintain adequate nutrition. Weather shocks and unpredictable precipitation and temperature patterns result in damage to infrastructure, economic disruption, and reduced productivity, which in turn affect political priorities, economic growth, and the broader sociocultural context (IFPRI 2015).

These setbacks disproportionately affect vulnerable communities because of differences in exposure, susceptibility, and coping capacities, amplifying socioeconomic disparities. People living in poverty tend to rely on climate-sensitive assets and have limited access to resources to cope and recover. Their increased vulnerability is mirrored on a larger scale by developing countries, which often lack the necessary resources and technologies needed for effective adaptation (UNDESA 2020). The communities and countries facing this enhanced susceptibility are also those most likely to be grappling with the highest burden of malnutrition, highlighting the role of climate change in exacerbating existing global inequalities.

Unpredictable weather shocks such as droughts and floods can disrupt both the food production system and supply-chain distribution. This can not only lead to price volatility, it can also negatively affect the availability, accessibility, and stability of nutritious and diverse diets (Gitz et al. 2016; Mirzabaev et al. 2023). Even in the absence of weather events, the anthropogenic (that is, derived from human activity) increases in air and water temperatures linked to the climate crisis can severely affect agrifood production, although the effects are nonlinear (Burke, Hsiang, and Miguel 2015). Rising temperatures have been found to affect livestock growth, production, reproduction, and health, which leads to reduced livestock, egg, and dairy production (Cheng, McCarl, and Fei 2022) and compromises crop yields (Tito, Hasconcelos, and Feeley 2018). Changes in ocean temperatures

Figure 4.1 Effects of Climate Change on Key Determinants of Nutrition and Nutrition Outcomes

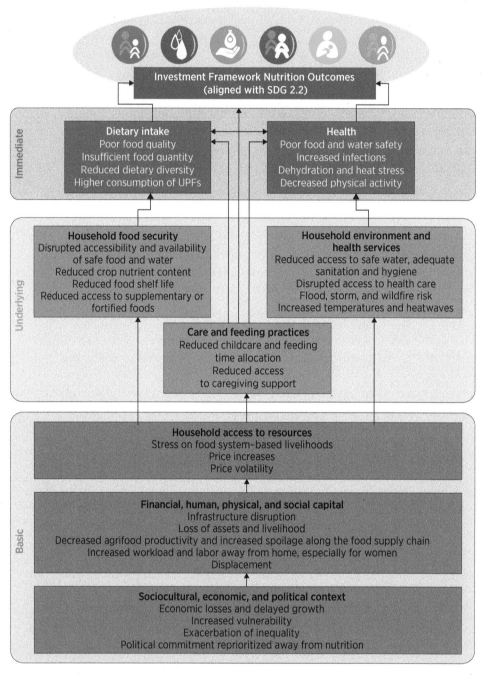

Source: World Bank, based on UNICEF 2013 and inspired by IFPRI 2015.
Note: SDG = Sustainable Development Goal; UPFs = ultraprocessed foods. The icons represent the six targets for SDG 2.2: stunting, anemia, low birthweight, childhood overweight, breastfeeding, and wasting.

and sea level rise also disrupt fisheries and aquaculture production, affecting the blue food system. Modeling studies project that the distribution of fish stocks or catch potential will change with climate change, favoring higher latitudes and negatively affecting tropical areas, where many populations rely on fish as the most accessible source of animal protein (FAO 2020). These effects on food production systems also affect the livelihoods and income of small-scale food producers and, through price hikes, of food buyers, causing financial hardship and leading to reduced dietary quantity and quality, among other poverty-related determinants of malnutrition. Furthermore, they can have wider catastrophic consequences, including triggering social unrest and conflict in politically unstable contexts. Examples include the conflict in Darfur and some of the Arab Springs, which were associated with food insecurity and rising prices driven or exacerbated by climate factors (Moon 2007; Soffiantini 2020).

Climate change has also been linked to increases in foodborne pathogens and increased concentrations of toxic compounds in crops, affecting food safety as well as having a negative effect on the quality of drinking and cooking water and on water-based ecosystems through droughts, heavy rainfall, and increased freshwater salinity (Deshpande, Chang, and Levy 2020; FAO 2018; Gitz et al. 2016; Vineis, Chan, and Khan 2011). Additionally, through its impact on rainfall and temperature, climate change can affect the spatial and seasonal distribution of infectious diseases (Wu et al. 2016). The resulting increase in incidences of diarrhea, malaria, and other infections further exacerbates nutritional outcomes, leading to increased health costs as well as indirect social costs on individuals, families, and communities. This is particularly concerning for populations with an already depleted nutritional status, because malnutrition operates in a vicious mutual synergism, increasing the risk of infection severity (Macallan 2009). These effects can become catastrophic in populations already burdened with limited access to health care services, safe water, sanitation, and hygiene, which are also threatened by climate shocks.

Climate change significantly affects biodiversity by altering habitats, shifting species distributions, and disrupting ecological interactions. Rising temperatures force many species to migrate to cooler areas, often leading to population declines or extinctions when they cannot adapt quickly enough. Melting ice and rising sea levels threaten the biodiversity of islands, submerging coastal habitats and endangering numerous endemic plant and animal species. Changes in phenology, such as earlier flowering or breeding times, can create mismatches between species and their food sources or pollinators. Additionally, ocean warming and acidification cause coral bleaching, disrupting marine ecosystems and threatening the habitat of thousands of species (Shivanna 2022). These effects on ecosystems and biodiversity negatively affect food production and food and nutrition security (Sunderland 2011). Agrodiversity has a direct relationship to improved dietary diversity (Luna-González and Sørensen 2018; Oduor et al. 2019). Loss of genetic diversity limits the genetic variation needed to breed crops that are resilient to climate change and decreases the variety of crops and livestock available to maintain a healthy diet (FAO 2021).

The increased greenhouse gases (GHGs) that are driving anthropogenic climate change can even worsen the nutritional quality of food. Elevated carbon dioxide (CO_2) has been found to decrease the protein and mineral concentrations in food by 5–15 percent and the amount of B vitamins by up to 30 percent (Ebi and Loladze 2019). Modeled projections show that, by 2050, increases in CO_2 could decrease growth in the global availability of key nutrients by approximately 20 percent for protein, 14 percent for iron, and 15 percent for zinc, relative to expected technology and market gains (Beach et al. 2019). This has important implications for health and socioeconomic development, because micronutrient deficiencies are linked to a number of negative health outcomes, impaired cognitive function, reduced work and school performance, and gender disparities (Darnton-Hill et al. 2005). Women tend to be more at risk of developing micronutrient deficiencies, especially iron-deficiency anemia. This not only has social and health costs for the women themselves, but it also has adverse effects on their reproductive outcomes. Smith, Golden, and Myers (2017) have estimated that, by 2050, 1.4 billion women and children will face increased iron deficiency risk due to climate change-mediated reductions in iron supply.

Although pathways between climate change and food and nutrition insecurity are mostly well documented, the evidence directly quantifying the impact of climate change on nutrition outcomes is limited. Global-level modeling studies have consistently linked undernutrition to climate change, highlighting that progress toward better nutrition is likely to be hindered by climate change (Ishida et al. 2014; Lloyd et al. 2018; Lloyd, Kovats, and Chalabi 2011). Climate-related changes in diets, which reduce overall food intake and vegetable and fruit consumption, are expected to lead to more than half a million additional deaths globally by 2050 (Springmann et al. 2016). Projected decreases in calorie availability because of climate change are forecast to lead to an additional 24 million undernourished children, with nearly half of them residing in Sub-Saharan Africa, compared with a scenario unaffected by climate change (Nelson et al. 2009). A systematic review of meta-analyses identified 17 of 22 studies reporting a significant relationship between climate change proxies (droughts, floods, and climate variability) and malnutrition, as well as highlighting that experiencing drought conditions raised the likelihood of both wasting and underweight by almost 50 percent (Lieber et al. 2022). Empirical evidence from Bangladesh documents a correlation between excessive heat in the month of birth and reduced mid-upper-arm circumference in children, highlighting, among possible causes, the negative impact of weather fluctuations on croplands and total rain-fed rice lands (Hanifi et al. 2022). Although their risk assessment model presents uncertainties, Lloyd, Kovats, and Chalabi (2011) have linked a high climate change scenario to a relative rise in severe stunting of 23 percent in Sub-Saharan Africa and 62 percent in South Asia by the 2050s. Another study has explored the role of wealth, estimating that stunting prevalence attributable to climate change in 2030 could range from 570,000 children living in prosperity in a low climate change scenario to more than 1 million children living in poverty in a high climate change scenario (Lloyd et al. 2018). Given the lifelong consequences of stunting for labor productivity and national economic development, these findings underscore the urgency of climate change mitigation on nutrition—especially in contexts in which resources are more limited.

Climate change is also believed to exacerbate obesity, through reduced availability and accessibility of fresh food products and a consequent dietary shift to less expensive ultraprocessed foods (UPFs; Cuschieri, Grech, and Cuschieri 2021). Climate change worsens and perpetuates poverty, constraining individuals' ability to make healthy choices, particularly when coupled with the obesogenic environments that often characterize low-income neighborhoods (Swinburn et al. 2019). A study looking at the effect of temperature on body mass index (BMI) across various age and gender groups found that—after controlling for agricultural production, trade, fertility rates, and gross domestic product per capita—a 1°C increase in temperature resulted in 5 percent and 2 percent increases in the BMI of girls and women, respectively, in developing countries (Trentinaglia et al. 2021). The effects of climate change are therefore expected to worsen the socioeconomic burden of obesity and noncommunicable diseases (NCDs), adding to the extremely high health care costs, lost productivity, and premature mortality that countries of all income levels are already facing as a result of them (Cuschieri, Grech, and Cuschieri 2021). High temperatures may also decrease physical activity, worsening overweight and obesity (Trentinaglia et al. 2021).

This climate crisis–driven added burden of undernutrition, overweight and obesity, and micronutrient deficiencies undermines the resistance of affected populations to further climate-related nutritional and health risks, resulting in a vicious cycle with significant negative implications for these communities.

Bearing the Brunt: Women, Climate Change, and Nutrition

Amid the complex interplay of climate change and its repercussions, various vulnerable groups bear the brunt of these impacts. Women, children, older persons, indigenous peoples, minoritized people, migrants, rural workers, people with disabilities or living in poverty, and those residing in vulnerable regions are all disproportionately burdened by the heightened effects of climate change (OHCHR 2016). Among these groups, women stand out because of their pivotal significance in both the climate and the nutrition spaces.

Women are particularly vulnerable to climate change because of their physiological differences from men, such as reduced heat dissipation through sweating, higher working metabolic rates, and thicker subcutaneous fat that impedes radiative cooling (Duncan 2006).

Furthermore, compared with men, women are more exposed to climate hazards. In addition to the outdoor exposure they face through their role in agriculture, more women than men collect water for their household in about 70 percent of countries. As climate shocks hinder the availability of safe water sources, they are forced to walk longer distances, often in extreme temperatures (Sellers 2016). During pregnancy, they are particularly vulnerable to extreme heat and infectious disease, which climate change exacerbates, leading to worsened maternal outcomes (Smith et al. 2014). Exposure to extreme heat in pregnancy has been associated with a 25.3 percent increased risk of LBW (Zhang et al. 2021). During climate-related disasters, women face higher mortality rates (WHO 2014) and decreased life expectancy (Neumayer and Plümper 2007), as well as increased risks of physical, sexual, and domestic violence (IFRC 2007). Additionally, they are more susceptible to mood disorders and economic hardship post-disaster, particularly those with lower socioeconomic status (WHO 2002). Forced migration disproportionately affects poorer populations and women, who are often overlooked in migration analyses (Norris et al. 2002). Women are also more susceptible to climate-mediated malnutrition, because they are likely to reduce their own food consumption relative to other household members when crop yields decrease or during food shortages (Sellers 2016), despite having higher and more urgent nutritional needs during adolescence, pregnancy, and lactation. This may affect their nutritional status and lead to worsened birth outcomes, perpetuating the intergenerational cycle of malnutrition.

Women also tend to face unique barriers when attempting to cope with the effects of climate change, which acts as a risk multiplier for gender-based health disparities. Because of their increased household and childcare responsibilities, as well as labor market discrimination, women are mostly confined to informal employment and face pay inequity (Sellers 2016). Women in developing countries, even more than in higher-income economies, are especially likely to be engaged in agriculture—where they represent at least 40 percent of the labor force (Palacios-Lopez, Christiaensen, and Kilic 2017)—and their livelihood is therefore particularly vulnerable to droughts, floods, and other climate shocks. Additionally, they tend to have limited access to information, aggravating social exclusion, even from accessing communal resources. Despite having an essential role in food production—women are estimated to produce more than 50 percent of the world's food (Nelson et al. 2012)—gender-biased land-tenure practices often prevent them from owning land, affecting their agency in decision-making and their ability to access collateral loans. The combination of reduced information, lack of control, and lack of land and capital ownership result in women's limited ability to access agricultural inputs and technology to improve their resilience to extreme weather events (Sellers 2016).

The disproportional effect of climate change on women has a negative effect not only on their own nutrition and health, but also on that of their entire household. Their role in the food system is not limited to food production: women tend to take care of food processing, purchasing, preparation, and overall family dietary management, thus serving as gatekeepers of food and nutrition security at the household level. Effects on livelihood and income are reflected in a family's nutrition and health. Because of their limited bargaining power, women adjust their spending, shifting to purchase cheaper, less diverse food for their household (Botreau and Cohen 2019). Additionally, by straining the already heavy workload of women living in rural areas, climate change indirectly impairs women's ability to provide appropriate care to children and implement appropriate child feeding practices, which are critical for child growth and nutrition (Nyantakyi-Frimpong 2021).

A Bidirectional Relationship through Food Systems

Climate change significantly affects the determinants of malnutrition, particularly for women living in developing countries, and these same determinants can also contribute to climate change. Food systems, in particular, both influence and are influenced by ecosystems and climate systems, as shown in figure 4.2. Food systems account for more than one-third of the overall anthropogenic footprint on GHG emissions, which are expected to increase because of urbanization and shifting food consumption patterns (Crippa et al. 2021; Xiong et al. 2022).

Figure 4.2 Interlinks among Climate Systems, Food Systems, and Natural Ecosystems

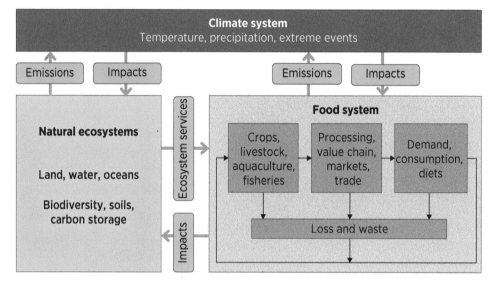

Source: Adapted from Mbow et al. 2019.

As detailed in figure 4.3, agriculture activities account for a sizable proportion (45.4 percent) of the food system's carbon footprint, and the remainder originates from land-use change and from the various supply-chain components of pre- and postproduction, including waste disposal, transportation, consumption, input manufacturing, retail, energy generation, industrial processing, and packaging (Sutton, Lotsch, and Prasann 2024).

Among agricultural activities, the livestock sector stands out as it accounts for 14.5 percent of total global anthropogenic emissions (Gerber et al. 2013), with cattle, specifically, contributing to almost two-thirds of all livestock GHGs (FAO 2023c). In addition to directly releasing GHG emissions into the atmosphere, agriculture-driven land-use changes degrade ecosystems—through, for example, deforestation and wetland drainage—which degrade carbon stores, causing additional CO_2 releases. Alarmingly, agriculture emissions are expected to continue to rise, because urbanization is driving a shift toward diets that are richer in animal products and poorer in healthier food items such as legumes, coarse grains, and other vegetables (Kovacs et al. 2021).

Figure 4.3 Breaking Down the Food System's Carbon Footprint

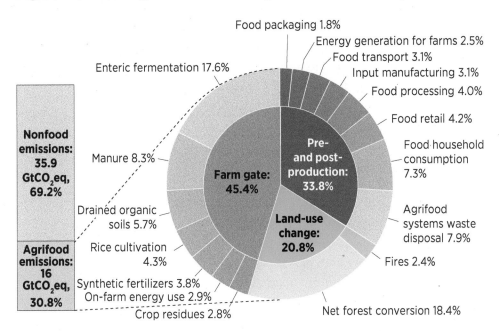

Source: World Bank analysis by Sutton et al, 2024, based on data from FAO 2023b.
Note: Enteric fermentation is a part of the digestive process of ruminant animals such as cattle, sheep, goats, and buffalo that produces various gases, including carbon dioxide and methane.

Contributions of emissions arising from food system processes beyond agriculture and land use—such as the manufacturing of inputs such as fertilizers, pesticides, and feed, as well as activities such as processing, storage, refrigeration, retail, waste management, food services, and transportation—have generally been less explored but are still deserving of attention. Notably, the production, industrial processing, packaging, and distribution of UPFs have been estimated to account for up to one-third of total diet-related GHG emissions in a range of high-income countries, generated primarily during the production and processing stages (Anastasiou et al. 2022). Globally, fresh, minimally processed foods and their culinary preparations are increasingly being displaced by UPFs (Monteiro et al. 2013). Brazil's experience underscores this trend as well as its environmental consequences: a 30-year study revealed a 21 percent increase in diet-related GHG emissions, largely attributed to the growing consumption of UPFs (da Silva et al. 2021). These hyperpalatable, cheap, ready-to-consume food products—often energy-dense and rich in sodium, sugar, and unhealthy fats—raise serious concerns for planetary and human health, as their rising consumption has been systematically associated with a higher risk of obesity and diet-related NCDs (Lane et al. 2024). As dietary patterns continue to shift around the world, the negative effects of UPF consumption are also expected to increase. Both a strong and sustained global commitment and context-specific policies and actions are essential to improve supply, food environments, and demands, facilitating sustainable healthy diets (Menon and Olney 2024).

Food loss and waste is an additional food system pathway that contributes to climate change: GHG emissions from food loss and waste are estimated to account for 8–10 percent of total anthropogenic emissions (Mbow et al. 2019). Food waste is defined as the disposal of food by consumers, and food loss refers to the reduction of edible food during production, postharvest, and processing. The latter tends to be particularly pronounced in developing countries because of inadequate infrastructure. Both food loss and waste also have significant consequences for food security, affecting both global and local food availability: collectively, food loss and waste amount to approximately 25–30 percent of total food produced.

In addition to contributing to obesity and NCDs, food overconsumption (generally defined as consuming food in excess of one's nutritional requirements) can be considered a form of food waste because it puts unnecessary pressure on food systems, generating GHG emissions beyond the need to sustain human health (Mbow et al. 2019). Similarly, the food system experiences "opportunity food losses" when people opt for resource-intensive, animal-based products over nutritionally equivalent plant-based alternatives (Mbow et al. 2019). This is particularly relevant for higher-income countries, where shifting to a planet-friendly diet would lead to the largest per capita carbon reductions (Sun et al. 2022). The EAT–Lancet Commission report calls for substantial global dietary shifts, including doubling the consumption of healthy plant-based foods and halving the intake of added sugar and red meat. At the same time, the report acknowledges that animal-sourced foods do play an important role in resource-constrained regions and that recommendations need to be contextualized to local realities (Willett et al. 2019). For example, in Bangladesh, where growing meat consumption over 16 years has driven an increase in GHG emissions, meeting the EAT–Lancet "ideal planetary diet" or even FAO's food-based dietary guidelines would further increase GHG emissions compared with the country's current dietary habits due to higher dairy consumption (Divya et al. 2022).

Box 4.1 highlights how three different dietary scenarios to meet India's national protein recommendations would impact GHG emissions.

Box 4.1

Greenhouse Gas Cost of Closing the Protein Gap in India

In a pioneering effort, a World Bank team is exploring the greenhouse gas (GHG) emission cost of achieving national dietary recommendations in different countries. On the basis of household consumption data from the 2011 Indian Household Survey, the team found that the population was consuming just 65.2 percent of the recommended amount of protein sources, such as pulses, meat, fish, and eggs. Using GHG emission coefficients, they modeled the GHG cost of the current Indian diet as well as the additional emissions that would arise from closing the protein gap. Three alternative pathways were then explored to highlight differences between food sources: meeting the protein dietary recommendations by increasing the intake of pulses, white meat, and red meat would increase GHG emissions by 56 percent, 63 percent, and 239 percent, respectively (refer to figure B4.1.1).

Figure B4.1.1 Modeled GHG Emission Estimates to Achieve the Recommended Protein Intake in India

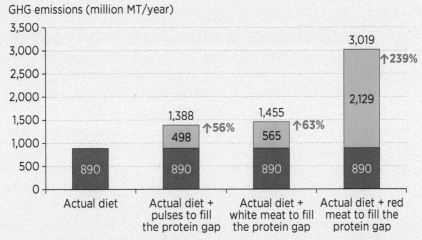

Source: Informal communications with Chris Jackson and Francis Addeah Darko, World Bank.
Note: See annex 4A for details on the methodology used in this study. GHG = greenhouse gas.

(continued)

Box 4.1

Greenhouse Gas Cost of Closing the Protein Gap in India (*continued*)

Red meat is rich in highly bioavailable vitamins and minerals—especially iron and vitamin B12—yet excess consumption has been associated with increased risk of noncommunicable diseases and is widely known to have a detrimental impact on the planet (WHO 2023). Robust empirical analysis of the emission cost of diets can play an important role in assisting policy makers in avoiding the risk of negative climate–nutrition trade-offs. Influencing consumption patterns of demand while considering the nutritional and environmental needs and risks in the local context is essential to achieve the win–win of sustainable and healthy diets that balance the needs of both people and planet.

Source: Informal communications with Chris Jackson and Francis Addeah Darko, World Bank.
Note: See annex 4A for details on the methodology used in this study.

Another form of opportunity loss is the use of commercial milk formulas (CMFs), such as infant and toddler formulas, as a replacement for breastfeeding. CMFs are a significant contributor to GHG emissions, with a carbon footprint over the full product life cycle estimated at 11–14 kg CO_2 per kilogram of CMF (Andresen et al. 2022; Karlsson et al. 2019; Pope et al. 2021). Globally, only 44 percent of infants younger than age 6 months are exclusively breastfed (WHO 2021). Meeting the global targets for breastfeeding would not only result in far larger decreases in GHG emissions than could be achieved from decarbonizing CMF manufacturing, but it would also aid adaptation and enhance resilience to disasters (Long et al. 2021; Smith 2019). This suggests that it is necessary to reframe breastfeeding as foundational to food and health security (Pérez-Escamilla 2017) and as a policy priority across multiple sectors, including climate mitigation (Tomori 2023). Investments in breastfeeding should be considered a carbon offset in global financing schemes aimed at fostering sustainable food, health, and economic systems (Smith et al. 2024). To highlight the environmental importance of breastfeeding, the Green Feeding Climate Action Tool (https://greenfeedingtool.org/#/) enables users to calculate the carbon and water footprint of CMFs at both country and global levels. Table 4.1 presents outcomes for two low- and middle-income countries, extracted from the table generated by the tool (see the complete table in annex 4B).

Table 4.1   Carbon and Water Footprints Associated with Consumption of CMFs among Infants Younger Than Six Months, Ghana and Mexico

Country examples	Breastfeeding practices with infants younger than 6 months			Carbon and water footprints associated with CMF consumption among infants younger than 6 months			
	EBF or pred. BF (%)	Partial BF (%)	Not BF (%)	No. of infants	Lost milk (million L)	Carbon footprint (CO$_2$ equiv., million kg)	Water footprint (million L)
Ghana	64	34	2	878,148	9	26–33	11,141
Mexico	32	42	26	1,902,031	81	167–213	72,391

Source: Green Feeding Climate Action Tool (https://greenfeedingtool .org/#/). Simplified version of table generated by the Green Feeding Climate Action Tool (see annex 4B for detailed version downloaded directly from the tool).

Note: These amounts are estimated on the basis of rates of breastfeeding and clinical assumptions about the percentage of mothers who can breastfeed (that is, who do not have a medical or physical barrier). CMFs = commercial milk formulas; EBF = exclusive breastfeeding, as with a child receiving no other food or drink except breast milk for the first 6 months of life; equiv. = equivalent; k = kilogram; L = liter; lost milk = difference between potential production of breastmilk minus actual annual production of breastmilk; partial BF = partial breastfeeding, meaning that the infant receives both breastmilk in addition to other sources of nourishment, including formula or solid foods; pred. BF = predominant breastfeeding, meaning that the infant's predominant source of nourishment has been breast milk, but the infant may also have received liquids such as water and water-based drinks and fruit juice.

Ensuring Climate Actions Are Nutrition-Sensitive and Nutrition Actions Are Climate-Sensitive

Until recently, climate change, undernutrition, and obesity were considered stand-alone crises to be addressed separately; yet, it is now well-established that they are tightly interconnected. For example, the Lancet Commission on Obesity has introduced the concept of a global syndemic of obesity, undernutrition, and climate change because these crises coincide in time and space, mutually influence each other, and result in compounded consequences. Their interconnectedness implies that numerous systemic interventions could function as dual- or even triple-purpose measures to simultaneously alter the course of all three "pandemics" (Swinburn et al. 2019). As highlighted by the Generation Nutrition coalition (2024, p. 45), "In climate, as in many other areas, nutrition is far too often missing from the agenda and opportunities for synergistic approaches are therefore missed." Decision-makers should therefore ensure that climate actions account for possible outcomes that affect nutrition and, conversely, that nutrition interventions are designed with climate sensitivity in mind. Synergies and trade-offs need to be considered. When designing policies and interventions for climate and nutrition, an integrated systems approach is needed not only to enhance their overall impact but also to prevent further deterioration of both climate and nutrition outcomes. Boxes 4.2 and 4.3 present examples of World Bank nutrition programs that integrate climate adaptation or mitigation activities (or both) within their strategies.

Box 4.2

Indonesia's Climate-Sensitive Actions to Reduce Stunting

The "Why"

To maintain the success of Stranas Stunting (National Strategy to Accelerate Stunting Prevention), Indonesia must address its climate vulnerabilities. Climate events such as El Niño and La Niña are increasingly affecting the agriculture sector in the country, especially rice production, affecting food and nutrition security among vulnerable populations. The government has identified both stunting reduction and nutrition as priorities.

The "What"

The World Bank has been supporting the Government of Indonesia's Stranas Stunting through the flagship Investing in Nutrition and Early Years (INEY) program for results (PforR). The new phase of the program, INEY 2, will tackle these interconnected challenges by

• Updating the National Action Plan for Food and Nutrition to include a Climate and Nutrition Adaptation Plan

• Establishing an integrated and climate-responsive monitoring and evaluation system to better inform the links between nutrition and climate

(continued)

Box 4.2

Indonesia's Climate-Sensitive Actions to Reduce Stunting (continued)

- Incentivizing immunization coverage for climate-sensitive diarrheal diseases

- Training community health workers on stunting prevention and climate adaptation and resilience, with a focus on the specific needs of women.

Source: Informal communications with Anne Marie Provo, Task Team Leader for the Indonesia INEY project.
Note: See annex 4C for details on the INEY program.

Box 4.3

Enhancing Climate and Nutrition Co-benefits in Madagascar

The "Why"

With one of the highest stunting rates globally and a unique geographic exposure to climate risks, Madagascar cannot afford to overlook the climate–nutrition nexus. Climate shocks have been intensifying food and nutrition insecurity, particularly in regions heavily dependent on small-scale rain-fed agriculture. After the 2021 drought, more than 1.1 million people faced food insecurity, and the number of malnourished children doubled. Projections indicate that intensified flooding will increase diarrheal disease and vector-borne and zoonotic diseases in affected areas of the country, which will further threaten the nutritional status of vulnerable populations.

The "What"

The Government of Madagascar has integrated several climate mitigation and adaptation activities into phase two of its Multiphase

(continued)

Box 4.3

Enhancing Climate and Nutrition Co-benefits in Madagascar (continued)

Programmatic Approach (MPA2) Improving Nutrition Outcomes, supported by the World Bank:

- Targeting health and nutrition support to areas of highest climate vulnerability

- Strengthening community health and nutrition sites to effectively address undernutrition

- Increasing access and quality of nutrition and basic health services for climate-sensitive vector-borne (transmitted to humans through insects) and waterborne diseases

- Incorporating climate-related indicators into results-based financing

- Training health workers and community health workers in climate shock preparedness and response

- Increasing access to biofortified, climate-resilient seeds and cuttings

- Improving monitoring and evaluation of nutrition and climate-related diseases; understanding the impact of climate on households; and integrating nutrition, food security, and meteorological data.

Source: Informal communications from Lisa Saldanha, World Bank.
Note: See annex 4C for details on the MPA2 initiative.

Climate risks should be assessed carefully, particularly when designing and formulating nutrition policies that involve the food system or dietary recommendations. The Paris Climate Agreement requires signatory countries and organizations to keep GHG emissions in line with a country's nationally determined contributions. Strategies that might lead to increased GHG emissions should ideally be discouraged, and shared opportunities for both nutrition improvement and climate adaptation and mitigation should instead be prioritized. This, however, does not suggest the adoption of cookie-cutter solutions.

This chapter has already touched on the importance of considering context-specific nutritional and environmental needs when looking at reducing food system GHG emissions from livestock. Strategies to curb overconsumption of harmful levels of red and processed meat could yield negative trade-offs in contexts in which animal product consumption is low and micronutrient deficiencies are prevalent. Livestock- and animal-derived food sources can play a pivotal role in enhancing nutrition, alleviating poverty, promoting gender equality, bolstering livelihoods, enhancing food security, and improving overall health (Adesogan et al. 2020). Yet, countries with low animal product consumption should implement appropriate measures to prevent reaching levels of meat overconsumption that are harmful for both their populations' health and the planet. This is especially important as the global demand for protein from livestock-based foods is projected to rise by 14 percent per person and by 38 percent overall between 2020 and 2050, with the fastest growth in demand anticipated to occur in South Asia and Sub-Saharan Africa (Komarek et al. 2021).

When animal-sourced food production is appropriately scaled and produced in harmony with local ecosystems, it can support circular and diverse agroecosystems and even yield environmental benefits (Beal et al. 2023). Additionally, other protein sources with a lower environmental footprint could be promoted as a suitable alternative to animal products. Edible insects, for example, are consumed as part of traditional diets worldwide and have been found to be suitable for farming and mass production, while using less space and fewer resources and producing far less GHGs than traditional livestock (Halloran et al. 2016, 2017, 2018). Overall, nutritional needs need to be assessed as carefully as environmental sustainability by both nutrition and climate decision-makers to achieve balanced and effective solutions for the people and the planet.

In addition to being climate sensitive, nutrition interventions must be tailored to enhance resilience and minimize the negative consequences of unexpected extreme weather events on nutrition, preserving food accessibility, availability, and stability, as well as ensuring food safety, access to safe water, and prevention and treatment of climate-sensitive diseases. The world needs to be prepared when climate change–related events hit: any strategy put in place is at risk of faltering if it does not account for shocks and changes in precipitation and temperature patterns.

Benefits of Investing in Both Nutrition and Climate Change Actions

Given the evident connection between climate and nutrition, investing in both can enhance health and sustainability and yield improved social and economic returns. The climate change crisis appears to have garnered substantial traction and large-scale funding from the international community, although most finance flow is directed to mitigation, leaving adaptation financing below current needs. Additionally, the benefits of investing in nutrition continue to be somewhat neglected, receiving only limited attention from the public and private sectors.

Malnutrition in all its forms imposes a staggering financial burden on the global economy, imposing unacceptably high costs on national governments. Investing in nutrition through a climate lens needs to be prioritized to achieve healthy, resilient, and empowered populations that are better equipped to support economies and effectively tackle the adverse consequences of climate change.

The past decade has seen a dramatic surge in climate finance flow, with public and private funds nearly quadrupling between 2011 and 2022 and reaching almost $1.3 trillion in 2021–22 (Buchner et al. 2023). Climate financing mechanisms are designed to channel funds toward projects mitigating or adapting to climate change, leveraging investments from various public or private sources at national or international levels and through bilateral or multilateral channels. The growing set of climate financing instruments—such as grants, green bonds, equities, debt swaps, guarantees, carbon markets, and concessional loans—represents a pivotal opportunity to holistically address interconnected global issues with benefits that extend beyond environmental concerns. Leveraging these instruments to positively affect climate and nutrition simultaneously enhances the resilience of vulnerable communities and reduces their vulnerability to further climate-related risks, ultimately protecting them from adverse socioeconomic consequences.

Although zero or near-zero net emission activities are ideal targets for capital investments with a climate mandate, they represent only a fraction of economic activities. Large GHG emitters that are committed to implementing transition pathways to meet sustainability goals can also present significant climate financing opportunities, broadening the scope of eligible activities, entities, and technologies across the global economy. The agrifood sector, as a major contributor to GHGs, offers an unparalleled opportunity to channel climate-related investments with far-reaching benefits. However, 2019–20 estimates indicate that the sector receives only 4.3 percent of total global climate financing; bridging this investment gap requires a substantial increase, ranging from sevenfold to 44-fold (Chiriac, Vishnumolakala, and Rosane 2023). One starting point involves repurposing the staggering annual allocation of public subsidies to agriculture and fisheries, which range from anywhere between $638 billion across 79 countries in 2016–18 to a post-COVID-19 (Coronavirus) estimate by OECD of $851 billion globally in 2020–22 (Damania et al. 2023; OECD 2023). Some of these funds are currently allocated to environmentally harmful practices and hold immense potential to bolster climate-resilient initiatives (World Bank 2023). This is discussed further in chapters 6 and 9.

The private sector could also have a prominent role in investing in the climate-resilient agricultural value chain—for instance, by introducing innovative technologies that improve efficiency and sustainability of food production or by supporting small-scale farmers. Blended financing combining capital from public and philanthropic institutions and private sector investments are instrumental to derisk and stimulate capital flow to high-impact projects. These investments could take the form of impact-focused funds to ensure that these opportunities not only generate financial return but also deliver social and environmental good (Van den Berg 2023). For example, the International Finance Corporation (IFC), as the leading global institution focused on crowding-in private financing for development, has recently launched a partnership with the rice business subsidiary of the key agribusiness player in Viet Nam. IFC will help the company develop an improved and sustainable rice supply chain, simultaneously decreasing production costs and halving the postharvest loss rate by 2030 (IFC 2023).

Agrifood entities could also become eligible to issue green and sustainable bonds by establishing strong transition plans that demonstrate a clear commitment to mitigation and adaptation efforts. The Climate Bonds Initiative (2020) has proposed a Transition Framework for assessing credible and ambitious transitions, ensuring transparency and effectiveness, thereby avoiding "greenwashing." Figure 4.4 displays how the Climate Bonds framework allows the categorization and labeling of "green" and "transition" activities to inform eligible climate investments. The figure presents two examples of transition activities from the agrifood sector that would unlock both climate and nutrition benefits.

Figure 4.4 Determining Climate Investment Eligibility through the Climate Bonds Transition Framework

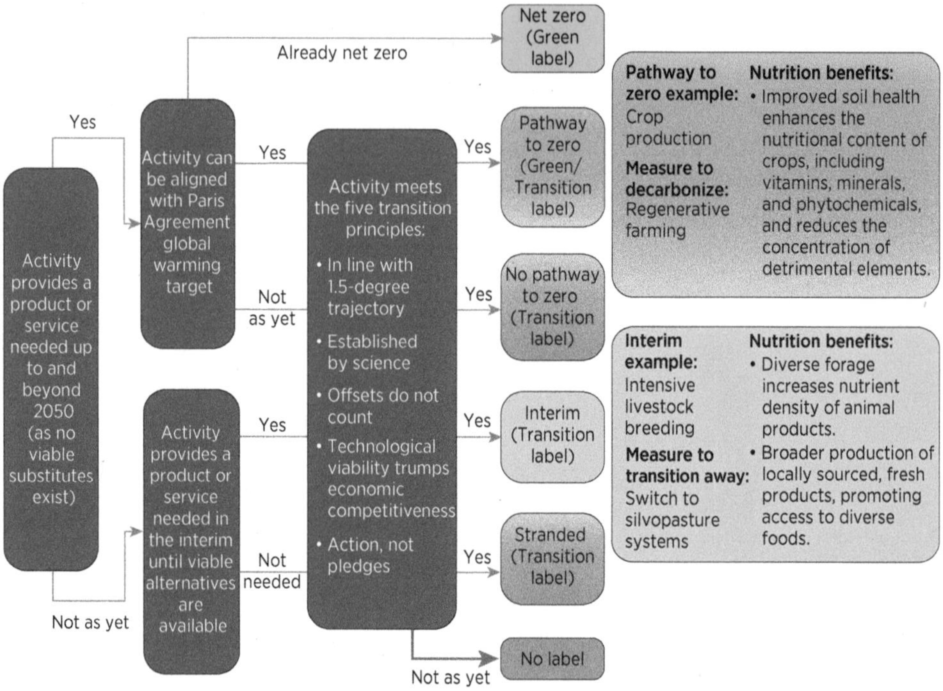

Source: Adapted from Climate Bonds Initiative 2020.

Additionally, the Climate Bonds Initiative recommends assessing entities against the hallmarks of credible transition, which allow a demonstration of the concrete ability and intent to transition through specific action plans and accountability systems. Brazilian agrifood companies Sygenta and Amaggi were assessed against the hallmarks in two case studies, setting a standard for how entities within this sector need to set ambitious yet feasible transition objectives, and restructure their operations, to realistically align with the Paris Agreement (Climate Bonds Initiative 2023).

Stakeholders should be ready to recognize these opportunities and encourage new investments beyond traditionally green activities. At the same time, we call on private agrifood companies with a focus on nutrition to embrace these guidelines to establish strong transition plans and attract climate financing.

Opportunities to leverage climate financing are further discussed in chapter 9, where table 9.1 presents examples of funds with the potential to finance impactful activities targeting both climate adaptation and nutrition.

Entry Points for Climate Change Adaptation and Mitigation Investments for Nutrition

Generally, climate change adaptation strategies consist of adjustments to respond to actual or expected climate change shocks, stressors, risks, or opportunities. Mitigation actions aim to reduce and stabilize the flow of heat-trapping GHG emissions in the atmosphere to prevent further anthropogenic changes. Strategies to promote adaptation often include mitigation components and vice versa. Because of the synergy between climate change and nutrition, climate change adaptation and mitigation investments can be potent avenues for promoting nutrition, allowing countries to simultaneously combat climate change and improve nutritional outcomes.

Climate Action and Nutrition: Pathways to Impact, prepared by the FAO for the Initiative on Climate Action and Nutrition, includes a useful collection of response options for integrated action on nutrition- and climate-relevant outcomes (FAO 2023a). Yet, careful review of nutrition-sensitive evidence identified a very limited number of experimental studies of climate-smart nutrition-sensitive interventions, all with an exclusive focus on adaptation, and only five that explicitly investigated the ability of nutrition-sensitive programs to buffer the effects of climate shocks on nutrition-related outcomes. Among these, targeted cash-transfer interventions were found to protect dietary diversity scores and calorie intake against climate shocks in both Pakistan and Zambia (Asfaw et al. 2017; Mustafa 2022). It is unclear, however, how these findings would translate to nutrition indicators: Ongudi and Thiam (2020) found positive, albeit nonsignificant, correlations between a cash-transfer program in Kenya and child anthropometric outcomes and no evidence showing that receiving the transfer would buffer the effects of drought on child nutrition.

In Chad, an integrated community resilience program that incorporated climate-adaptation measures may have prevented an increase in acute malnutrition, and it had a positive impact on stunting and child illness. The multisectoral intervention included climate-smart agriculture practices such as dry-season vegetable gardens; water, sanitation, and hygiene promotion; health nutrition and behavior change; and food distribution based on an early warning system (Marshak, Young, and Radday 2017).

Finally, a study in Guatemala evaluated a program targeting an area affected by repeated droughts by providing households with high-yield heat-resistant chickens and training in raising poultry. The intervention was associated with large positive effects on anthropometric indicators among girls ages six months to five years; nonsignificant effects were found among boys (Mullally 2018).

The study in Guatemala offers an interesting example of an intervention that could leverage the key role of women in household food and nutrition security. Chickens and small livestock are often controlled by women in poor households (Wong et al. 2017) and are believed to offer income potential and empowerment through asset control (Roy et al. 2015). To formulate meaningful strategies, decision-makers should recognize and harness the role of women in food systems, empower them to achieve better climate and nutrition outcomes, and enhance their resilience to climate-related challenges. Figure 4.5 displays a set of entry points for climate mitigation and adaptation strategies that have the potential to positively affect nutritional outcomes and can be tailored to target women as they are the ideal recipients of climate- and nutrition-smart interventions.

Figure 4.5 Climate Change Mitigation and Adaptation Entry Points for Improved Nutrition Targeted to Women

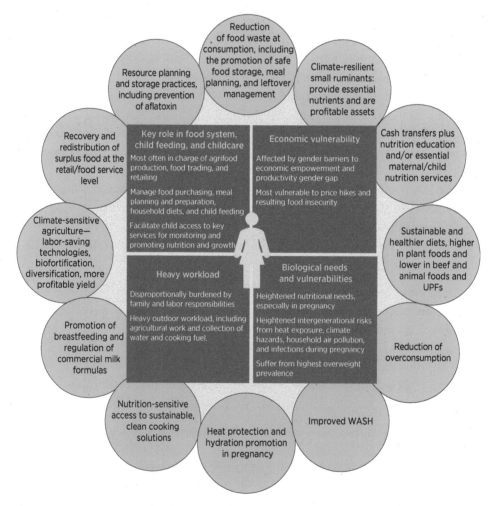

Source: Original figure for this publication.
Note: UPFs = ultraprocessed foods; WASH = water, sanitation, and hygiene.

Targeting women also offers the opportunity and added benefit of reaching their children. Children represent another key population that is uniquely susceptible to nutrition and climate risks while also having the potential to become agents of change. Yet, only 2.4 percent of the key multilateral climate fund investments are currently supporting child-responsive activities (UNICEF 2023). UNICEF's Children's Climate Risk Index is a helpful tool to identify countries where children are most threatened by climate change (Rees 2021), allowing the prioritization of protective actions. Climate investments that are intentional in targeting both women and children are best placed to achieve maximum returns on nutrition and health outcomes and consequently improve human capital. Breastfeeding, with its unparalleled health and nutrition benefits to mothers and children; the ability to strengthen infant resilience to floods, cyclones, and other climate shocks; and being waste-free and extremely resource-efficient, is an example of a climate-smart, child-responsive practice targeting women with significant gains and co-benefits for human and planetary health (Smith et al. 2024). To promote breastfeeding, cash transfers combined with behavior change communication have been effective in multiple contexts, as discussed in chapter 5. Additionally, they have been found to positively affect dietary diversity (Manley, Alderman, and Gentilini 2022), which in turn supports healthy breastfeeding.

Finally, women-centered investments align with the principles of locally led adaptation (LLA), an approach recognized for its effectiveness, efficiency, and equity in delivering adaptation actions, by ensuring that efforts incorporate local priorities and channel funding to local actors (GCA 2022). By adhering to the LLA paradigm and its principles, we can achieve a climate-resilient future characterized by inclusion, participation, justice, and equity (Soanes et al. 2021). Investments based on LLA are anticipated to enhance resilience and mitigation capacities, improve efficiency through better returns on investment, and ensure equitable distribution of the positive impacts (GCA 2022).

Although a focus on women and their children is crucial in the climate and nutrition space, it is important to recognize other populations that may also be vulnerable to both nutrition and climate challenges or have a significant role in climate change and food systems. Indigenous populations are another example of this dual vulnerability because they are susceptible to climate hazards and rising malnutrition levels while also contributing valuable and proven knowledge to the transition toward more sustainable food systems (FAO, Alliance of Biodiversity International, and CIAT 2021). Decision-makers should explore their local contexts to identify other vulnerable and marginalized groups that should be targeted by climate–nutrition initiatives.

References

Adesogan, Adegbola T., Arie H. Havelaar, Sarah L, McKune, Marjatta Eilittä, and Geoffrey E. Dahl. 2020. "Animal Source Foods: Sustainability Problem or Malnutrition and Sustainability Solution? Perspective Matters." *Global Food Security* 25: 100325. https://doi.org/10.1016/j.gfs.2019.100325.

Anastasiou, K., P. Baker, M. Hadjikakou, G. A. Hendrie, and M. Lawrence. 2022. "A Conceptual Framework for Understanding the Environmental Impacts of Ultra-Processed Foods and Implications for Sustainable Food Systems." *Journal of Cleaner Production* 368: 933155. https://doi.org/10.1016/j.jclepro.2022.133155.

Andresen, Ellen C., Anne-Grete R. Hjelkrem, Anne K. Bakken, and Lene F. Andersen. 2022. "Environmental Impact of Feeding with Infant Formula in Comparison with Breastfeeding." *International Journal of Environmental Research and Public Health* 19 (11): 6397. https://doi.org/10.3390/ijerph19116397.

Asfaw, Solomon, Alessandro Carraro, Benjamin Davis, Sudhanshu Handa, and David Seidenfeld. 2017. *Cash Transfer Programmes for Managing Climate Risk: Evidence from a Randomized Experiment in Zambia.* Rome: Food and Agriculture Organization of the United Nations. https://doi.org/10.13140/RG.2.2 .33167.59048.

Beach, Robert H., Timothy B. Sulser, Allison Crimmins, Nicola Cenacchi, Jefferson Cole, Naomi K. Fukagawa, Daniel Mason-D'Croz, et al. 2019. "Combining the Effects of Increased Atmospheric Carbon Dioxide on Protein, Iron, and Zinc Availability and Projected Climate Change on Global Diets: A Modelling Study." *The Lancet Planetary Health* 3(7): e307–17. https://doi.org/10.1016 /S2542-5196(19)30094-4.

Beal, Ty, Christopher D. Gardner, Mario Herrero, Lora L. Iannotti, Lutz Merbold, Stella Nordhagen, and Anne Mottet. 2023. "Friend or Foe? The Role of Animal-Source Foods in Healthy and Environmentally Sustainable Diets." *Journal of Nutrition* 153 (2): 409–25. https://doi.org/10.1016/j.tjnut.2022.10.016.

Botreau, Hélène, and Marc J. Cohen. 2019. *Gender Inequalities and Food Insecurity: Ten Years after the Food Price Crisis, Why Are Women Farmers Still Food-Insecure?* Nairobi: Oxfam. https://reliefweb.int/report/world/gender-inequalities-and-food -insecurity-ten-years-after-food-price-crisis-why-are-women.

Buchner, Barbara, Baysa Naran, Rajashree Padmanabhi, Sean Stout, Costanza Strinati, Dharshan Wignarajah, Gaoyi Miao, et al. 2023. *Global Landscape of Climate Finance.* San Francisco: Climate Policy Initiative. https://www .climatepolicyinitiative.org/wp-content/uploads/2023/11/Global-Landscape-of -Climate-Finance-2023.pdf.

Burke, Marshall, Solomon Hsiang, and Edward Miguel. 2015. "Global Non-Linear Effect of Temperature on Economic Production." *Nature* 527: 235–39. https://doi.org/10.1038/nature15725.

Cheng, Muxi, Bruce McCarl, and Chengcheng Fei. 2022. "Climate Change and Livestock Production: A Literature Review." *Atmosphere* 13 (1): 140. https://doi.org/10.3390/atmos13010140.

Chiriac, Daniela, Harsha Vishnumolakala, and Paul Rosane. 2023. *Landscape of Climate Finance for Agrifood Systems.* San Francisco: Climate Policy Initiative.

Climate Bonds Initiative. 2020. *Financing Credible Transitions: How to Ensure the Transition Label Has Impact.* White Paper. London: Climate Bonds Initiative. https://www.climatebonds.net/transition-finance/fin-credible-transitions.

Climate Bonds Initiative. 2023. *Investment Opportunities: Agri-Food Sector in Brazil.* London: Climate Bonds Initiative. https://www.climatebonds.net/files/reports/investment_opportunity_report_brazil_.pdf.

Crippa, M., E. Solazzo, D. Guizzardi, F. Monforti-Ferrario, F. N. Tubiello, and A. Leip. 2021. "Food Systems Are Responsible for a Third of Global Anthropogenic GHG Emissions." *Nature Food* 2: 198–209.

Cuschieri, Sarah, Elizabeth Grech, and Andrea Cuschieri. 2021. "Climate Change, Obesity, and COVID-19—Global Crises with Catastrophic Consequences. Is This the Future?" *Atmosphere* 12 (10): 1292. https://doi.org/10.3390/atmos12101292.

Damania, Richard, Esteban Balseca, Charlotte de Fontaubert, Joshua Gill, Kichan Kim, Jun Rentschler, Jason Russ, et al. 2023. *Detox Development: Repurposing Environmentally Harmful Subsidies.* Washington, DC: World Bank. https://doi.org/10.1596/978-1-4648-1916-2.

Darnton-Hill, Ian, Patrick Webb, Philip W. J. Harvey, Joseph M. Hunt, Nita Dalmiya, Mickey Chopra, Madeleine J. Ball, et al. 2005. "Micronutrient Deficiencies and Gender: Social and Economic Costs." *American Journal of Clinical Nutrition* 81(5): 1198S–205S. https://doi.org/10.1093/ajcn/81.5.1198.

da Silva, Jacqueline Tereza, Josefa María Fellegger Garzillo, Fernanda Rauber, Alana Kluczkovski, Ximena Schmidt Rivera, Gabriela Lopes da Cruz, Angelina Frankowska, et al. 2021. "Greenhouse Gas Emissions, Water Footprint, and Ecological Footprint of Food Purchases According to Their Degree of Processing in Brazilian Metropolitan Areas: A Time-Series Study from 1987 to 2018." *The Lancet Planetary Health* 5(11): e775–85. https://doi.org/10.1016/S2542-5196(21)00254-0.

Deshpande, Aniruddha, Howard Chang, and Karen Levy. 2020. "Heavy Rainfall Events and Diarrheal Diseases: The Role of Urban–Rural Geography." *American Journal of Tropical Medicine and Hygiene* 103(3): 1043–49.

Divya, Mehra, Junying Tong, Felipe Dizon, and Saskia De Pee. 2022. *Healthy and Sustainable Diets in Bangladesh.* Policy Research Working Paper 10160, World Bank, Washington, DC.

Duncan, K. 2006. "Global Climate Change, Air Pollution, and Women's Health." *WIT Transactions on Ecology and the Environment* 99(10). https://doi.org/10.2495/RAV060611.

Ebi, Kristie L., and Irakli Loladze. 2019. "Elevated Atmospheric CO_2 Concentrations and Climate Change Will Affect Our Food's Quality and Quantity." *The Lancet Planetary Health* 3(7): e283–84.

FAO (Food and Agriculture Organization of the United Nations). 2018. *The State of Agricultural Commodity Markets 2018.* Rome: FAO. https://www.fao.org/documents/card/en/c/I9542EN.

FAO (Food and Agricultural Organization of the United Nations). 2020. *The State of World Fisheries and Aquaculture 2020: Sustainability in Action.* Rome: FAO. https://doi.org/10.4060/ca9229en.

FAO (Food and Agricultural Organization of the United Nations). 2021. *Climate Change, Biodiversity and Nutrition Nexus—Evidence and Emerging Policy and Programming Opportunities.* Rome: FAO.

FAO (Food and Agricultural Organization of the United Nations). 2023a. *Climate Action and Nutrition: Pathways to Impact.* Rome: FAO.

FAO (Food and Agricultural Organization of the United Nations). 2023b. FAOSTAT: Emissions Totals (data set). Accessed March 30, 2024. https://www.fao.org/faostat/en/#data/Gt.

FAO (Food and Agriculture Organization of the United Nations). 2023c. *Global Livestock Environmental Assessment Model (GLEAM).* Rome: FAO. https://www.fao.org/gleam/en.

FAO (Food and Agricultural Organization of the United Nations), Alliance of Bioversity International, and CIAT (International Center for Tropical Agriculture). 2021. *Indigenous Peoples' Food Systems: Insights on Sustainability and Resilience in the Front Line of Climate Change.* Rome: FAO.

GCA (Global Center on Adaptation). 2022. "Section 3, Cross Sectoral Themes." In *State and Trends in Adaptation Reports 2021 and 2022,* 358–470. Rotterdam and Abidjan: Global Center on Adaptation.

Generation Nutrition. 2024. *Rethinking the EU's ODA Investments in Nutrition: Catalyzing Transformative Change.* Paris: Global Health Advocates. https://www.ghadvocates.eu/app/uploads/2024-06_Generation-Nutrition-Report-EU-ODA-funding.pdf.

Gerber, P. J., H. Steinfeld, B. Henderson, A. Mottet, C. Opio, J. Dijkman, A. Falcucci, and G. Tempio. 2013. *Tackling Climate Change through Livestock: A Global Assessment of Emissions and Mitigation Opportunities.* Rome: Food and Agriculture Organization of the United Nations. https://www.fao.org/4/i3437e/i3437e.pdf.

Gitz, Vincent, Alexandre Meybeck, Leslie Lipper, Cassandra de Young, and Susan Braatz. 2016. *Climate Change and Food Security: Risks and Responses.* Food and Agriculture Organization of the United Nations. https://www.fao.org/3/i5188e/I5188E.pdf.

Halloran, Afton, Roberto Flore, Paul Vantomme, and Nanna Roos. 2018. *Edible Insects in Sustainable Food Systems.* Edinburgh: Springer.

Halloran, A., Y. Hanboonsong, N. Roos, and S. Bruun. 2017. "Life Cycle Assessment of Cricket Farming in North-Eastern Thailand." *Journal of Cleaner Production* 156: 83–94. https://doi.org/10.1016/j.jclepro.2017.04.017.

Halloran, Afton, Nanna Roos, Jørgen Eilenberg, Allessandro Cerutti, and Sander Bruun. 2016. "Life Cycle Assessment of Edible Insects for Food Protein: A Review." *Agronomy for Sustainable Development* 36: 57. https://doi.org/10.1007/s13593-016-0392-8.

Hanifi, S. M. Manzoor Ahmed, Nidhiya Menon, and Agnes Quisumbing. 2022. "The Impact of Climate Change on Children's Nutritional Status in Coastal Bangladesh." *Social Science & Medicine* 294: 114704. https://doi.org/10.1016/j.socscimed.2022.114704.

IFC (International Finance Corporation). 2023. "IFC Regional Vice President Visits Viet Nam to Focus on Nation's Transition to a Low-Carbon Growth Model." Press release, November 13, 2023. https://pressroom.ifc.org/all/pages/PressDetail.aspx?ID=27865.

IFPRI (International Food Policy Research Institute). 2015. *Global Nutrition Report 2015: Actions and Accountability to Advance Nutrition and Sustainable Development.* Washington, DC: IFPRI.

IFRC (International Federation of the Red Cross and Red Crescent). 2007. *World Disasters Report.* Geneva: IFRC. https://www.preventionweb.net/publication/world-disasters-report-2007-focus-discrimination.

Ishida, Hiroyuki, Shota Kobayashi, Shinjiro Kanae, Tomoko Hasegawa, Shinichiro Fujimori, Yonghee Shin, Kiyoshi Takahashi, et al. 2014. "Global-Scale Projection and Its Sensitivity Analysis of the Health Burden Attributable to Childhood Undernutrition under the Latest Scenario Framework for Climate Change Research." *Environmental Research Letters* 9 (6): 064014. https://doi.org/10.1088/1748-9326/9/6/064014.

Karlsson, Johann O., Tara Garnett, Nigel C. Rollins, and Ellin Roos. 2019. "The Carbon Footprint of Breastmilk Substitutes in Comparison with Breastfeeding." *Journal of Cleaner Production* 222: 436–45. https://doi.org/10.1016/j.jclepro.2019.03.043.

Komarek, Adam M., Shahnila Dunston, Dolapo Enahoro, H. Charles J. Godfray, Mario Herrero, Daniel Mason-D'Croz, Karl M. Rich, et al. 2021. "Income, Consumer Preferences, and the Future of Livestock-Derived Food Demand." *Global Environmental Change* 70: 102343. https://doi.org/10.1016/j.gloenvcha.2021.102343.

Kovacs, Brittany, Lindsay Miller, Martin C. Heller, and Donald Rose. 2021. "The Carbon Footprint of Dietary Guidelines around the World: A Seven Country Modeling Study." *Nutrition Journal* 20 (15): 1–10.

Lane, Melissa M., Elizabeth Gamage, Shutong Du, Deborah N. Ashtree, Amelia J. McGuinness, Sarah Gauci, Phillip Baker, et al. 2024. "Ultra-Processed Food Exposure and Adverse Health Outcomes: Umbrella Review of Epidemiological Meta-Analyses." *BMJ* 384: e077310. https://doi.org/10.1136/bmj -2023-077310.

Lieber, Mark, Peter Chin-Hong, Knox Kelly, Madhavi Dandu, and Sheri D. Weister. 2022. "A Systematic Review and Meta-Analysis Assessing the Impact of Droughts, Flooding, and Climate Variability on Malnutrition." *Global Public Health* 17 (1): 68–82. https://doi.org/10.1080/17441692.2020 .1860247.

Lloyd, Simon J., Mook Bangalore, Zaid Chalabi, R. Sari Kovats, Stèphane Hallegatte, Julie Rozenberg, Hugo Valin, et al. 2018. "A Global-Level Model of the Potential Impacts of Climate Change on Child Stunting Via Income and Food Price in 2030." *Environmental Health Perspectives* 126 (9): 097007. https://doi .org/10.1289/EHP2916.

Lloyd, Simon J., R. Sari Kovats, and Zaid Chalabi. 2011. "Climate Change, Crop Yields, and Undernutrition: Development of a Model to Quantify the Impact of Climate Scenarios on Child Undernutrition." *Environmental Health Perspectives* 119 (12): 1817–23. https://doi.org/10.1289/ehp.1003311.

Long, Aoife, Kian Mintz-Woo, Hannah Daly, Maeve O'Connell, Beatrice Smyth, and Jerry D. Murphy. 2021. "Infant Feeding and the Energy Transition: A Comparison between Decarbonising Breastmilk Substitutes with Renewable Gas and Achieving the Global Nutrition Target for Breastfeeding." *Journal of Cleaner Production* 324:129280. https://doi .org/10.1016/j.jclepro.2021.129280.

Luna-González, Diana V., and Marten Sørensen. 2018. "Higher Agrobiodiversity Is Associated with Improved Dietary Diversity, but not Child Anthropometric Status, of Mayan Achí People of Guatemala." *Public Health Nutrition* 21 (11): 2128–41. https://doi.org/10.1017/S1368980018000617.

Macallan, Derek. 2009. "Infection and Malnutrition." *Medicine* 37 (10): 525–28. https://doi.org/10.1016/j.mpmed.2009.07.005.

Manley, James, Harold Alderman, and Ugo Gentilini. 2022. "More Evidence on Cash Transfers and Child Nutritional Outcomes: A Systematic Review and Meta-Analysis." *BMJ Global Health* 7: e008233.

Marshak, Anastasia, Helen Young, and Anne Radday 2017. "Water, Livestock, and Malnutrition Findings from an Impact Assessment of Community Resilience to Acute Malnutrition Programme in Chad." *Field Exchange* 54: 64–65.

Mbow, Cheikh, Cynthia Rosenzweig, Luis Gustavo Barioni, Tek Sapkota, Tim G. Benton, Emma Liwenga, Francesco N. Tubiello, et al. 2019. "Food Security." In *Climate Change and Land: An IPCC Special Report on Climate Change, Desertification, Land Degradation, Sustainable Land Management, Food Security, and Greenhouse Gas Fluxes in Terrestrial Ecosystems*, edited by P. R. Shukla, J. Skea, E. Calvo Buendia, V. Masson-Delmotte, H.-O. Pörtner, D. C. Roberts, P. Zhai, et al., 437–550. New York: Cambridge University Press.

Menon, P., and D. Olney, D. 2024. "Transforming Food Systems for Sustainable Healthy Diets: A Global Imperative." *World Bank Blogs,* May 30, 2024. https://blogs.worldbank.org/en/agfood/transforming-food-systems-for-sustainable-healthy-diets--a-globa.

Mirzabaev, Alisher, Rachel Bezner Kerr, Toshihiro Hasegawa, Prajal Pradhan, Anita Wreford, Maria Cristina Tirado von der Pahlen, and Helen Gurney-Smith. 2023. "Severe Climate Change Risks to Food Security and Nutrition." *Climate Risk Management* 39 (100473).

Monteiro, C. A, J.-C. Moubarac, G. Cannon, S. W. Ng, and B. Popkin. 2013. "Ultra-Processed Products Are Becoming Dominant in the Global Food System." *Obesity Reviews* 14 (Supplement 2): 21–28. https://doi.org/10.1111/obr.12107.

Moon, Ban Ki. 2007. "A Climate Culprit in Darfur." *Washington Post,* June 15, 2007. https://www.washingtonpost.com/archive/opinions/2007/06/16/a-climate-culprit-in-darfur/8ffc62ad-14f2-412f-80ed-103545fe5697/.

Mullally, Conner C. 2018. "Livestock Transfers and Resilience: Evidence from a Randomized Trial in Guatemala." Paper presented at the 2018 Agricultural & Applied Economics Association Annual Meeting, Washington, DC, August 5, 2018.

Mustafa, Ghulam. 2022. "Weather Shocks, Unconditional Cash Transfers and Household Food Outcomes." PIDE Working Papers No. 2022: 8, Pakistan Institute of Development Economics, Islamabad.

Nelson, Gerald C., Mark W. Rosegrant, Jawoo Koo, Richard Robertson, Timothy Sulser, Tingju Zhu, Claudia Ringler, et al. 2009. *Climate Change: Impact on Agriculture and Costs of Adaptation.* Washington, DC: International Food Policy Research Institute.

Nelson, Sybil, Ilaria Sisto, Eve Crowley, and Marcela Villarreal. 2012. "Women in Agriculture: Closing the Gender Gap for Development." In *Feeding a Thirsty World: Challenges and Opportunities for a Water and Food Secure*, edited by A. Jägerskog and T. Jønch Clausen, 25–30. Stockholm: Stockholm International Water Institute.

Neumayer, Eric, and Thomas Plümper. 2007. "The Gendered Nature of Natural Disasters: The Impact of Catastrophic Events on the Gender Gap in Life Expectancy, 1981–2002." *Annals of the Association of American Geography* 97 (3): 551–66. https://doi.org/10.1111/j.1467-8306.2007.00563.x.

Norris, Fran H., Matthew J. Friedman, Patricia J. Watson, Christopher M. Byrne, Eolia Diaz, and Krzysztof Kaniasty. 2002. "60,000 Disaster Victims Speak: Part I. An Empirical Review of the Empirical Literature, 1981–2001." *Psychiatry* 65 (3): 207–39. https://doi.org/10.1521/psyc.65.3.207.20173.

Nyantakyi-Frimpong, Hanson. 2021. "Climate Change, Women's Workload in Smallholder Agriculture, and Embodied Political Ecologies of Undernutrition in Northern Ghana." *Health & Place* 68: 102536.

Oduor, Francis Odhiambo, Julia Boedecker, Gina Kennedy, and Céline Termote. 2019. "Exploring Agrobiodiversity for Nutrition: Household On-Farm Agrobiodiversity Is Associated with Improved Quality of Diet of Young Children in Vihiga, Kenya." *PLOS ONE* 14 (8): e0219680.

OECD (Organisation for Economic Co-operation and Development). 2023. *Agricultural Policy Monitoring and Evaluation 2023: Adapting Agriculture to Climate Change*. Paris: OECD.

OHCHR (Office of the United Nations High Commissioner for Human Rights). 2016. *Discussion Paper: The Rights of Those Disproportionately Impacted by Climate Change*. Geneva: OHCHR. https://www.ohchr.org/sites/default/files/Documents/Issues /ClimateChange/EM2016/DisproportionateImpacts.pdf.

Ongudi, Silas, and Djiby Racine Thiam. 2020. "Prenatal Health and Weather-Related Shocks under Social Safety Net Policy in Kenya." ERSA Working Paper No. 831, Economic Research Southern Africa, Cape Town, South Africa.

Palacios-Lopez, Amparo, Luc Christiaensen, and Talip Kilic. 2017. "How Much of the Labor in African Agriculture Is Provided by Women?" *Food Policy* 67: 52–63. https://doi.org/0.1016/j.foodpol.2016.09.017.

Pérez-Escamilla, Rafael. 2017. "Food Security and the 2015–2030 Sustainable Development Goals: From Human to Planetary Health: Perspectives and Opinions." *Current Developments in Nutrition* 1 (7): e000513.

Pope, Daniel H., Johann O. Karlsson, Philip Baker, and David McCoy. 2021. "Examining the Environmental Impacts of the Dairy and Baby Food Industries: Are First-Food Systems a Crucial Missing Part of the Healthy and Sustainable Food Systems Agenda Now Underway?" *International Journal of Environmental Research and Public Health* 18 (23): 12678.

Rees, N. 2021. *The Climate Crisis Is a Child Rights Crisis: Introducing the Children's Climate Risk Index*. New York: UNICEF.

Roy, Shalini, Jinnat Ara, Narayan Das, and Agnes R. Quisumbing. 2015. "'Flypaper Effects' in Transfers Targeted to Women: Evidence from BRAC's 'Targeting the Ultra Poor' Program in Bangladesh." *Journal of Development Economics* 117: 1–19.

Sellers, Sam. 2016. *Gender and Climate Change: A Closer Look at Existing Evidence*. New York: Global Gender and Climate Alliance.

Shivanna, K. R. 2022. "Climate Change and Its Impact on Biodiversity and Human Welfare." *Proceedings of the Indian National Science Academy* 88 (2): 160–71.

Smith, Julia Patricia, Phillip Baker, Roger Mathisen, Aoife Long, Nigel Rollins, and Marilyn Waring. 2024. "A Proposal to Recognize Investment in Breastfeeding as a Carbon Offset." *Bulletin of the World Health Organization* 102 (5): 336–43. https://doi.org/10.2471/BLT.23.290210.

Smith, Julie P. 2019. "A Commentary on the Carbon Footprint of Milk Formula: Harms to Planetary Health and Policy Implications." *International Breastfeed Journal* 14: 49.

Smith, Kirk R., Alistair Woodword, Diarmid Campbell-Lendrum, Dave D. Chadee, Yasushi Honda, Qiyong Liu, Jane M. Olwoch, et al. 2014. "Human Health: Impacts, Adaptation, and Co-benefits." In *Climate Change 2014: Impacts, Adaptation, and Vulnerability. Part A: Global and Sectoral Aspects. Contribution of Working Group II to the Fifth Assessment Report of the Intergovernmental Panel on Climate Change*, edited by Christopher B. Field and Vicente R. Barros, 709–53. Cambridge and New York: Cambridge University Press.

Smith, M. R., C. D. Golden, and S. S. Myers. 2017. "Potential Rise in Iron Deficiency Due to Future Anthropogenic Carbon Dioxide Emissions." *GeoHealth* 1 (6): 248–57. https://doi.org/10.1002/2016GH000018.

Soanes, Marek, Aditya Bahadur, Clare Shakya, Barry Smith, Sejal Patel, Cristina Rumbaitis del Rio, Tamara Coger et al. 2021. "Principles for Locally Led Adaptation." International Institute for Environment and Development, London.

Soffiantini, Giulia. 2020. "Food Insecurity and Political Instability during the Arab Spring." *Global Food Security* 26: 100400.

Springmann, Marco, Daniel Mason-D'Croz, Sherman Robinson, Tara Garnett, H. Charles J. Godfray, Douglas Gollin, Mike Rayner, et al. 2016. "Global and Regional Health Effects of Future Food Production under Climate Change: A Modelling Study." *The Lancet* 387 (10031): 1937–46. https://doi.org/10.1016/S0140-6736(15)01156-3.

Sun, Zhongxiao, Laura Scherer, Arnold Tukker, Seth A. Spawn-Lee, Martin Bruckner, Holly K. Gibbs, and Paul Behrens. 2022. "Dietary Change in High-Income Nations Alone Can Lead to Substantial Double Climate Dividend." *Nature Food* 3: 9–37.

Sunderland, T. C. H. 2011. "Food Security: Why Is Biodiversity Important?" *International Forestry Review* 13 (3): 265–74.

Sutton, William R., Alexander Lotsch, and Ashesh Prasann. 2024. *Recipe for a Livable Planet: Achieving Net Zero Emissions in the Agrifood System*. Agriculture and Food Series. Conference Edition. Washington, DC: World Bank. https://hdl.handle.net/10986/41468.

Swinburn, Boyd A., Vivica I. Kraak, Steven Allender, Vincent J. Atkins, Jessica R. Bogard, Hannah Brinsden, Alejandro Calvillo, et al. 2019. "The Global Syndemic of Obesity, Undernutrition, and Climate Change: The Lancet Commission Report." *The Lancet* 393 (10173): 791–846. https://doi.org/10.1016/S0140-6736(18)32822-8.

Tito, Richard, Heraldo L. Hasconcelos, and Kenneth J. Feeley. 2018. "Global Climate Change Increases Risk of Crop Yield Losses and Food Insecurity in the Tropical Andes." *Global Change Biology* 24 (2): e592–602. https://doi.org/10.1111/gcb.13959.

Tomori, Cecília. 2023. "Protecting, Promoting and Supporting Breastfeeding in All Policies: Reframing the Narrative." *Frontiers in Public Health* 11: 1149384.

Trentinaglia, Maria Teresa, Marco Parolini, Franco Donzelli, and Alessandro Olper. 2021. "Climate Change and Obesity: A Global Analysis." *Global Food Security* 29: 100539.

UNDESA (United Nations Department of Economic and Social Affairs). 2020. "Chapter 3: Climate Change: Exacerbating Poverty and Inequality." In *World Social Report: Inequality in a Rapidly Changing World*, 81–107. New York: UNDESA. https://www.un.org/development/desa/dspd/wp-content/uploads/sites/22/2020/02/World-Social-Report-2020-Chapter-3.pdf.

UNICEF (United Nations Children's Fund). 2013. *Improving Child Nutrition: The Achievable Imperative for Global Progress*. New York: UNICEF.

UNICEF (United Nations Children's Fund. 2023. "Falling Short: Addressing the Climate Finance Gap for Children. Available at https://www.unicef.org/media/142181/file/Falling-short-Addressing-the-climate-finance-gap-for-children-June-2023.pdf.

Van den Berg, M. 2023. "Five Reasons the Private Sector Should Invest in the Potential of Smallholder Farmers." *Fairer Economies* (blog), June 28, 2023. https://www.weforum.org/agenda/2023/06/five-reasons-the-private-sector-should-invest-in-the-potential-of-smallholder-farmers/.

Vineis, Paolo, Queenie Chan, and Aneire Khan. 2011. "Climate Change Impacts on Water Salinity and Health." *Journal of Epidemiology and Global Health* 1 (1): 5–10.

Willett, Walter, Johann Rockström, Brent Loken, Marco Springmann, Tim Lang, Sonja Vermeulen, Tara Garnett, et al. 2019. "Food in the Anthropocene: The EAT–*Lancet* Commission on Healthy Diets from Sustainable Food Systems." *The Lancet* 393 (10170): 447–92.

WHO (World Health Organization). 2002. *The World Health Report 2002: Reducing Risks, Promoting Healthy Life*. Geneva: WHO.

WHO (World Health Organization). 2014. *Gender, Climate Change and Health*. Geneva: WHO. http://apps.who.int/iris/bitstream/10665/144781/1/9789241508186_eng.pdf.

WHO (World Health Organization). 2021. *Global Exclusive Breastfeeding Scorecard 2021.* Geneva: WHO.

WHO (World Health Organization). 2023. *Red and Processed Meat in the Context of Health and the Environment: Many Shades of Red and Green.* WHO information brief. Geneva: WHO.

Wong, J. T., J. de Bruyn, B. Bagnol, H. Grieve, M. Li, R. Pym, and R. G. Alders. 2017. "Small-Scale Poultry and Food Security in Resource-Poor Settings: A Review." *Global Food Security* 15: 43–52.

World Bank. 2023. *Detox Development: Repurposing Environmentally Harmful Subsidies.* Washington, DC: World Bank. https://www.worldbank.org/en/topic /climatechange/publication/detox-development.

Wu, Xiaoxu, Yongmei Lu, Sen Zhou, Lifan Chen, and Bing Xu. 2016. "Impact of Climate Change on Human Infectious Diseases: Empirical Evidence and Human Adaptation." *Environment International* 86: 14–23.

Xiong, Xin, Lixiao Zhang, Yan Hao, Pengpeng Zhang, Zhimin Shi, and Tingting Zhang. 2022. "How Urbanization and Ecological Conditions Affect Urban Diet-Linked GHG Emissions: New Evidence from China." *Resources, Conservation and Recycling* 176: 105903.

Zhang, Jun Xi, Meng Yang, Peng Hui Ji, Qin Yang Li, Jian Chai, Pan Pan Sun, Xi Yan, et al. 2021. "The Association between Outdoor Ambient Temperature and the Risk of Low Birth Weight: A Population-Based Cohort Study in Rural Henan, China." *Biomedical Environmental Sciences* 34 (11): 905–9. https://doi .org/10.3967/bes2021.124.

5

Interventions That Address All Forms of Malnutrition

Mireya Vilar-Compte, Hoa Thi Mai Nguyen, Kyoko Shibata Okamura, and Mia Blakstad

KEY MESSAGES

Interventions Targeting Pregnant and Lactating Mothers

- Iron and iron–folic acid (I/IFA) supplementation during pregnancy is linked to significant reductions (49 percent) in maternal anemia. Multiple micronutrient supplements (MMS) outperform I/IFA in reducing low birthweight (LBW) by 12–15 percent and small-for-gestational-age births by 7–12 percent. In addition, evidence suggests that MMS significantly decrease stillbirths by 9 percent. Calcium supplementation in low- and middle-income countries (LMICs) during pregnancy has a pronounced effect on reducing the risk of preeclampsia by 48 percent and on birth outcomes, including reductions in LBW (by 16 percent) and preterm births (by 47 percent).

- Intermittent preventive treatment for malaria in pregnancy remains effective and has positive impacts, including reductions in maternal anemia (10 percent) and risk of LBW (21 percent).

- Maternity leave is a nutrition intervention associated with increased breastfeeding duration and increased probability of exclusive breastfeeding. For women employed in the informal sector who are commonly excluded from such benefits, a maternity cash transfer seems a feasible strategy, with costs representing less than 0.08 percent of gross domestic product.

Interventions Targeting Children

- Delayed cord clamping at birth is associated with increased total hemoglobin after birth (from 1.6 to 2.4 grams per deciliter [g/dL] higher) among infants and significant reductions in anemia

(8 percent) among children ages 6 months to 12 months, but more research is needed to understand its long-term protection and implementation in LMICs.

- Kangaroo mother care significantly reduces neonatal mortality by 32 percent, all-cause mortality (35 percent by two months, 25 percent by six months), and severe infection and sepsis by 15 percent. It improves early breastfeeding initiation (2.6 days earlier), exclusive breastfeeding (52 percent at discharge or at 28 days), and growth. Adequate health care support and access are crucial for correct implementation, particularly in LMICs.

- Vitamin A supplementation among children ages 6 months to 59 months leads to notable reductions in all-cause mortality (by 12 percent) and diarrhea incidence (by 15 percent). Prophylactic zinc reduces the incidence of diarrhea by 9 percent among children in LMICs ages 1 month to 59 months.

- Small-quantity lipid-based nutrient supplements (SQ-LNS) are strongly associated with reductions in stunting (by 12 percent), severe stunting (by 17 percent), wasting (by 14 percent), severe wasting (by 31 percent), anemia (by 16–34 percent), and all-cause mortality (by 27 percent) among children ages 6 months to 24 months. Ready-to-use therapeutic foods (RUTF) are important for treating severe acute malnutrition; when compared with a dietary approach, they are associated with an improved recovery of weight (by 33 percent).

- Interventions focused on breastfeeding counseling and education significantly increase reported rates of early initiation (by 20 percent) and are linked to a twofold improvement in reported exclusive breastfeeding rates, with corresponding reductions in projected diarrhea incidence rates.

- When iron-fortified products or iron supplements are provided, school feeding and nutrition interventions can significantly reduce anemia prevalence among vulnerable (that is, displaced, rural, or low-income) schoolchildren.

Interventions Targeting the General Population

- Cash-plus-nutrition interventions (that is, cash transfers and other components, such as nutritional education, behavior change communications, and supplements) can, if designed carefully, reduce the odds of stunting. Evidence of the effects of cash transfers on wasting is inconclusive, and further research is needed.

Various programs, such as integrated agriculture and nutrition, vegetable gardens and homestead food production, and livestock interventions, may have positive effects on dietary diversity. There is also an association between homestead food production and vegetable garden programs and reductions in anemia. Further studies are needed in this area, especially considering its importance in climate change adaptation and mitigation.

- Evidence suggests that water, sanitation, and hygiene (WASH) interventions combined with nutrition services have the potential to improve height for age (0.13–0.15 standardized mean difference); WASH interventions can also reduce the risk of diarrhea among children by 30–50 percent and all-cause child mortality by about 30 percent.

- Iron-fortified foods with or without other micronutrients effectively reduce the overall prevalence of anemia; fortification of wheat flour, soy sauce, and condiments and double-fortified salt show significant impacts. Biofortification of staple crops has been shown to reduce micronutrient deficiencies and is being scaled up in many countries. School-based deworming programs can also significantly reduce the risk of anemia among children.

Framework for Achieving Optimum Nutrition

Accelerating improvements in the nutritional status of children and mothers requires a holistic approach, with actions across multiple sectors and levels of intervention. The 2013 update to *The Lancet*'s series on maternal and child nutrition described a framework of multilevel and multisectoral actions to effectively address risk factors that can contribute to poor child nutrition outcomes (Black et al. 2013) and tackle the immediate, underlying, and enabling determinants of malnutrition, as described in the United Nations Children's Fund conceptual framework (UNICEF 2021). Interventions to address risk factors at the immediate level were classified as nutrition-specific interventions and implied direct actions, such as provision of micronutrient supplements. At the underlying level, nutrition-sensitive interventions were brought to address indirect causes of malnutrition and included the integration of nutrition goals into the design and implementation of programs in other sectors, such as social protection, agriculture, and water (Ruel and Alderman 2013). The change in nomenclature from nutrition-specific and nutrition-sensitive to direct and indirect interventions has not yet been universally accepted by agencies. To avoid the dissonance associated with both nomenclatures and to align with country-level implementation platforms, the following sections are organized according to target groups (prenatal, perinatal, children, and general population) and delivery platforms across health, social protection, agriculture, water and sanitation, and education, as well as the private sector in the production and delivery of nutrition-oriented services and commodities (refer to figure 5.1).

A growing body of evidence has also contributed to an emerging global consensus on the best buys to address obesity and diet-related challenges.

Figure 5.1 Multisectoral and System-Geared Framework for Nutrition

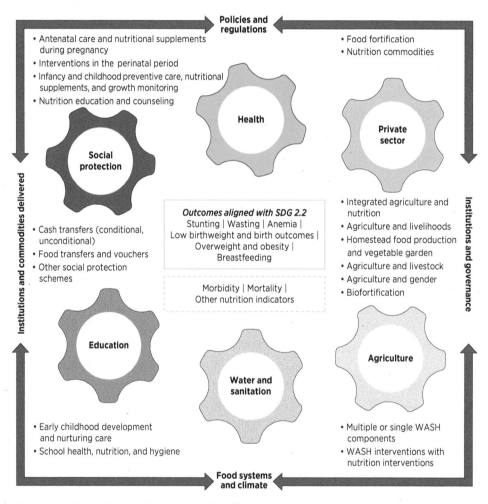

Source: Original figure for this publication.
Note: SDG = Sustainable Development Goal; WASH = water, sanitation, and hygiene.

Recommended actions on unhealthy diets and physical activity in the World Health Organization's (WHO) revised best buys include reformulation policies for healthier food and beverage products; front-of-package labeling; publicly funded food procurement and service policies for facilitating healthy diets; behavioral change communication and mass media campaigns; policies to protect children from harmful food marketing; and population-wide communication campaigns to promote physical activity, which include links to community-based programs and environmental improvements (WHO 2023b). These actions fall in the policy space and are elaborated on further in chapter 6.

High-Impact Nutrition Interventions Delivered through the Health Sector

A targeted systematic review was conducted to update the findings of the 2021 *Lancet Maternal and Child Health Series* with the latest published evidence. The review focused on high-impact nutrition interventions (that is, those with moderate or strong evidence) delivered through the health sector. It included meta-analyses, systematic reviews, and randomized controlled trials (RCTs) published in 2018–23 in English or Spanish and focused on interventions in low- and middle-income countries (LMICs), with evidence on the effects on the Sustainable Development Goal (SDG) 2.2 nutrition targets (more specifics about the methodology of the review can be found in the PROSPERO protocol CRD42024529609 [Vilar-Compte and Nguyen 2024] as well as in annex 5A). The review summarizes the evidence across four thematic areas: (1) prenatal interventions, (2) perinatal and neonatal interventions, (3) interventions for children younger than age five years, and (4) infant and young child nutrition education and counseling interventions. Figure 5.2 provides more specific information about the interventions included in each of these thematic areas, and annex 5B presents evidence summary tables.

Prenatal Interventions

For more than a decade, the WHO (2012, 2016) has recommended a daily intake of 30–60 milligram (mg) of elemental iron and 400 micrograms (µg) of folic acid during pregnancy to reduce maternal anemia and low birthweight (LBW). Daily iron and iron–folic acid (I/IFA) supplementation in pregnancy—compared with supplements without iron or placebo—is consistently associated with a reduced risk of maternal anemia and LBW. Recent reviews are in line with prior evidence (Keats et al. 2021; Oh, Keats, and Bhutta 2020) in documenting a significant reduction in maternal

Figure 5.2 Overview of Nutrition Interventions Delivered through the Health Sector in LMICs

	Intervention	How is it delivered?	To whom?	What is delivered?
Prenatal interventions	Antenatal multiple micronutrient supplementation	Antenatal care provided in different settings (such as clinical, community)	Pregnant women	Supplements containing more than three micronutrients
	Iron/iron–folic acid supplementation		Pregnant women	30–60 mg of elemental iron, 400 μg of folic acid
	Calcium supplements		Pregnant women with low calcium intake	Generally, a high dose of ≥ 1 g per day
	Balanced energy protein supplementation		Undernourished pregnant women living under the poverty line	Supplements in which protein accounts for less than 25 percent of the total caloric content
	Malaria preventive treatment		Pregnant women living in malaria-endemic areas	Sulfadoxine-pyrimethamine administered after week 13 and doses administered at least one month apart
Perinatal and neonatal interventions	Delayed cord clamping	Delayed cord clamping	Delivery services and maternity guards	Newborns
	Kangaroo mother care	Kangaroo mother care	Neonatal intensive care services, newborn nursery, and continued at home	Mothers and/or caregivers, low-birthweight and preterm babies
Interventions for children under five years of age	Vitamin A supplementation	Routine primary care visits and community-based programs	Children 6–59 months living in areas with prevalence of vitamin A deficiency	100,000 IU for infants 6–11 months and 200,000 IU for children 12–59 months; every 4–6 months
	Preventive zinc supplementation		Children 2–59 months	Usually, a syrup with 10 mg and 15 mg daily, 24–26 weeks
	Therapeutic zinc supplementation		Children 6 months and older with acute diarrhea	20 mg zinc daily, 10–14 days
	Small-quantity lipid-based nutrient supplementation		Children 6–23 months	Lipid-based nutrient supplements, typically 100–120 kcal/d, highly nutrient-dense and fortified
	Multiple micronutrient powders for point-of-use fortification		Children 6–59 months	Ready-to-use sachets with a dry mixture of micronutrients
	Ready-to-use therapeutic foods	Mostly community-based management as outpatient	Children 6–59 months with uncomplicated severe acute malnutrition	High energy, fortified, ready to eat, non water based food, typically ≥ 500 kcal/d
Infant and young child nutrition education and counseling interventions	Breastfeeding counseling/education	Peer counselors, community health workers, and/or health care providers Facility-based, community-based, home-based, and/or online One-on-one and/or group-based	Mothers, families, and/or caregivers of infants and young children	Skilled guidance and support to mothers, family, and/or caregivers on • how to breastfeed effectively and address any challenges they may encounter • complementary feeding and/or responsive feeding
	Complementary feeding counseling/education			

Source: Original figure for this publication.
Note: g = gram; IU = international units; kcal/d = kilocalories per day; LMICs = low- and middle-income countries; μg = microgram.

anemia of about 49 percent (Hansen et al. 2023). As for LBW, evidence suggests a reduced risk of 12 percent when comparing IFA with folic acid (Oh, Keats, and Bhutta 2020) and, potentially, an even larger reduction when assessing I/IFA versus placebo (Hansen et al. 2023). Furthermore, a recent meta-analysis suggests a potential effect of IFA on babies born small for gestational age (SGA) as well (Hansen et al. 2023). From an implementation perspective, tolerance and adherence to daily I/IFA supplementation have been recognized as sizable challenges (Desta et al. 2019). In addition, iron deficiency is often associated with the presence of other micronutrient deficiencies; hence, there may be a need for additional supplementation involving enriched diets or multiple micronutrient supplements (MMS).

Recent years have seen a shift toward recommending MMS (Keats, Das, et al. 2021; WHO 2020). Meta-analyses are consistent in documenting that, when compared with I/IFA, MMS are associated with significantly larger reductions in LBW of 12–17 percent (Gomes et al. 2023; Hofmeyr et al. 2023; Keats et al. 2019; Kinshella et al. 2021; Oh et al. 2020) and in SGA infants of 7–12 percent (Keats et al. 2019; Kinshella et al. 2021; Oh, Keats, and Bhutta 2020). For preterm births, evidence shows a consistent reduction, but not a statistically significant one (4–10 percent; Gomes et al. 2023; Hofmeyr et al. 2023; Keats et al. 2019; Kinshella et al. 2021; Oh, Keats, and Bhutta 2020). The evidence also suggests a significant 9 percent decrease in stillbirths (Hofmeyr et al. 2023; Oh, Keats, and Bhutta 2020). Findings are consistent across different methodological approaches, when accounting for gestational age assessed through different measures (Gomes et al. 2023), and for subgroup analyses (Keats et al. 2022). When limited to trials using MMS formulations containing more than four micronutrients, the findings indicate even larger reductions (Oh, Keats, and Bhutta 2020). On the basis of this evidence, MMS is now gradually being introduced in several countries, with a clear strategy to switch from I/IFA to MMS and updating of national guidelines and local production efforts in some countries, such as Bangladesh and Indonesia.

Calcium supplementation among healthy pregnant women with low calcium intake leads to better pregnancy and birth outcomes. For example, recent evidence from LMICs shows that, when compared with placebo, calcium supplements are strongly associated with a 48 percent reduction in the risk of preeclampsia (Kinshella et al. 2021). When pooling data from high-income countries (HICs) and LMICs, similar associations between calcium supplementation and reduced risk of preeclampsia have been documented (Gunabalasingam et al. 2023; Hofmeyr et al. 2018). Recent evidence also confirms a strong association between calcium supplementation and a reduction in the risk of preterm births even larger than prior estimates (47 percent versus 24 percent; Hofmeyr et al. 2018, 2023; Kinshella et al. 2021). Past studies had reported some evidence regarding the association between calcium supplementation and a reduced risk of LBW (Hofmeyr et al. 2018). A recent meta-analysis reports a significant 16 percent risk reduction (Kinshella et al. 2021), although there are some contradictions between studies (Hofmeyr et al. 2018; Kinshella et al. 2021). Findings on LBW are likely to be correlated with the impacts of calcium supplementation on preterm births. Calcium supplementation has not, however, been scaled up in most countries because of implementation challenges with providing women with three separate 500 mg calcium supplements daily. New evidence suggests that a single dose of 500 mg is noninferior to the standard of 1,500 mg in preventing preeclampsia and preterm birth (Dwarkanath et al. 2024), which will simplify some of the cost and implementation challenges.

Balanced energy supplementation (BEP) is another intervention targeted to pregnant women. BEP involves food supplements in which the proteins account for less than 25 percent of the total caloric content. Some older reviews suggest that when compared with control participants (that is, those receiving no supplementation with either food or micronutrients), BEPs decreased the risk of LBW by 40 percent, SGA babies by 29 percent, stillbirths by 61 percent, and perinatal mortality by 50 percent (Lassi, Padhani, and Rabbani 2021). Despite such large and statistically significant associations, evidence is limited and based primarily on outdated studies. Moreover, the context has changed, because the current standard of care generally includes I/IFA and, increasingly, MMS. Therefore, the relevant control group today should be women given I/IFA or MMS rather than no supplementation at all. The evidence on the effects of BEP versus IFA or MMS is, however, insufficient. Updated research is needed, especially considering the high costs and the integration of new interventions.

Intermittent preventive treatment of malaria in pregnancy (IPTp) is a public health intervention recommended by the WHO (2023c) for pregnant women living in malaria-endemic areas. The intervention involves giving pregnant women full therapeutic courses of antimalarial medication at specified times during pregnancy, regardless of whether they are infected with malaria. Recent studies of IPTp report significant reductions in maternal anemia (by 10 percent; Moorthy et al. 2020) and LBW (by 21 percent; van Eijk et al. 2019). However, concerns about resistance to sulfadoxine–pyrimethamine (SP)—the antimalarial medication recommended by the WHO—have increased recently, motivating reviews to assess whether the reductions in anemia and LBW are sustained when using other antimalarials. Findings suggest that, despite reduced effectiveness in high-resistance areas (van Eijk et al. 2019), IPTp-SP continues to be an effective intervention (Gutman et al. 2021). Using azithromycin as part of IPTp has also shown positive impacts on LBW, preterm births, and neonatal deaths (Hume-Nixon et al. 2021).

Perinatal and Neonatal Interventions

The care provided during the prenatal and neonatal period is crucial for the health outcomes of both the mother and the child, and some interventions have the potential to influence nutrition-related outcomes.

Evidence suggests that delayed cord clamping to allow additional blood flow from the placenta to the newborn can increase the infant's iron stores and contribute to better nutritional status and health outcomes. The WHO published some 2014 guidelines (WHO 2014), but they have not been updated since then. A more recent Cochrane review covering HICs and LMICs found that delayed rather than immediate or early cord clamping reduced the risk of neonatal death by 27 percent and of intraventricular hemorrhage by 17 percent among preterm babies (Rabe et al. 2019). Such findings have been for the most part confirmed in studies involving full-term babies. There is also significant evidence associating delayed cord clamping with reductions in the risk of anemia among full-term and preterm babies (Li et al. 2021; Zhao et al. 2019), as well as increased total hemoglobin during the initial days after birth (ranging from 1.6 g/dL for full-term babies to 2.4 g/dL for preterm babies; Moorthy et al. 2020; Persad et al. 2021). Delayed cord clamping has also been associated with significant reductions of 18–42 percent in blood transfusions until discharge (Jasani et al. 2021; Moorthy et al. 2020; Persad et al. 2021). However, evidence suggests the existence of knowledge gaps in how delayed clamping is implemented and understood, presupposing an important challenge for decision-makers (McDonald 2023). In addition, the literature that focuses exclusively on LMICs is limited, which is a substantial aspect to consider because obstetric and perinatal health care services can vary greatly.

Another intervention promoted by the WHO is kangaroo mother care (KMC), a method of care for infants that involves skin-to-skin contact with a parent to promote infant health and bonding. Although it is beneficial for any newborn—because it promotes bonding, regulates body temperature, and supports breastfeeding—it has traditionally been recommended for preterm and LBW newborns, and evidence for its benefits is strong. Recent evidence from LMICs highlights a 32 percent reduction in neonatal mortality (Sivanandan and Sankar 2023), as well as reductions in all-cause mortality measured at different points during the first year (Guo 2023; Sivanandan and Sankar 2023). Findings also suggest a significant 15 percent reduction in severe infection and sepsis (Sivandandan and Sankar 2023). Other significant benefits include improvements in exclusive breastfeeding at discharge or at 28 days (52 percent; Sivandandan and Sankar 2023) and in children ages one month to six months (51 percent). Furthermore, evidence also associates KMC with gains in height (0.21 centimeters per week [cm/week]) and weight (4.08 grams per day [g/day]; Sivanandan and Sankar 2023), as well as in growth velocity (Park et al. 2020). Despite these benefits, correct implementation of KMC requires adequate managerial support at relevant health care facilities, adequately trained health care personnel, and guidelines and protocols at the clinic level. The WHO (2023d) published updated guidelines that address some of these implementation challenges.

Children Younger Than Age Five Years

This section addresses single and multiple micronutrients and food supplementation interventions for infants and children younger than age five years that were previously found to have strong to moderate evidence for their implementation (Keats, Das, et al. 2021; Keats, Oh, et al. 2021).

Vitamin A is essential for children's healthy growth and development. There is indirect evidence that it can reduce stunting by limiting diarrhea incidence and mortality (Imdad et al. 2010), and on that basis the WHO recommends providing 100,000 international units (IU) of vitamin A to children ages 6 months to 11 months and 200,000 IU every four to six months for children ages 12–59 months in settings in which the prevalence of night blindness is 1 percent or higher among children ages 24–59 months or where vitamin A deficiency is 20 percent or higher among infants and children. An updated review of vitamin A supplementation in children ages 6 months to 59 months shows a strong and significant reduction of 12 percent, compared with placebo, in all-cause mortality, as well as in diarrhea-specific mortality (Imdad et al. 2022). The review also documents a significant 15 percent reduction in diarrhea-specific incidence.

Zinc is another essential micronutrient that supports immune function, cell growth, and neurodevelopment among infants and children. Earlier reviews documented that preventive zinc supplementation in healthy children ages 1 month to 59 months in LMICs was associated with a significant 11 percent reduction in the incidence of diarrhea but showed no effect on mortality, anemia, stunting, or wasting (Tam et al. 2020). Updated reviews confirm these findings (Imdad et al. 2022; Lassi, Kurji, et al. 2020) but report a significant 9 percent reduction in the risk of diarrhea incidence (Imdad et al. 2023). Despite such benefits, prior studies have highlighted that adoption of preventive zinc supplementation remains low, with challenges linked to consistent supply, distribution, and delivery (Gupta, Brazier, and Lowe 2020). Currently, there are no available platforms for delivery of prophylactic zinc supplements. Zinc could potentially be added to micronutrient powders, especially considering that the scale-up of prophylactic zinc as a single-nutrient strategy does not seems feasible. Zinc supplementation for treatment of diarrhea in children older than six months has been associated with the shortening of the average duration of diarrhea and a significant 27 percent reduction in the risk of diarrhea persisting until day seven (Lazzerini and Wanzira 2016). Oral rehydration solution combined with zinc has also shown a significant 24 percent reduction in diarrhea mortality (Scott et al. 2020).

Small-quantity lipid-based nutrient supplements (SQ-LNS) are used to address nutrient gaps and prevent malnutrition in vulnerable populations of young children through supplements that are highly dense and fortified. Preventive use of SQ-LNS has been extensively evaluated over the past two decades. Prior evidence involving populations in LMICs has documented that, when provided during complementary feeding among children ages 6 months to 24 months and compared with no intervention, SQ-LNS significantly reduced the prevalence of severe stunting, moderate stunting, and moderate wasting (Das et al. 2019). More recent reviews confirm these findings, documenting a significant reduction in the prevalence of stunting (by 12 percent), severe stunting (by 17 percent), wasting (by 14 percent), and severe wasting (by 31 percent; Dewey et al. 2021, 2022). In addition, recent studies comparing medium-quantity lipid-based nutrient supplements (MQ-LNS) and SQ-LNS have found no significant differences in effects on weight for length or prevalence of wasting; MQ-LNS did not significantly improve height for age or reduce stunting, whereas SQ-LNS had significant effects on these outcomes (Dewey et al. 2023). Evidence has also associated SQ-LNS with a reduced prevalence of anemia (by 16 percent) and iron deficiency anemia (by 64 percent; Wessells et al. 2021). Moreover, other studies suggest that for children between the ages of 6 months and 24 months, SQ-LNS can reduce the risk of all-cause mortality by 27 percent (Stewart et al. 2020). Although the evidence for SQ-LNS is strong, it is essential to contextualize it in broader efforts to improve the diets of infants and young children (UNICEF 2023). As stressed in the most recent WHO (2023e) wasting prevention and management guidelines, SQ-LNS can be considered for the prevention of wasting for a limited duration, while continuing "to enable access to adequate home diets for the whole family and providing infant and young child feeding counselling." SQ-LNS has been found to be beneficial in operational research settings;

however, the fundamental challenge is to bring SQ-LNS to scale. Achieving this goal requires identifying at-risk children, providing SQ-LNS through already existing nutrition programs, and working with other sectors, such as health and social protection. Other effective implementation recommendations include securing consistent supply and distribution, addressing cultural acceptance of the products, training the health care workforce, and tracking product usage to avoid under- or overuse (Kodish et al. 2017).

Micronutrient powders (MNPs), a dry mixture of iron and other micronutrients, have previously been associated with a 24 percent reduced risk of anemia among children ages 1 month to 59 months living in LMICs (Tam et al. 2020). Recent evidence indicates reductions in anemia ranging between 18 percent and 31 percent (Moorthy et al. 2020; Suchdev et al. 2020). Despite these positive impacts, there is some potential for increased risk of diarrhea (Suchdev et al. 2020; Tam et al. 2020). Therefore, it is important to integrate MNPs into broader nutrition and health programs (for example, community counseling) to minimize potential problems (Pelletier and DePee 2019). Evidence also shows inconsistent effects of MNPs on stunting and wasting; such findings might be influenced by factors such as the nutritional status of the population and the presence of infections and inflammation.

Management of severe acute malnutrition (SAM) in children younger than age five years involves stabilization and/or rehabilitation. Stabilization includes, among other interventions, treatment for dehydration and potential infections, whereas rehabilitation among children with uncomplicated SAM focuses on catch-up growth through ready-to-use therapeutic food (RUTF) provided at the community level and through outpatient services to help recovery. As highlighted in the most recent WHO guidelines (WHO 2023e), this treatment should always be delivered along with medical and psychosocial support, such as counseling on preventive health actions such as breastfeeding. Prior evidence has shown that standard RUTF, when compared with an alternative dietary approach, is associated with an improved recovery of weight (by 33 percent) and has suggested an increase in the mean rate of weight gain during the intervention of about 1.12 grams per kilogram per day (g/kg/day) day (Schoonees et al. 2019). A more recent review found that, when compared with energy-dense home food, RUTFs were associated with a likely improvement in the mean rate of height gain of about 0.7 mm/day (Das et al. 2020). The same review converged with prior research in supporting the parallel use of broad-spectrum oral amoxicillin for children with uncomplicated SAM. When compared with no antibiotic, it increased recovery and possible weight gain (0.67 g/kg/day) and reduced all-cause mortality (by 26 percent). As highlighted in the updated WHO guidelines (2023e), programs that deliver RUTF require constant monitoring of children and, ideally, integration into existing health systems; this can be challenging, particularly in areas with weak and underfunded health infrastructure. Furthermore, a note of caution is necessary regarding the use of RUTF supplements; their use should not displace breastfeeding or undermine the use of local and sustainable solutions.

Infant and Young Child Nutrition Education and Counseling

Optimal nutrition for infants and young children includes breastfeeding and complementary feeding, which are considered fundamental to ensure long-term child nutrition and well-being.

The 2023 *Lancet Series on Breastfeeding* offers policy and programmatic recommendations to support mothers who want to breastfeed (Pérez-Escamilla et al. 2023), including investments in breastfeeding public awareness and education, skilled counseling, and both prenatal and postnatal support. Breastfeeding, skilled counseling, and peer counseling during the prenatal and postpartum periods are included as high-impact interventions in the 2021 *Lancet Series on Maternal and Child Health* (*The Lancet* 2021). Although counseling and education vary in terms of their timing, frequency, platform delivery, and settings (refer to figure 5.2), there is strong evidence from LMICs that breastfeeding counseling and education is associated with increased rates of early initiation of breastfeeding and exclusive breastfeeding (Lassi, Rind, et al. 2020). Prior studies highlight a twofold improvement in exclusive breastfeeding rates at less than one month and at one month to five months when interventions were delivered at either the home or community level (Sinha et al. 2017). The same study suggested that continued breastfeeding after age six months had a slightly lower increase when education and counseling strategies were delivered in combined settings (that is, home or community and health services). Some potential factors in the effects of breastfeeding counseling and education are the intensity of contacts and the need to have an adequately trained workforce (Pérez-Escamilla et al. 2023).

According to WHO guidelines (2023f), complementary feeding, the process of providing foods in addition to milk when breast milk or milk formula alone are no longer adequate to meet nutritional requirements, generally starts at age 6 months and continues until age 23 months. This is a critical period in child development, and inappropriate complementary feeding practices are associated with future adverse health consequences.

Interventions to improve complementary feeding practices often consist of education and counseling aimed at informing and shaping caregivers' decisions on proper feeding practices and can also include food supplements. Evidence reviews assessing education and counseling interventions generally find no significant effects on growth (that is, no evidence of impact on stunting or wasting) but did find significant associations with feeding practices, including age at introduction of semisolid foods, hygiene practices, and duration of breastfeeding (Arikpo et al. 2018; Janmohamed et al. 2020; Mahumud et al. 2022). Some studies have examined whether the effects of complementary feeding education and counseling are modified by food security (Lassi, Rind, et al. 2020), but more research in this area is needed.

Caution should be exercised in interpreting estimates of the impact of education on infant and young child nutrition on breastfeeding outcomes, such as early initiation of breastfeeding and exclusive breastfeeding, because of the possibility of social desirability bias in maternal reported breastfeeding practices. Mothers in the intervention group may be more likely to report the promoted practices because they are more aware of the desired responses than mothers in the control group, as illustrated in a recent analysis in Kenya (Stewart et al. forthcoming). Educational interventions can clearly improve caregivers' knowledge of breastfeeding recommendations, but high-quality social and behavior change communication and support are needed to translate that knowledge into actual improvements in practices. In addition, it is important to recognize the deleterious effect of commercial determinants in shaping caregivers' decisions regarding infant and young child feeding. The industry that produces foods targeted to this age group spends billions of dollars in marketing. If counseling and education interventions are not adequately designed, implemented, funded, and accompanied by other interventions, such as those highlighted in chapter 6, it will be difficult to counterbalance such commercial determinants (Pérez-Escamilla et al. 2023).

Nutrition Interventions Delivered through the Social Protection Sector

The social protection sector is a critical player in the fight against poverty and vulnerability, offering a broad spectrum of interventions that directly target the social determinants of health and have the potential to contribute to the delivery of nutrition interventions. In addition, social protection systems provide national platforms that allow overlaying of interventions targeting the most vulnerable segments of the population. These interventions, which include conditional and unconditional cash transfers, adaptive safety nets, asset transfers, livelihood programs, and in-kind assistance, among others, are essential to address malnutrition. Social protection interventions can enhance food security and dietary diversity, which are pivotal for nutrition outcomes (deGroot et al. 2017; Kumar et al. 2018). Labor market regulations, such as maternity leave, can overlap with social protection programs, especially among informally employed individuals, and they are critically important for maternal and child health.

To underscore the contributions of the social protection sectors in achieving better nutrition, a systematic review was conducted. The review included scientific literature published in 2013–23 in English and Spanish, focused on cash transfers (conditional and unconditional), food transfers and vouchers, and maternity leave implemented in LMICs. More information is available in the PROSPERO protocol (CRD42024552449) (Nguyen et al 2024), as well as in annex 5A. Figure 5.3 summarizes specific information about the social protection interventions included, and annex 5C presents the evidence summary tables.

Cash Transfers

Cash transfers amount to an estimated $240 billion annually (based on information from 98 low-income, middle-income, and high-income economies) and cover an estimated 795 million individuals globally, with an average daily benefit of $1 in low-income countries and up to $10 in HICs (Gentilini et al. 2023). Unconditional cash transfers provide beneficiaries the choice to spend cash as they prefer without having to comply with specific behaviors. However, some unconditional cash transfers do include some nudges (or co-responsibilities) with minimal monitoring or enforcement, such as messages about the importance of education or food expenditures (Baird et al. 2014). Conditional cash transfers make disbursements of cash contingent on certain behaviors, such as regular attendance at health promotion or child growth promotion sessions. Previous evidence from systematic reviews suggests that both conditional and unconditional cash transfers have the potential to improve short-term food consumption and dietary quality (Ruel and Alderman 2013). Some cash transfer programs also take into account malnutrition prevalence or risk, typically by targeting households with children in the first 1,000 days of life (refer to box 5.1). In addition, many countries have child allowance programs, which are generally unconditional cash transfers that are categorically targeted to pregnant or lactating women with children younger than age two years. Implementers also often combine cash transfers with behavior change communication and the delivery of nutrition-specific commodities or other nutrition-specific interventions (refer to box 5.2) to improve the nutritional status of children in the first 1,000 days of life.

Figure 5.3 Overview of Nutrition Interventions Delivered through the Social Protection Sector in LMICs

	Intervention	How is it delivered?	To whom?	What is delivered?
Cash transfers	**Unconditional cash transfers**	Variable depending on the context and infrastructure, including direct bank deposits, mobile money transfers, or physical cash	Vulnerable populations, such as low-income or labor-constrained households, pregnant women and mothers, or caregivers	Direct financial support to beneficiaries to cover basic needs and provide a safety net without requiring compliance with specific behaviors
	Conditional cash transfers			Direct financial support to beneficiaries to cover basic needs and provide a safety net contingent on certain behaviors
	Cash transfers + behavior change communication			Direct financial support to beneficiaries to cover basic needs and provide a safety net combined with behavior change communication
Food transfers and vouchers	**Food transfers**	Direct distribution to beneficiaries at designated distribution centers or door to door	Targeted at • Households facing food insecurity, vulnerabilities linked to poverty, conflict, or crises • Vulnerable pregnant mothers, infants, and young children	Staple foods and food items to promote a balanced diet
	Vouchers	Direct distribution of paper-based vouchers or electronic transfers (such as cards, mobile money)		Vouchers with a monetary value to purchase foods
Maternity leave	**Maternity leave**	Social security and/or employer; growing interest in alternative delivery mechanisms to cover women employed in the informal sector	Women before, during, and after childbirth and mothers of infants	Protected leave of at least 14 weeks (fully or partially paid)

Source: Original table for this publication.
Note: LMICs = low- and middle-income countries.

Box 5.1

Rwanda's Nutrition-Sensitive Direct Support Program

The Nutrition-Sensitive Direct Support (NSDS) program, a component of Rwanda's World Bank–supported Strengthening Social Protection Project, was designed to address demand-side constraints faced by poor households in accessing nutritious foods and engaging in activities that promote appropriate health and nutrition practices in the first 1,000 days of a child's life. Households are targeted using a community-based classification of household socioeconomic status, now being transitioned to a national social registry. The NSDS program is a pillar of the government's multisectoral stunting reduction strategy. The cash transfers are coupled with co-responsibilities for beneficiaries to participate in prenatal care and postnatal care visits, as well as to attend growth monitoring and promotion activities with their targeted child younger than age two years. During the COVID-19 pandemic, the program enabled the government to mitigate the effect of economic shocks for the most vulnerable households through a significant and rapid expansion of enrolled beneficiary households. Early experience from the program has catalyzed additional resources for scale-up through a $400 million Development Policy Operation on Human Capital.

Source: Informal consultation with Jonathan Kweku Akuoku, World Bank.

Box 5.2

A Cash-Transfer Program in Niger

As part of the national safety net system, the government of Niger set up an unconditional cash transfer program that reached 100,000 households by 2019, providing small monthly transfers of CFAF 10,000 (about $20) to women in poor households for a period of 24 months. The program combines cash transfers with behavior change measures to promote early childhood development. The behavior change component includes parental training activities to encourage health, nutrition, psychosocial stimulation, and child protection practices. It is implemented through monthly village assemblies, community meetings, and household visits delivered by

(continued)

Box 5.2

A Cash-Transfer Program in Niger *(continued)*

trained nongovernmental organization operators and community workers. Participation is encouraged and monitored but is not a formal condition to receive the cash transfers.

A cluster randomized controlled trial of the program showed positive effects on dietary diversity but not on anthropometric outcomes. The evaluation did not indicate any improvements in either stunting or wasting. The cash-transfer program improved adults' but not children's dietary diversity, whereas the behavioral change communication improved children's but not adults' dietary diversity (Premand and Barry 2022).

The World Bank worked with the government to introduce additional interventions as part of a graduation program. These interventions included a group savings promotion, coaching and entrepreneurship training, and psychosocial interventions to improve the livelihoods of program participants. An evaluation of the graduation program suggested positive effects on economic outcomes and psychosocial well-being, especially among program participants who received psychosocial interventions. The evaluation of the graduation program did not assess impacts on dietary diversity or nutritional outcomes (Bossuroy et al. 2022).

Source: Correspondence with the American Institute for Research.

Although some evidence suggests that cash-only programs may have an impact on stunting and height for age (Durao et al. 2020; Manley, Alderman, and Gentilini 2022), more studies point to the effect of cash-plus-nutrition interventions (programs that provide cash but also include components such as nutritional education, behavior change communication, or supplements). For example, a recent meta-analysis reports an odds ratio of 0.85, indicating that the odds of stunting among children are 15 percent lower when cash-plus-nutrition programs are implemented in South Asia (de Hoop et al. 2024). Recent RCTs confirm these findings (Ahmed, Hoddinott, and Roy 2024; Carneriro et al. 2021; Field and Maffioli, forthcoming) and report significant postintervention reductions in stunting of about 5 percentage points. For wasting, the evidence is more limited. The most recent WHO guidelines (2023e) establish that among "infants and children with severe wasting and/or nutritional oedema, cash transfers in addition to routine care may be provided to decrease relapse and improve overall child health" but acknowledge that more evidence is needed. The current review found small and inconclusive effects of cash transfers on wasting and weight for height (de Hoop et al. 2024; Durao et al. 2020).

There is strong evidence on the effect of cash transfers in improving dietary diversity (refer to box 5.2). Consistent with prior studies (Manley, Alderman, and Gentilini 2022), recent meta-analyses report that cash-only interventions positively affect dietary diversity (average effect of 0.14 standard deviation), with a larger effect in Sub-Saharan Africa (average effect of 0.26 standard deviation; de Hoop et al. 2024). The impact of cash-only programs on dietary diversity seems to be irrespective of conditionality (Durao et al. 2020; Pega et al. 2022). However, evidence from meta-analyses report stronger effects of cash-plus programs on dietary diversity (average effect of 0.41 standard deviation), which is consistent with evidence from recent RCTs that report improvements in the likelihood of children meeting minimum dietary diversity (Ahmed, Hoddinott, and Roy 2024) and child food diversity scores (Field and Maffioli forthcoming).

Although cash transfers have also been associated with reductions in LBW (Glassman et al. 2013; Lisboa et al. 2023) and childhood anemia (Durao et al. 2020; Segura-Pérez, Grajeda, and Pérez-Escamilla 2016), as well as with improvements in breastfeeding indicators (Ahmed, Hoddinott, and Roy 2024), more research is needed.

Food Transfers and Vouchers

Other nutrition-sensitive social protection programs include food transfers and vouchers. Evaluations of these programs often show positive effects on outcomes such as dietary diversity. However, because nutrition is a secondary consideration in many of the program designs, evidence from existing systematic reviews and meta-analyses remains limited.

Food transfers and vouchers primarily aim to improve food security and nutrition by providing food assistance to poor households or by providing households with vouchers that they can use to purchase food. School feeding programs are a form of in-kind food transfer that, when properly designed, can optimize food provision. However, in this document we identify it as an education sector intervention, discussed later.

Studies on food-transfer or voucher interventions generally include other components, such as behavioral change or counseling, supplements, and promotion of health services use. The evidence suggest that food-transfer (plus other components) interventions may reduce stunting and improve dietary diversity (Durao et al. 2020; Leroy, Olney, and Ruel 2018; Leroy et al. 2020). Only one study reported significant anemia-protective effects among children and mothers (Leroy, Olney, and Ruel 2016).

Similar effects were reported for food vouchers (plus other components) (Ara et al. 2022; Durao et al. 2020). Studies comparing food transfers or cash transfers with controls suggest that both interventions can be effective in improving nutrition outcomes and dietary diversity (Ahmed, Hoddinott, and Roy 2024; Ramírez-Luzuriaga et al. 2016).

Implementation of food transfers and food vouchers in LMICs can face several key challenges, including the definition and adequate targeting of the beneficiaries and ensuring that the transfers or vouchers reach them in a timely manner (Alderman, Gentilini, and Yemtsov 2017). Food transfers also require adequate quality and consumption. Another aspect that emerges in the literature is the fragility of such programs during crises such as ethnic conflicts, climate events, and so forth. Careful planning, strong governance, and community involvement tend to minimize some of these challenges. In addition, although food transfers and vouchers can be important social protection interventions, they should ideally not create dependence, as has been the case in recent designs for adaptive safety nets. This requires designing parallel interventions to encourage self-sufficiency in the longer term.

Maternity Leave

Maternity leave allows employed women to take advantage of a protected leave of absence around the time of childbirth. The International Labour Organization convention on this topic stipulates a leave period of at least 14 weeks, and maternity leave should ideally be fully or partially paid (ILO 1998). Such leave is a social protection intervention that supports the health and nutrition of both the mother and the child during a critical period of development. Although there are important gaps in the literature, research suggests that it can contribute to better breastfeeding practices (Chai, Nandi, and Heyman 2018), timely vaccinations (Hajizadeh et al. 2015), and improved childcare (Heymann et al. 2017), all of which are essential for the child's physical and cognitive development.

There is evidence that improvements in breastfeeding duration and prevalence of exclusive breastfeeding are associated with maternity leave. For example, maternity leave of at least three months is associated with a three times higher likelihood of maintaining breastfeeding at three months (Navarro-Rosenblatt and Garmendia 2018). Maternity leave has also been associated with a 52 percent increase in exclusive breastfeeding practices (Sinha et al. 2015). Despite not being included in the systematic review because of its design, one multicountry longitudinal study of LMICs (Chai, Nandi, and Heyman 2018) provides convergent evidence for the association of maternity leave with positive results on a variety of breastfeeding indicators. For example, a one-month paid maternity leave policy is associated with an increase of 7.4 percentage points in the prevalence of early initiation of breastfeeding, a 5.86 percentage point increase in the prevalence of exclusive breastfeeding for children younger than six months, and a 2.21-month increase in average breastfeeding duration.

Evidence also documents the role of early return to work as a barrier to optimal breastfeeding. Although prior evidence has mainly emerged from HICs, recent evidence highlights similar results for LMICs. For example, a meta-analysis in Ethiopia (Wake and Mittiku 2021) estimates that mothers who returned to work within the first six months after giving birth had significantly lower odds of practicing exclusive breastfeeding. Similarly, a systematic review of barriers to and facilitators of exclusive breastfeeding among employed mothers in LMICs highlights extended maternity leave mandates as a fundamental facilitator (Gebrekidan et al. 2020).

Maternity leave often works through social security and employment-based platforms that can exclude self-employed and informally employed women. This is concerning because in many LMICs, women of reproductive age in the workforce disproportionately hold such jobs. Hence, there is an urgent need to respond to this challenge. Maternity cash transfers have been suggested as an alternative, and implementation costs have been estimated for Brazil, Ghana, Indonesia, Mexico, and the Philippines (Carroll et al. 2022; Siregar et al. 2021; Ulep et al. 2021; Vilar-Compte et al. 2019). On average, these costs would amount to less than 0.08 percent of gross domestic product, whereas their returns can be substantial. In the Philippines, discussions have progressed to the stage at which legislative bills are currently under consideration (refer to box 5.3).

Box 5.3

Maternity Cash Transfers for Women Employed in the Informal Sector in the Philippines

Maternity protection policies are critical nutrition-sensitive interventions that address the structural barriers at the nexus of maternal health, infant and young child nutrition, gender equity in the labor sector, and women's rights. The enactment of the Expanded Maternity Leave Law Republic Act 11210 (Official Gazette 2019) in the Philippines in 2019 marked a significant

(continued)

Box 5.3

Maternity Cash Transfers for Women Employed in the Informal Sector in the Philippines *(continued)*

legislative milestone by increasing paid maternity leave from 60 days to 105 days, among other vital measures. Although it falls short of Viet Nam's six-month paid maternity leave, it still brings the Philippines' legislation in line with the standards of the International Labour Organization's Conventions 183 and 191. However, a substantial proportion of the female workforce, particularly those in the informal economy who cannot contribute to the Social Security System, remain excluded from this law's benefits. Studies from various countries, including the Philippines, suggest that a publicly financed, noncontributory maternity cash transfer (MCT) is the appropriate modality for providing maternity support. The financing need to implement an MCT in the Philippines has been quantified using a robust economic model (Ulep et al. 2021). Building on this research, the Maternity Benefit for Women in the Informal Economy (Senate Bill 148; 2022) was filed by the same legislator who championed the Extended Maternity Leave Law. This bill aims to extend MCT to informal sector workers, drawing on Ulep et al.'s (2021) study and additional research on the economic impacts of suboptimal breastfeeding practices in the Philippines (Alive & Thrive 2022). Submitted to the Senate Committee on Women, Children, Family Relations and Gender Equality in July 2022, the bill is currently under review. The filing of the bill was welcomed by champions and advocates of women's rights and rights of informal sector workers, as well as the Commission on Human Rights. Two counterpart bills, titled "An Act Granting Maternity Benefits to Women Workers in the Informal Economy, Amending for This Purpose Republic Act No. 11210, Appropriating Funds Therefore, and for Other Purposes" (House Bills 4759 and 10070) were filed in the House of Representatives on September 2022 and March 2024, respectively. Both bills are currently awaiting committee review.

Source: Based on Roger Mathisen and Paul Zambran, Alive & Thrive, https://www.aliveandthrive.org/en/the-new-cost-of-not-breastfeeding-tool.

Nutrition Interventions Delivered through the Agriculture Sector

Nutrition-oriented agricultural practices can increase dietary diversity and improve other nutrition outcomes through pathways such as increases in food access resulting from own production, agricultural sales, changes in food prices, increases in women's control over resources, and women's time allocation to agricultural production (Ruel, Quisumbing, and Balagamwala 2018). Many agriculture programs with nutrition considerations are part of larger packages, which makes it hard to disentangle their relative contribution. To contribute to filling such gaps, a systematic review was conducted. The review included scientific literature published in 2013–23 in English and Spanish and focused on agriculture programs with nutrition-specific information, agriculture programs targeted at increasing commodity sales using livelihood interventions, agriculture programs aiming to improve food access through homestead food production and vegetable gardens, agriculture and livestock interventions (including small animals, livestock, and fisheries), and agriculture programs seeking to improve nutrition through improvements in women's agency. Although biofortification was not part of the systematic review, some general findings are also presented.

More information is available in the PROSPERO protocol (CRD42024552449) (Nguyen et al. 2024) as well as in annex 5A. Figure 5.4 summarizes specific information about the nutrition and agriculture interventions, and annex 5C presents the evidence summary tables.

Nutrition and Agriculture Programs

Two recent meta-analyses indicate that agriculture interventions may result in moderate yet positive effects on dietary diversity (de Hoop et al. 2024; Margolies et al. 2022). For example, programs that deliver agriculture training, provision of agricultural inputs, irrigation support, and other agriculture interventions and combine them with nutrition interventions, including behavior change communication and the provision of supplements, significantly improve dietary diversity by about 0.14 standard mean deviation (de Hoop et al. 2024; Margolies et al. 2022). According to de Hoop et al. (2024), a similar effect size is reported by livelihoods programs and livestock interventions. Consistent with prior research (Berretta et al. 2023; Ruel, Quisumbing, and Balagamwala 2018), larger effects on dietary diversity are reported for homestead food production and vegetable garden interventions (0.24 standardized mean difference [SMD]) and gender-based interventions (0.23 SMD).

The results from de Hoop et al. (2024) suggest that agriculture programs can also generate reductions in growth indicators, but the effects are small, and the evidence is inconclusive. For example, agricultural livelihood programs; homestead food production and vegetable garden programs; and programs that focus on small animals, livestock, and fisheries report small reductions in stunting (ranging between 7 percent and 9 percent reduction in the odds of stunting). Agricultural livelihoods programs and homestead food production and vegetable garden programs can also reduce the odds of wasting by about 11 percent and 14 percent, respectively.

Figure 5.4 Overview of Nutrition Interventions Delivered through the Agriculture Sector in LMICs

	Intervention	How is it delivered?	To whom?	What is delivered?
Agriculture programs	Integrated agriculture and nutrition programs	Delivery mechanisms vary greatly depending on the local context, resources available, and targeted outcomes of the intervention.	Farmers and primary caregivers	Training on agricultural practices combined with other nutrition interventions (such as infant, youth, and child nutrition supplements)
	Agricultural livelihoods programs			Training on agricultural practices combined with livelihoods or activities to improve market access for agricultural sales
	Homestead food production and vegetable garden programs			Training for primary caregivers in homestead food production related to livestock or vegetable gardens
	Agricultural livestock programs			Training on livestock practices or livestock transfers
	Integrated agriculture and gender programs			Training on agricultural practices combined with gender integration (such as women's group programming)
Biofortification	Biofortification	Delivered through the cultivation and consumption of nutrient-enriched crops	Distributed to farmers; benefit populations that consume the crops	Addition of nutrients to food crops prior to harvesting to tackle micronutrient deficiencies

Source: Original figure for this publication.
Note: LMICs = low- and middle-income countries.

Several studies included in the review reported significant associations between food production and vegetable garden interventions and reductions in anemia prevalence, hemoglobin concentration, or both. For example, a plant-based enhanced homestead food production intervention in Cambodia reported reductions in anemia of about 14 percentage points (Michaux et al. 2019). A similar program in Cambodia but based on home gardens (with or without a behavior change component) also found reductions in anemia rates. Likewise, a study on an enhanced homestead food production intervention plus behavior change communication in Nepal found improvements in hemoglobin levels and 24 percent less likelihood of children being anemic (Osei et al. 2017). Another study in Burkina Faso linked to an enhanced homestead food production intervention plus behavior change communication components reported significant improvements in children's levels of anemia, but only when the behavior components were provided by health committees (Dillon, Bliznashka, and Olney 2020; Heckert, Olney, and Ruel 2019; Olney et al. 2015).

The evidence suggests a need for further research, because considerable evidence gaps still exist. Further rigorous studies to clarify the impact that agricultural interventions can have on nutrition outcomes—and how to maximize that impact—need to be prioritized, especially in light of the important role that these kinds of interventions can play in climate adaptation and mitigation.

Biofortification

Biofortification is an agricultural nutrition strategy that aims at increasing the nutritional value of food crops to improve their micronutrient content (such as zinc, iron, and vitamin A). Biofortified products should be commonly consumed by populations in which there is a high prevalence of malnutrition and micronutrient deficiencies. Biofortification differs from conventional fortification because it focuses on making food more nutritious as it grows, rather than by adding nutrients during processing (Lowe 2021). Key crops that have been targeted for biofortification include rice, wheat, beans, sweet potatoes, cassava, and maize (Bouis, Saltzman, and Birol 2019).

According to a recent systematic review (Ofori et al. 2022), Harvest Plus, the Biocassava project, and the National Agricultural Research Organization are some of the major biofortification projects (Sheoran et al. 2022). Although each country context requires a unique approach to successfully implement and scale biofortification in the food system, evidence suggests that biofortification could be an approach to improve nutrition. For example, a six-month study of preschool children ages three years to five years was conducted in Nigeria, showing that biofortified cassava versus unfortified cassava resulted in a significant improvement in vitamin A (Afolami et al. 2021). Similarly, a review of iron-fortified crops in India, the Philippines, and Rwanda suggested significant increases in ferritin concentrations (Finkelstein, Haas, and Mehta 2017). However, there have also been some criticisms, including the fact that biofortification ignores the role of dietary diversity in delivering adequate nutrition and diverts scarce funding away from research into more diverse diets (van Ginkel and Chefras 2023). This places more emphasis on nutritious rather than diverse diets, for which implementation and behavior change might be more difficult. From a more operational perspective, some of the challenges of biofortification include seed distribution, policy support, and continued research to ensure that the biofortification process results in meaningful improvements in nutritional status.

Nutrition Interventions Delivered through the Water Sector

Water is fundamental to promoting equitable maternal and child nutrition. Lack of safe water and sanitation contributes to global malnutrition and negatively affects optimal human capital accumulation. There are different pathways through which water and sanitation contribute to maternal and child nutrition, including drinking water supply and sanitation; agriculture and food security, which encompass food systems; and water resources and ecosystems that are influenced by aspects such as climate change (refer to figure 5.5). Although acknowledging such diverse pathways, this section focuses on the contribution of water, sanitation, and hygiene (WASH) to nutrition outcomes, morbidity, and mortality. According to global estimates from 2019, poor WASH conditions contributed to 1.4–4.2 million deaths and 74–204 million disability-adjusted life years (DALYs) due to diarrhea, acute respiratory infections, undernutrition, and soil-transmitted helminthiases (WHO 2023a). Hence, public interventions to improve water access and safety have the potential to support maternal and child nutrition and reduce human capital disparities (Zhang and Borja-Vega 2024), especially considering that access to water resources and services during the early stages of life can have long-lasting effects (Damania et al. 2017). However, around 70 percent of the population of low-income countries and 40 percent of lower-middle-income countries lack access to safely managed drinking water facilities (Ritchie and Roser 2021).

Figure 5.5 Overview of Nutrition Interventions Delivered through the Water Sector in LMICs

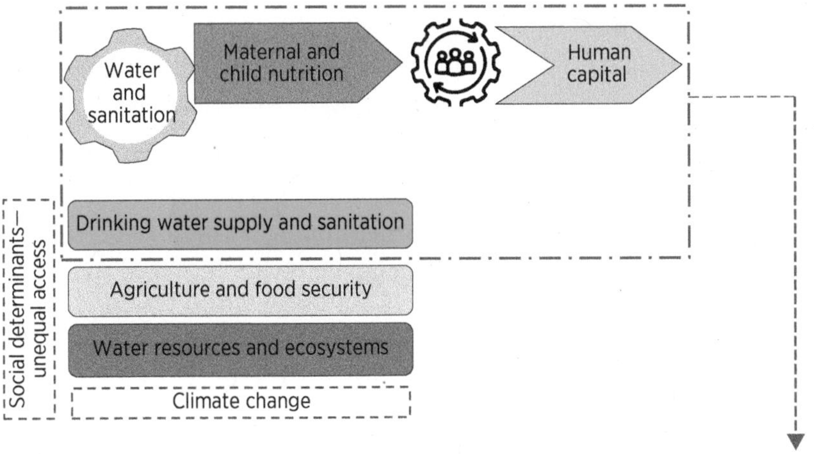

Intervention	How is it delivered?	To whom?	What is delivered?
Interventions with multiple or single WASH components alone	Infrastructure development at the community level, school based	Open population, community level	WASH interventions alone (such as improved quality, improved supply, introduction of sanitation, drinking-water disinfection, latrine renovation or construction)
WASH interventions with nutrition-specific programming			WASH interventions combined with infant, youth, and child nutrition education/counseling, supplementation, or deworming

(Left side label spanning both rows: Water, sanitation, and hygiene (WASH))

Source: Original figure for this publication.
Note: LMICs = low- and middle-income countries.

Recognizing the role of water-related interventions in addressing malnutrition, a systematic review was conducted, which included scientific literature published in 2013–23 in English and Spanish and was complemented by inputs from experts in the field. More information is available in the PROSPERO protocol (CRD42024552449) (Nguyen et al. 2024) and in annex 5A. The related evidence summary table is provided in annex 5C.

WASH interventions that include nutrition-specific services may result in improvements in height-for-age *z* scores (HAZ) of 0.13 SMD (Bekele, Rawstorne, and Rahman 2020), as can interventions that provide sanitation and hygiene services in addition to water (improvements in HAZ of 0.15 SMD; Gizaw and Worku 2019). Coverage of sanitation interventions is also fundamental (Augsburg and Rodríguez-Lesmes 2018). A recent at-scale cluster (village) RCT of sanitation interventions in four countries estimated that going from no coverage to 100 percent coverage could yield a 0.43 standard deviation significant increase in child height (Cameron et al. 2022). The same study reported that at coverage lower than 50 percent, there appear to be no gains in height.

Evidence from a recent meta-analysis underscores the role of WASH interventions in reducing the risk of diarrhea among children (Wolf et al. 2022). More specifically, it reports that, compared with untreated water source interventions supplying water filtered at point-of-use and higher quality significantly reduced the risk of diarrhea among children in LMICs by about 50 percent. Compared with unimproved sanitation, providing basic sanitation with a sewer connection reduced the risk of diarrhea among children by 47 percent, and promotion of handwashing with soap reduced this risk by 30 percent. Moreover, the impacts on diarrhea can be larger if programs integrate different WASH components. Interventions focusing on a sole component neglect the complementarity across them. For example, providing a village with universal access to both hygienic latrines and in-home piped water led to significant reductions in severe cases of diarrhea (Duflo et al. 2015). These findings are highly relevant in the context of nutrition because persistent diarrhea in the early stages of life creates a condition called gut dysfunction, which prevents children from absorbing nutrients and hence increases the risk of stunting (Budge et al. 2019; Zhang and Borja-Vega 2024).

A novel meta-analysis (Kremer et al. 2023) pooled evidence from several RCTs to assess the effect of water treatment on child mortality; it estimated that water treatment reduced the odds of all-cause child mortality by about 30 percent. Furthermore, this study profited from costing and coverage data from an actual project in Kenya and calculated a cost per DALY averted due to water treatment of $39. Given these findings, water treatment should be prioritized as an investment for health and nutrition. WASH investments and nutrition complement one another; although both independently play an important role in early childhood development, the interaction between them plays an additional significant role (Abramovsky et al. 2019). This calls for the need to design and implement interventions targeting both nutrition and WASH. Some promising advancements can be observed in empirical research testing packages that have integrated agriculture, nutrition, and WASH services (Wegmüller et al. 2022), as well as in measurement of water dimensions relative to the human-relative experience (refer to box 5.4). However, more research is needed to determine the optimal design and implementation.

Box 5.4

Water and Nutrition: New Monitoring Opportunities to Trigger Better Action

The recognition of the interconnectedness of water, food security, and nutrition has been growing, in part because of advances in the ability to measure water insecurity, defined as the inability to reliably access and use water to meet basic domestic needs. The Water Insecurity Experience (WISE) Scales bring a new, user-centered perspective to the water sector (www.WISEscales.org). Although prior global indicators measured only supply-side characteristics (for example, water availability or infrastructure), the WISE Scales capture how people experience and interact with water in their daily lives. The WISE Scales consist of 12 questions about universal experiences with issues of water for consumption (for example, drinking, cooking) and hygiene (for example, handwashing), as well as the psychological burden of water insecurity (for example, worry, anger). The WISE Scales have been validated globally and been used by scores of organizations in more than 55 countries.

One of the strengths of WISE Scales is that they are better predictors of many nutrition and health outcomes than water infrastructure or water availability indicators. For example, there is growing evidence about the effect of water insecurity on child well-being, including duration of breastfeeding, quality of complementary foods, and dietary diversity. For these and other reasons, the WISE Scales are important measures to consider when designing and implementing nutrition-sensitive water interventions. In fact, the WISE Scales have already served the needs of local and national organizations for guiding investment decisions and understanding impact.

Source: Pablo Gaitan-Rossi (EQUIDE - Universidad Iberoamericana) and Sera Young (Northwestern University).

Nutrition Interventions Delivered through the Education Sector

The education sector plays a pivotal role in delivering health and nutrition interventions for children and adolescents. Early childhood development (ECD) programs (delivered through either home visits or community centers), preschools, and schools serve as critical platforms for nutrition promotion, where children spend a significant portion of their day and can be taught healthy behaviors (refer to figure 5.6). Such educational institutions can provide nutritious meals, supplements, or both. Moreover, they can integrate health promotion through nutrition education and physical activity programs for both caregivers and pupils. Some of these institutions might also have health services that can be instrumental in delivering some medications (for example, deworming), supplements (for example, IFA), or immunizations. These actions can also improve cognitive function, thereby supporting the overall development and future potential of young individuals (Xu et al. 2021).

Figure 5.6 Overview of Nutrition Interventions Delivered through the Education Sector in LMICs

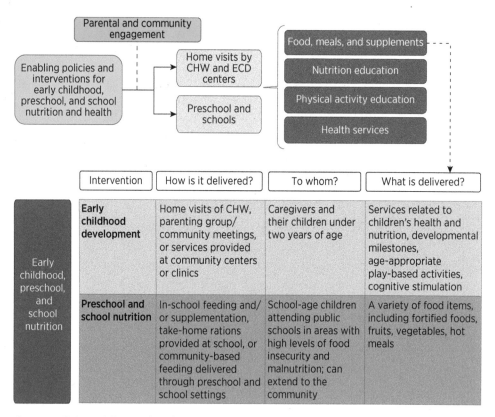

Source: Original figure for this publication.
Note: CHW = community health workers; ECD = early childhood development; LMICs = low- and middle-income countries.

Although all of these interventions are relevant, only food, meals, and supplements provided through ECD programs, preschools, and schools are addressed in the findings of the systematic review presented here. The review included ECD, preschool, and school programs providing foods, meals, and supplements to children and assessed their impact on the SDG 2.2 indicators. It included scientific literature published in 2013–23 in English and Spanish. More information is available in the PROSPERO protocol (CRD42024552449) (Nguyen et al. 2024) and in annex 5A. The related evidence summary table is provided in annex 5C.

Early Childhood Development Programs

ECD interventions aim to provide a strong foundation for the well-being, growth, and development of children, which can lead to improved health, education, and economic outcomes throughout the life course. These interventions are especially critical in LMICs, where children are often at higher risk of developmental delays due to poverty, poor health, and less access to high-quality services and healthful foods. They are often categorized at the intersection between education and social protection and are typically targeted at infants and young preschool children.

The aggregate literature is inconclusive regarding the impacts of ECD on SDG 2.2 indicators. The review did not find significant improvements in height for age and stunting as a result of ECD programs (Attanasio et al. 2014, 2022; Galasso et al. 2019; Premand and Barry 2022). However, interventions that combined several components, such as health, nutrition, WASH, or agriculture, with ECD reported significant reductions in stunting and other growth indicators (Gelli et al. 2018; Taneja et al. 2022). These findings seem consistent with the nurturing care framework, which states that for children to reach their full potential, interventions need five interrelated components: good health, adequate nutrition, responsive caregiving, security and safety, and opportunities for early learning (WHO, UNICEF, and World Bank 2018).

School Nutrition Programs

Preschool and school nutrition programs generally aim to improve the nutritional status, health, and educational outcomes of children. These programs typically deliver a variety of food items, such as fortified biscuits, fruits and vegetables, and sometimes hot meals, to school-age children attending public schools in rural and urban areas, where food insecurity and malnutrition are prevalent. The delivery of these programs can take different forms, including in-school feeding and take-home rations. In some cases, they can even extend beyond the school setting to provide food to the broader community, especially in areas where moderate and severe food insecurity prevail.

The evidence emerging from synthesis studies on children ages 5 years to 19 years suggests a possible association between school nutrition programs and weight for age (Kyere et al. 2020; Wang and Fawzi 2020). For anemia-related indicators, the results are mixed; for body mass index, study results were mainly consistent in finding no association with school nutrition programs (Choedon et al. 2024; Kyere et al. 2020).

On one hand, there is more specific evidence regarding school feeding programs that use fortified products that show significant associations with anemia prevalence and hemoglobin levels among particularly vulnerable populations such as displaced groups (Adelman et al. 2019), rural populations (Finkelstein et al. 2019), and low-income populations (Krämer, Kumar, and Vollmer 2021). On the other hand, studies linked to the provision of school meals were varied in their aims and outcomes. Among the studies that measured HAZ, all found significant associations with improved outcomes (Anitha et al. 2019; Gelli et al. 2019; Murayama et al. 2018), and several found improvements in hemoglobin concentrations (Baliki et al. 2023; Murayama et al. 2018). None reported adverse effects related to increased risk of overweight and obesity. Studies assessing preschool and school feeding programs providing micronutrient supplements reported an improvement in anemia-related indicators (Batra et al. 2016; Iannotti et al. 2015, 2016), but no effects on anthropometry. These studies suggest that although school nutrition programs may provide a useful platform for nutrition education and for delivering IFA supplements or deworming medicines, their impact on child stunting, wasting, or other SDG 2.2 targets remains elusive, at least in part because they miss the most critical first 1,000-day window for nutritional impacts.

Multisectoral Delivery of Nutrition Interventions

As shown earlier in figure 5.1, nutrition is commonly delivered in a multisectoral manner because of its complex interactions with various sectors such as health, agriculture, education, and social protection. This integrated approach is essential to address the multifaceted determinants of nutrition. This section outlines two examples of multisectoral interventions.

Deworming

Periodic deworming, also known as preventive chemotherapy, is recommended to control soil-transmitted helminth infections in at-risk populations (such as school-age children, adolescent girls, and women of reproductive age), particularly in areas where such infections are widely spread. Deworming is associated with significant reductions in anemia among school-age children (12 percent; Moorthy et al. 2020) and pregnant women (15 percent; Salam, Das, and Bhutta 2021), as well as with improvements in hemoglobin among nonpregnant populations (Byrne et al. 2021). Other benefits among school-age children that might be related to deworming are gains in height and weight (Taylor-Robinson et al. 2019), although more evidence is needed.

Deworming is considered a multisectoral nutrition intervention because it involves at least three sectors: (1) the health sector, which plays a crucial role in administering the treatments and educating communities about its importance; (2) the education sector, which serves as a platform for mass deworming programs, reaching a large number of children in an efficient manner; and (3) the water sector, because WASH programs are an integral part of preventing reinfection by improving access to safe water and sanitation measures.

Food Fortification Targeted to the General Population

Large-scale food fortification (LSFF) is a proven intervention to prevent micronutrient deficiencies by adding essential vitamins and minerals to foods that are commonly consumed by the general population. LSFF is often divided into three groups: (1) foods for which there are WHO guidelines, such as salt, wheat flour, maize flour, and rice; (2) foods under consideration for WHO guidelines, such as oil, sugar, and milk; and (3) condiments such as soy sauce, bouillon, and fish sauce for which there are currently no WHO guidelines. In the 2021 *Lancet Series on Maternal and Child Health* (*The Lancet* 2021), LSFF was identified as an intervention with strong evidence for its implementation, although no specific evidence of its effect was detailed. Recent studies suggest that food fortification is an important strategy to reduce anemia. For example, when compared with unfortified products, iron-fortified products are associated with reductions in anemia prevalence, 27 percent for wheat flour (Field and Maffioli forthcoming), 75 percent for soy sauce (Da Silva Lopes et al. 2021), and 66 percent for condiments (Jalal et al. 2023), although further evidence is needed. Evidence also suggests that fortified foods are associated with improvements in hemoglobin levels (mean differences range between 2.75 grams per liter (g/L) and 14.81 grams per liter (g/L), depending on the product; Da Silva Lopes et al. 2021; Field and Maffioli forthcoming; Larson et al. 2021). Similar results are reported in synthesis research focused on products fortified with iron plus other micronutrients. For instance, there is strong evidence linking double fortification of salt with iron and iodine to significant reductions in anemia prevalence (reductions ranging between 16 percent and 21 percent) and hemoglobin levels (mean differences ranging between 0.44 g/L and 30.1 g/L; Larson et al. 2021; Ramírez-Luzuriaga et al. 2018). Although similar findings have been reported for double-fortified rice (Peña-Rosas et al. 2019) and condiments (Jalal et al. 2023), more evidence is still needed.

LSFF is a multisectoral nutrition intervention that requires the collaboration of (1) the health sector in identifying nutrient deficiencies in the community (a critical step to guarantee that fortified foods are delivered to the intended recipients); providing guidelines for the micronutrients needed; and helping set coherent nutrition standards as well as limiting the promotion and distribution of low-quality fortified ultraprocessed foods; (2) the private sector, the government, or both in producing fortified staples and establishing delivery mechanisms; (3) the agriculture sector, which can support the integration of sustainable and scalable fortification into food systems; and (4) the social protection and education sectors in bringing public awareness to fortified products and making sure that these products are accepted and regularly consumed (Mkambula et al. 2020; Sarma et al. 2021). Some of these elements are addressed in more detail in chapter 6.

Summary of the Evidence and Implications for Scale-Up

Although several of the interventions highlighted in this chapter are likely to enhance well-being, the strength of evidence regarding their impact on SDG 2.2–related outcomes varies. Recognizing the need for stakeholders and decision-makers to adopt, design, and implement interventions at scale and within limited budget envelopes, chapter 7 leverages the updated evidence to develop global scenarios for investment and optimization. These scenarios are informed by a rigorous process of evidence assessment, availability of coverage and cost data, and consultation with experts in the field, and the interventions and effect sizes are summarized in table 5.1.

Table 5.1   Summary of the Nutrition Interventions and Effect Sizes

Intervention	Target population	Effects	Effect size	Source
Children				
Cash transfers (conditional)	Children below the poverty line	Reduces stunting 12–59 months	OR = 0.808 (0.395, 0.956)	Field and Maffioli forthcoming
Delayed umbilical cord clamping	Pregnant women (at birth, but impact is for children ages <1 month)	Reduces anemia 0–5 months	RR = 0.92 (0.87, 0.99)	Zhao et al. 2019 This estimate does not correspond to the age bracket; there are no recent estimates, and the assumption is that the effect would be at least the same as for children ages ≥6 months
		Reduces anemia 6–12 months	≥6 months, RR = 0.92 (0.87, 0.99)	Zhao et al. 2019
IYCN education and counseling	For children ages <1 month	Increases exclusive breastfeeding (home or community settings)	OR = 2.17 (1.84, 2.56)	Sinah et al. 2017
	For children ages <6 months	Increases exclusive breastfeeding (home or community settings)	OR = 2.48 (1.99, 3.09)	Sinah et al. 2017
	For children ages 6–23 months	Increases age-appropriate partial breastfeeding (combined delivery: home or community settings and health systems and services)	OR = 1.82 (1.36, 2.45)	Sinah et al. 2017

(continued)

Table 5.1 Summary of the Nutrition Interventions and Effect Sizes (*continued*)

Intervention	Target population	Effects	Effect size	Source
Kangaroo mother care	Ages 1–5 months	Increases exclusive breastfeeding	OR = 1.39 (1.11, 1.74)	Boundy et al. 2016
	Ages <1 month	Reduces neonatal prematurity	Neonatal RR = 0.68 (0.53, 0.86)	Sivanandan and Sankar 2023
Micronutrient powders (i.e., iron sprinkles)	Children ages 6–59 months, not already receiving LNS	Reduces anemia	RR = 0.69 (0.62, 0.77)	Moorthy et al. 2020
CRS + zinc	Children ages 0–59 months (different quantity by age)	Reduces diarrhea mortality	RR = 0.24 (0.15, 0.38)	Munos, Walker, and Black 2010; calculated as RR = 0.31 (0.20–0.49) for ORS, with additional RR of 0.77 due to the addition of zinc Walker and Black 2010
SQ-LNS	Children ages 6–23 months old living in households below the poverty line	Reduces the odds of stunting	PR = 0.88 (0.85, 0.91)	Dewey et al. 2021
		Reduces the incidence of SAM	PR = 0.69 (0.55, 0.86)	Dewey et al. 2022
		Reduces the incidence of MAM	PR = 0.86 (0.80, 0.93)	Dewey et al. 2021
		Reduces iron-deficiency anemia	PR = 0.36 (0.30, 0.44)	Wessells et al. 2021

(continued)

Table 5.1   Summary of the Nutrition Interventions and Effect Sizes (continued)

Intervention	Target population	Effects	Effect size	Source
Treatment of SAM	Children experiencing SAM	Increases recovery from episode	RR 1.33 (1.16, 1.54) Recovery RR = 1/1.33 (1/1.54, 1/1.16)	Schoonees et al. 2019
Vitamin A supplementation	Children ages 6–59 months	Reduces diarrhea incidence	RR = 0.85 (0.82, 0.87)	Imdad et al. 2022
		Reduces diarrhea mortality	RR = 0.88 (0.79, 0.98)	Imdad et al. 2022
Zinc supplementation (prophylactic)	Children ages 1–59 months	Reduces diarrhea incidence	RR = 0.91 (0.90, 0.93)	Imdad et al. 2023
Pregnant women				
Calcium supplementation	Pregnant women	Reduces maternal mortality (hypertensive disorders)	RR = 0.17 (0.02, 1.39)	Hofmeyr et al. 2018
		Reduces preterm births	RR = 0.76 (0.60, 0.97)	Hofmeyr et al. 2023 All women
Iron and folic acid supplementation	Women of reproductive age (pregnant and nonpregnant)	Reduces anemia	RR = 0.51 (0.38, 0.70)	Hansen et al. 2023 Anemia in pregnant women
			RR = 0.73 (0.56, 0.95)	Fernández-Gaxiola and De-Regil 2011 Anemia in nonpregnant women
		Reduces SGA birth outcomes	RR = 0.39 (0.17, 0.86)	Hansen et al. 2023

(continued)

Table 5.1 Summary of the Nutrition Interventions and Effect Sizes *(continued)*

Intervention	Target population	Effects	Effect size	Source
Intermittent preventative treatment of malaria during pregnancy	Pregnant women in areas where there is malaria risk	Reduces anemia	RR = 0.90 (0.84, 0.95)	Moorthy et al. 2020
		Reduces SGA birth outcomes	RR = 0.65 (0.55, 0.77)	Eisele et al. 2010
Multiple micronutrient supplementation	Pregnant women	Reduces anemia	RR = 0.51 (0.38, 0.70)	Hansen et al. 2023 Anemia in pregnant women
		Reduces risk of SGA birth outcomes	RR = 0.90 (0.84, 0.96)	Hofmeyr et al. 2023, MMS vs. IFAS
		Reduces risk of stillbirths	RR = 0.91 (0.86, 0.98)	Hofmeyr et al. 2023, MMS vs. IFAS
General				
Iron and folic acid fortification (wheat, maize, or rice)	Everyone (except children ages <6 months)	Reduces anemia	PR = 0.976 (0.975, 0.978)	Barkley, Wheeler, and Pachón 2015
Iron and iodine fortification of salt	Everyone (except children ages <6 months)	Reduces anemia	RR = 0.79 (0.66, 0.94)	Baxter et al. 2022
		Reduces neonatal mortality	PR = 0.976 (0.975, 0.978)	Barkley, Wheeler, and Pachón 2015

Source: Original table for this publication.

Note: For interventions without updated evidence, the one used in the original model was kept. Values in parentheses are 95% confidence intervals; IFAS = Iron and folic acid supplementation; IYCN = infant and young child nutrition; LNS = lipid-based nutrient supplements; MAM = moderate acute malnutrition; MMS = multiple micronutrient supplements; OR = odds ratio; ORS = oral rehydration solution; PR = prevalence ratio; RR = risk ratio; SAM = severe acute malnutrition; SGA = small for gestation age; SQ-LNS = small-quantity lipid-based nutrition supplements.

References

Abramovsky, Laura, Britta Augsburg, Pamela Jervis, Bansi Malde, and Angus Phimister. 2019. "Complementarities in the Production of Child Health." Working Paper W19/15, Institute for Fiscal Studies, London.

Adelman, Sarah, Daniel O. Gilligan, Joseph Konde-Lule, and Harold Alderman. 2019. "School Feeding Anemia Prevalence in Adolescent Girls and Other Vulnerable Household Members in a Cluster Randomized Controlled Trial in Uganda." *Journal of Nutrition* 149 (4): 659–66.

Afolami, Ibukun, Martin N. Mwangi, Folake Samuel, Erick Boy, Paul Ilona, Elise F. Talsma, Edith Feskens, et al. 2021. "Daily Consumption of Pro-Vitamin A Biofortified (Yellow) Cassava Improves Serum Retinol Concentrations in Preschool Children in Nigeria: A Randomized Controlled Trial." *American Journal of Clinical Nutrition* 113 (1): 221231. https://doi.org/10.1093/ajcn/nqaa290.

Ahmed, Akhter, John Hoddinott, and Shalini Roy. 2024. "Food Transfers, Cash Transfers, Behavior Change Communication and Child Nutrition: Evidence from Bangladesh." *World Bank Economic Review* lhae023. https://doi.org/10.1093/wber/lhae023.

Alderman, Harold, Ugo Gentilini, and Ruslan Yemtsov, eds. 2017. *The 1.5 Billion People Question: Food, Vouchers, or Cash Transfers?* Washington, DC: World Bank.

Alive & Thrive. 2022. "The New Cost of Not Breastfeeding Tool." Washington, DC: Alive & Thrive. https://www.aliveandthrive.org/en/the-new-cost-of-not-breastfeeding-tool.

"An Act Granting Maternity Benefits to Women Workers in the Informal Economy, Amending for This Purpose Republic Act No. 11210, Appropriating Funds Therefore, and for Other Purposes," or House Bills 4759 and 10070.

Anitha, Seetha, Joanna Kane-Potaka, Takuji W. Tsusaka, Deepti Tripathi, Shweta Upadhyay, Ajay Kavishwar, Ashok Jalagam, et al. 2019. "Acceptance and Impact of Millet-Based Mid-Day Meal on the Nutritional Status of Adolescent School Going Children in a Peri Urban Region of Karnataka State in India." *Nutrients* 11 (9): 2077. https://doi.org/10.3390/nu11092077.

Ara, Gulshan, Kazi Istiaque Sanin, Mansura Khanam, Md. Shafiqul Alam Sarker, Fahmida Tofail, Baitun Nahar, Imran Ahmed Chowdhury, et al. 2022. "A Comprehensive Intervention Package Improves the Linear Growth of Children under 2-Years-Old in Rural Bangladesh: A Community-Based Cluster Randomized Controlled Trial." *Scientific Reports* 12 (1): 21962.

Arikpo, Dachi, Ededet Sewanu Edet, Moriam T. Chibuzor, Friday Odey, and Deborah M. Caldwell. 2018. "Educational Interventions for Improving Primary Caregiver Complementary Feeding Practices for Children Aged 24 Months and Under." *Cochrane Database of Systematic Reviews* 5 (5): CD011768. https://doi.org/10.1002 /14651858.CD011768.pub2.

Attanasio, Orazio, Helen Baker-Cunningham, Raquel Bernal, Costas Meghir, Diana Pineda, and Marta Rubio-Codina. 2022. "Early Stimulation and Nutrition: The Impacts of a Scalable Intervention." *Journal of the European Economic Association* 20 (4): 1395–1432. https://doi.org/10.1093/jeea/jvac005.

Attanasio, Orazio P., Camila Fernández, Emla O. A. Fitzsimmons, Sally M. Grantham-McGregor, Costas Meghir, and Marta Rubio-Codina. 2014. "Using the Infrastructure of a Conditional Cash Transfer Program to Deliver a Scalable Integrated Early Child Development Program in Colombia: Cluster Randomized Controlled Trial." *BMJ* 349: g5785. https://doi.org/10.1136 /bmj.g5785.

Augsburg, Britta, and Paul Andrés Rodríguez-Lesmes. 2018. "Sanitation and Child Health in India." *World Development* 107: 22–39.

Baird, Sarah, Francisco H. G. Ferreira, Berk Özler, and Michael Woolcock. 2014. "Conditional, Unconditional and Everything in Between: A Systematic Review of the Effects of Cash Transfers on Schooling Outcomes." *Journal of Development Effectiveness* 6 (1): 1–43. https://doi.org/10.1080/19439342.2014.890362.

Baliki, Ghassan, Dorothee Weiffen, Pepijn Schreinemachers, Akina Shrestha, Rachana Manandhar Shrestha, Monika Schreiner, and Tilman Brück. 2023. "Effect of an Integrated School Garden and Home Garden Intervention on Anemia among School-Aged Children in Nepal: Evidence from a Cluster Randomised Controlled Trial." *Food and Nutrition Bulletin* 44 (3): 195–206. https://doi.org/10.1177/03795721231194124.

Barkley, Jonathan S., Kathleen S. Wheeler, and Helena Pachón. 2015. "Anaemia Prevalence May Be Reduced among Countries That Fortify Flour." *British Journal of Nutrition* 114 (2): 265–73.

Batra, Payal, Nina Schlossman, Ionela Balan, William Pruzensky, Adrian Balan, Carrie Brown, Madeleine G. Gamache, et al. 2016. "A Randomized Controlled Trial Offering Higher- Compared with Lower-Dairy Second Meals Daily in Preschools in Guinea-Bissau Demonstrates an Attendance-Dependent Increase in Weight Gain for Both Meal Types and an Increase in Mid-Upper Arm Circumference for the Higher-Dairy Meal." *Journal of Nutrition* 146 (1): 124–32. https://doi.org/10.3945/jn.115.218917.

Baxter, Jo-Anna B., Bianca Carducci, Mahdis Kamali, Stanley H. Zlotkin, and Zulfiqar A. Bhutta. 2022. "Fortification of Salt with Iron and Iodine versus Fortification of Salt with Iodine Alone for Improving Iron and Iodine Status." *Cochrane Database of Systematic Reviews* 2022 (4): CD013463. https://doi.org /10.1002/14651858.CD013463.pub2.

Bekele, Tolesa, Patrick Rawstorne, and Bayzidur Rahman. 2020. "Effect of Water, Sanitation and Hygiene Interventions Alone and Combined with Nutrition on Child Growth in Low and Middle Income Countries: A Systematic Review and Meta-Analysis." *BMJ Open* 10 (7). https://doi.org/10.1136/bmjopen -2019-034812.

Berretta, Miriam, Meital Kupfer, Shannon Shisler, and Charlotte Lane. 2023. "Rapid Evidence Assessment on Women's Empowerment Interventions within the Food System: A Meta-Analysis." *Agriculture & Food Security* 12: 13.

Black, Robert E., Cesar G. Victora, Susan P. Walker, Zulfiqar A. Bhutta, Parul Christian, Mercedes de Onis, Majid Ezzati, et al., 2013. "Maternal and Child Undernutrition and Overweight in Low-Income and Middle-Income Countries." *The Lancet* 382 (9890): 427–51. https://doi.org/10.1016/S0140-6736(13)60937-X.

Bossuroy, Thomas, Markus Goldstein, Bassirou Karimou, Dean Karlan, Harounan Kazianga, William Parienté, Patrick Premand, et al. 2022. "Tackling Psychosocial and Capital Constraints to Alleviate Poverty." *Nature* 605 (7909): 291–97.

Bouis, Howarth E., Amy Saltzman, and Ekin Birol. 2019. "Improving Nutrition through Biofortification." In *Agriculture for Improved Nutrition: Seizing the Momentum*, eds. Shenggen Fan, Sivan Yoseff, and Rajul Pandy-Lorch, 47–57. Wallingford, UK: International Food Policy Research Institute.

Boundy, Ellen O., Roya Dastjerdi, Donna Spiegelman, Wafaie W. Fawzi, Stacey A. Missmer, Ellice Lieberman, Sandhya Kajeepeta, et al. 2016. "Kangaroo Mother Care and Neonatal Outcomes: A Meta-Analysis." *Pediatrics* 137 (1).

Budge, Sophie, Alison H. Parker, Paul T. Hutchings, and Camila Garbutt. 2019. "Environmental Enteric Dysfunction and Child Stunting." *Nutrition Reviews* 77 (4): 240–53. https://doi.org/10.1093/nutrit/nuy068.

Byrne, Aisling, Giselle Manalo, Naomi E. Clarke, and Susana Vaz Nery. 2021. "Impact of Hookworm Infection and Preventive Chemotherapy on Haemoglobin in Non-Pregnant Populations." *Tropical Medicine & International Health* 26 (12): 1568–92. https://doi.org/10.1111/tmi.13681.

Cameron, Lisa, Paul Gertler, Manisha Shah, Maria Laura Alzua, Sebastian Martinez, and Sumeet Patil. 2022. "The Dirty Business of Eliminating Open Defecation: The Effect of Village Sanitation on Child Height from Field Experiments in Four Countries." *Journal of Development Economics* 159: 102990. https://doi.org/10.1016/j.jdeveco .2022.102990.

Carneiro, P., L. Kraftman, LG. Mason, L. Moore, I. Rasul, and M. Scott. 2021. "The Impacts of a Multifaceted Prenatal Intervention on Human Capital Accumulation in Early Life." *American Economic Review*, 111 (8): 2506–49.

Carroll, Grace, Mireya Vilar-Compte, Graciela Teruel, Meztli Moncada, David Aban-Tamayo, Heitor Werneck, Ricardo Montes de Moraes, et al. 2022. "Estimating the Costs for Implementing a Maternity Leave Cash Transfer Program for Women Employed in the Informal Sector in Brazil and Ghana." *International Journal for Equity in Health* 21: 20.

Chai, Yan, Arijit Nandi, and Jody Heyman. 2018. "Does Extending the Duration of Legislated Paid Maternity Leave Improve Breastfeeding Practices? Evidence from 38 Low-Income and Middle-Income Countries." *BMJ Global Health* 3 (5): e001032.

Choedon, Tashi, Eilise Brennan, William Joe, Natasha Lelijveld, Oliver Huse, Christina Zorbas, Kathryn Backholer, et al. 2024. "Nutritional Status of School-Age Children (5–19 Years) in South Asia: A Scoping Review." *Maternal & Child Nutrition* 20 (2): e13607. https://doi.org/10.1111/mcn.13607.

Damania, Richard, Sébastien Desbureaux, Marie Caitriona Hyland, Asif Mohammed Islam, Scott Michael Moore, Aude-Sophie Rodella, and Esha Dilip Zaveri. 2017. *Uncharted Waters: The New Economics of Water Scarcity and Variability*. Washington, DC: World Bank.

Da Silva Lopes, Katharina, Noyuri Yamaji, Md Obaidur Rahman, Maiko Suto, Yo Takemoto, Maria Nieves Garcia-Casal, and Erika Ota. 2021. "Nutrition-Specific Interventions for Preventing and Controlling Anaemia throughout the Life Cycle: An Overview of Systematic Reviews." *Cochrane Database of Systematic Reviews* 9 (9): CD013092. https://doi.org/10.1002/14651858.CD013092.pub2.

Das, Jai K., Rehana A. Salam, Yousuf Bashir Hadi, Sana Sadiq Sheikh, Afsah Z. Bhutta, Zita Weise Prinzo, and Zulfiqar A. Bhutta. 2019. "Preventive Lipid-Based Nutrient Supplements Given with Complementary Foods to Infants and Young Children 6 to 23 Months of Age for Health, Nutrition, and Developmental Outcomes." *Cochrane Database of Systematic Reviews* 5 (5): CD012611. https://doi.org/10.1002/14651858.CD012611.pub3.

Das, Jai K., Rehana A. Salam, Marwah Saeed, Faheem Ali Kazmi, and Zulfiqar A. Bhutta. 2020. "Effectiveness of Interventions for Managing Acute Malnutrition in Children under Five Years of Age in Low-Income and Middle-Income Countries: A Systematic Review and Meta-Analysis." *Nutrients* 12 (1): 116. https://doi.org/10.3390/nu12010116.

de Groot, Richard, Tia Palermo, Sudhanshu Handa, Luigi Peter Ragno, and Amber Peterman. 2017. "Cash Transfers and Child Nutrition: Pathways and Impacts." *Development Policy Review* 35 (5): 621–43. https://doi.org/10.1111/dpr.12255.

de Hoop, Thomas, Adria Molotsky, Amos Laar, Averi Chakrabarti, Garima Siwach, Rebecca Walcott, Varsha Ranjit, and Torben Behmer. 2024. *Synthesis of Evidence on the Impacts of Nutrition-Sensitive Interventions on Maternal and Children's Nutrition Outcomes*. Internal report. Washington, DC: World Bank.

Desta, Melaku, Bekalu Kassie, Habtamu Chanie, Henok Mulugeta, Tadess Yirga, Habtamu Temesgen, Cheru Tesema Leshargie, et al. 2019. "Adherence of Iron and Folic Acid Supplementation and Determinants among Pregnant Women in Ethiopia: A Systematic Review and Meta-Analysis." *Reproductive Health* 16 (1): 182. https://doi.org/10.1186/s12978-019-0848-9.

Dewey, Kathryn G., Charles D. Arnold, K. Ryan Wessells, Elizabeth L. Prado, Souheila Abbeddou, Seth Adu Afarwuah, Hasmot Ali, et al. 2022. "Preventive Small-Quantity Lipid-Based Nutrient Supplements Reduce Severe Wasting and Severe Stunting among Young Children: An Individual Participant Data Meta-Analysis of Randomized Controlled Trials." *American Journal of Clinical Nutrition* 116 (5): 1314–33. https://doi.org/10.1093/ajcn/nqac232.

Dewey, Kathryn G., Charles D. Arnold, K. Ryan Wessells, and Christine P. Stewart. 2023. "Lipid-Based Nutrient Supplements for Prevention of Child Undernutrition: When Less May Be More." *American Journal of Clinical Nutrition* 118 (6): 1133–44. https://doi.org/10.1016/j.ajcnut.2023.09.007.

Dewey, Kathryn G., K. Ryan Wessells, Charles D. Arnold, Elizabeth L. Prado, Souheila Abbeddou, Seth Adu-Afarwuah, Hasmot Ali, et al. 2021. "Characteristics that Modify the Effect of Small-Quantity Lipid-Based Nutrient Supplementation on Child Growth: An Individual Participant Data Meta-Analysis of Randomized Controlled Trials." *American Journal of Clinical Nutrition* 114: 15S–42S.

Dillon, Andrew, Lilia Bliznashka, and Deanna Olney 2020. "Experimental Evidence on Post-Program Effects and Spillovers from an Agriculture-Nutrition Program." *Economics & Human Biology* 36: 100820. https://doi.org/10.1016/j.ehb.2019.100820.

Duflo, Esther, Michael Greenstone, Raymond Guiteras, and Thomas Clasen. 2015. "Toilets Can Work: Short and Medium Run Health Impacts of Addressing Complementarities and Externalities in Water and Sanitation." Working Paper No. 21521, National Bureau of Economic Research, Cambridge, MA.

Durao, Solange, Marianne E. Visser, Vundli Ramokolo, Julicristie M. Oliveira, Bey-Marrié Schmidt, Yusentha Balakrishna, Amanda Brand, et al. 2020. "Community-Level Interventions for Improving Access to Food in Low- and Middle-Income Countries." *Cochrane Database of Systematic Reviews* 7 (7): CD011504. https://doi.org/10.1002/14651858.CD011504.pub2.

Dwarkanath, Pratibha, Alfa Muhihi, Christopher R. Sudfeld, Blair J. Wylie, Molin Wang, Nandita Perumal, Tinku Thomas, et al. 2024. "Two Randomized Trials of Low-Dose Calcium Supplementation in Pregnancy." *New England Journal of Medicine* 390 (2): 143–53.

Eisele, Thomas P., David Larsen, and Richard W. Steketee. 2010. "Protective Efficacy of Interventions for Preventing Malaria Mortality in Children in *Plasmodium falciparum* Endemic Areas." *International Journal of Epidemiology* 39 (suppl 1): i88–i101.

Fernández-Gaxiola, Ana C., and Luz Maria De-Regil. 2011. "Intermittent Iron Supplementation for Reducing Anaemia and Its Associated Impairments in Menstruating Women." *Cochrane Database of Systematic Reviews* 12.

Field, Erica M., and Elissa M. Maffioli. Forthcoming. "Are Behavioral Change Interventions Needed to Make Cash Transfers Work for Children? Experimental Evidence from Myanmar." *Economic and Cultural Change.*

Finkelstein, Julia L., Jere D. Haas, and Saurabh Mehta. 2017. "Iron-Biofortified Staple Food Crops for Improving Iron Status: A Review of the Current Evidence." *Current Opinion in Biotechnology* 44: 138–45. https://doi.org/10.1016/j .copbio.2017.01.003.

Finkelstein, Julia L., Saurabh Mehta, Salvador Villalpando, Veronica Mundo-Rosas, Sarah V. Luna, Maike Rahn, Teresa Shamah-Levy, et al. 2019. "A Randomized Feeding Trial of Iron-Biofortified Beans in School Children in Mexico." *Nutrients* 11 (2): 381. https://doi.org/10.3390/nu11020381.

Galasso, Emanuela, Ann M. Weber, Christine P. Stewart, Lisy Ratsifandrihamanana, and Lia C. H. Fernald. 2019. "Effects of Nutritional Supplementation and Home Visiting on Growth and Development in Young Children in Madagascar: A Cluster-Randomised Controlled Trial." *The Lancet Global Health* 7 (9): e1257–68.

Gebrekidan, Kahsu, Ensieh Fooladi, Virginia Plummer, and Helen Hall. 2020. "Enablers and Barriers of Exclusive Breastfeeding among Employed Women in Low and Lower Middle-Income Countries." *Sexual and Reproductive Healthcare* 25 (2020): 100514. https://doi.org/10.1016/j.srhc.2020.100514.

Gelli, Aulo, Elisabetta Aurino, Gloria Folson, Daniel Arhinful, Clement Adamba, Isaac Osei-Akoto, Edoardo Masset, et al. 2019. "A School Meals Program Implemented at Scale in Ghana Increases Height-for-Age During Midchildhood in Girls and in Children from Poor Households: A Cluster Randomized Trial." *Journal of Nutrition* 149 (8): 1434–42. https://doi .org/10.1093/jn/nxz079.

Gelli, Aulo, Amy Margolies, Marco Santocroce, Natalie Roschnik, Aisha Twalibu, Mangani Katundu, Helen Moestue, et al. 2018. "Using a Community-Based Early Childhood Development Center as a Platform to Promote Production and Consumption Diversity Increases Children's Dietary Intake and Reduces Stunting in Malawi: A Cluster-Randomized Trial." *Journal of Nutrition* 148 (10): 1587–97. https://doi.org/10.1093/jn /nxy148.

Gentilini, Ugo, Mohamed Bubaker Alsafi Almenfi, Hrishikesh T. M. M. Iyengar, Giorgia Valleriani, Yuko Okamura, Emilio Raul Urteaga, Sheraz Aziz, et al. "Global Social Protection Responses to Inflation." Living Paper v.5. Social Protection & Jobs Discussion Paper Series. Washington, DC: World Bank.

Gizaw, Zemichael, and Alemayehu Worku. 2019. "Effects of Single and Combined Water, Sanitation and Hygiene (WASH) Interventions on Nutritional Status of Children. A Systematic Review and Meta-Analysis." *Italian Journal of Pediatrics* 45 (1): 77. https://doi.org/10.1186/s13052-019-0666-2.

Glassman, Amanda, Denizhan Duran, Lisa Fleisher, Daniel Singer, Rachel Sturke, Gustavo Angeles, Jodi Charles, et al. 2013. "Impact of Conditional Cash Transfers on Maternal and Newborn Health." *Journal of Health, Population, and Nutrition* 31 (4, Supplement 2): 48–66.

Gomes, Filomena, Sufia Askari, Robert E. Black, Parul Christian, Kathryn G. Dewey, Martin N. Mwangi, Ziaul Rana, et al. 2023. "Antenatal Multiple Micronutrient Supplements versus Iron-Folic Acid Supplements and Birth Outcomes: Analysis by Gestational Age Assessment Method." *Maternal & Child Nutrition* 19 (3): e13509. https://doi.org/10.1111/mcn.13509.

Gunabalasingam, Sowmiya, Daniele De Almeida Lima Slizys, Ola Quotah, Laura Magee, Sara L. White, Jessica Rigutto-Farebrother, Lucilla Poston, et al. 2023. "Micronutrient Supplementation Interventions in Preconception and Pregnant Women at Increased Risk of Developing Pre-Eclampsia: A Systematic Review and Meta-Analysis." *European Journal of Clinical Nutrition* 77 (7): 710–30.

Guo, W. 2023. "Evaluation of the Impact of Kangaroo Mother Care on Neonatal Mortality and Hospitalization: A Meta-Analysis." *Advances in Clinical and Experimental Medicine* 32 (2): 175–83.

Gupta, S., A. K. M. Brazier, and N. M. Lowe. 2020. "Zinc Deficiency in Low- and Middle-Income Countries: Prevalence and Approaches for Mitigation." *Journal of Human Nutrition and Dietetics* 33 (5): 624–43.

Gutman, Julie R., Carole Khairallah, Kasia Stepniewska, Harry Tagbor, Mwayiwawo Madanitsa, Matthew Cairns, Anne Joan L'lanziva, et al. 2021. "Intermittent Screening and Treatment with Artemisinin-Combination Therapy versus Intermittent Preventive Treatment with Sulphadoxine-Pyrimethamine for Malaria in Pregnancy: A Systematic Review and Individual Participant Data Meta-Analysis of Randomised Clinical Trials." *eClinicalMedicine* 41: 101160. https://doi.org/10.1016/j.eclinm.2021.101160.

Hajizadeh, Mohammad, Jody Heymann, Erin Strumpf, Sam Harper, and Ariji Nandi. 2015. "Paid Maternity Leave and Childhood Vaccination Uptake: Longitudinal Evidence from 20 Low-and-Middle-Income Countries." *Social Science & Medicine* 140: 104–17. https://doi.org/10.1016/j.socscimed.2015.07.008.

Hansen, Rebekah, Emilie P. F. Sejer, Charlotte Holm, and Jeppe B. Schroll. 2023. "Iron Supplements in Pregnant Women with Normal Iron Status: A Systematic Review and Meta-Analysis." *Acta Obstetricia et Gynecologica Scandinavica* 102 (9): 1147–58.

Heckert, Jessica, Deanna K. Olney, and Marie T. Ruel. 2019. "Is Women's Empowerment a Pathway to Improving Child Nutrition Outcomes in a Nutrition-Sensitive Agriculture Program? Evidence from a Randomized Controlled Trial in Burkina Faso." *Social Science & Medicine* 233 (C): 93–102. https://doi.org/10.1016/j.socscimed.2019.05.016.

Heymann, Jody, Aleta R. Sprague, Arijit Nandi, Alison Earle, Priya Batra, Adam Schickedanz, Paul J. Chung, et al. 2017. "Paid Parental Leave and Family Wellbeing in the Sustainable Development Era." *Public Health Review* 38: 21.

Hofmeyr, G. Justus, Robert E. Black, Ewelina Rogozińska, Austin Heuer, Neff Walker, Per Ashorn, Ulla Ashorn, et al. 2023. "Evidence-Based Antenatal Interventions to Reduce the Incidence of Small Vulnerable Newborns and Their Associated Poor Outcomes." *The Lancet* 401 (10389): 1733–44. https://doi .org/10.1016/S0140-6736(23)00355-0.

Hofmeyr, G. Justus, Theresa A. Lawrie, Álvaro N. Atallah, Álvaro N. Atallah, and Maria Regina Torloni. 2018. "Calcium Supplementation during Pregnancy for Preventing Hypertensive Disorders and Related Problems." *Cochrane Database of Systematic Reviews* 2018 (10): CD001059. https://doi.org/10.1002/14651858.CD001059.pub5.

Hume-Nixon, Maeve, Alicia Quach, Rita Reyburn, Cattram Nguyen, Andrew Steer, and Fiona Russell. 2021. "A Systematic Review and Meta-Analysis of the Effect of Administration of Azithromycin during Pregnancy on Perinatal and Neonatal Outcomes." *Eclinical Medicine* 40: 101123. https://doi.org/10.1016/j.eclinm .2021.101123.

Iannotti, Lora, Sherlie Jean-Louis Dulience, Saminetha Joseph, Charmayne Cooley, Teresa Tufte, Katherine Cox, Jacob Eaton, et al. 2016. "Fortified Snack Reduced Anemia in Rural School-Aged Children of Haiti: A Cluster-Randomized, Controlled Trial." *PloS One* 11 (12): e0168121. https://doi.org/10.1371/journal .pone.0168121.

Iannotti, Lora L., Nicole M. Henretty, Jacques Raymond Delnatus, Windy Previl, Tom Stehl, Susan Vorkoper, Jaime Bodden, et al. 2015. "Ready-to-Use Supplementary Food Increases Fat Mass and BMI in Haitian School-Aged Children." *Journal of Nutrition* 145 (4): 813–22. https://doi.org/10.3945/jn .114.203182.

ILO (International Labour Organization). 1998. "More than 120 Nations Provide Paid Maternity Leave." ILO News, February 16, 1998. https://www.ilo.org /resource/news/more-120-nations-provide-paid-maternity-leave.

Imdad, Aamer, Kurt Herzer, Evan Mayo-Wilson, Mohammad Yawar Yakoob, and Zulfiqar A. Bhutta. 2010. "Vitamin A Supplementation for Preventing Morbidity and Mortality in Children from 6 Months to 5 Years of Age." *Cochrane Database of Systematic Reviews* 2010, issue 12, art. no. CD008524. https://doi.org/10.1002 /14651858.CD008524.pub2.

Imdad, Aamer, Evan Mayo-Wilson, Maya R. Haykal, Allison Regan, Jasleen Sidhu, Abigail Smith, and Zulfiqar A. Bhutta. 2022. "Vitamin A Supplementation for Preventing Morbidity and Mortality in Children from Six Months to Five Years of Age." *Cochrane Database of Systematic Reviews* 3 (3): CD008524. https://doi .org/10.1002/14651858.CD008524.pub4.

Imdad, Aamer, Jaimie Rogner, Rida N. Sherwani, Jasleen Sidhu, Allison Regan, Maya R. Haykal, Olivia Tsistinas, et al. 2023. "Zinc Supplementation for Preventing Mortality, Morbidity, and Growth Failure in Children Aged 6 Months to 12 Years." *Cochrane Database of Systematic Reviews* 2023 (3): CD009384. https://doi.org//10.1002/14651858.CD009384.pub3.

Jalal, Chowdhury S. B., Luz Maria De-Regil, Vanessa Pike, and Prasanna Mithra. 2023. "Fortification of Condiments and Seasonings with Iron for Preventing Anaemia and Improving Health." *Cochrane Database of Systematic Reviews* 2023 (9): CD009604. https://doi.org/10.1002/14651858.CD009604.pub2.

Janmohamed, Amynah, Nazia Sohani, Zohra S. Lassi, and Zulfqar A. Bhutta. 2020. "The Effects of Community Home Visit and Peer Group Nutrition Intervention Delivery Platforms on Nutrition Outcomes in Low and Middle-Income Countries: A Systematic Review and Meta-Analysis." *Nutrients* 12 (2): 440. https://doi.org/10.3390/nu12020440.

Jasani, Bonny, Ranjit Torgalkar, Xiang Y. Ye, Sulaiman Syed, and Prakesh S. Shah. 2021. "Association of Umbilical Cord Management Strategies with Outcomes of Preterm Infants: A Systematic Review and Network Meta-Analysis." *JAMA Pediatrics* 175 (4): e210102. https://doi.org/10.1001/jamapediatrics.2021.0102.

Keats, Emily C., Nadia Akseer, Pravheen Thurairajah, Simon Cousens, and Zulfqar A. Bhutta; Global Young Women's Nutrition Investigators' Group. 2022. "Multiple-Micronutrient Supplementation in Pregnant Adolescents in Low- and Middle-Income Countries: A Systematic Review and a Meta-Analysis of Individual Participant Data." *Nutrition Reviews* 80 (2): 141–56. https://doi.org/10.1093/nutrit/nuab004.

Keats, Emily C., Jai K. Das, Rehana A. Salam, Zohra S. Lassi, Aamer Imdad, Robert E. Black, and Zulfiqar A. Bhutta. 2021. "Effective Interventions to Address Maternal and Child Malnutrition: An Update of the Evidence." *The Lancet Child & Adolescent Health* 5 (5): 367–84. https://doi.org/10.1016/S2352-4642(20)30274-1.

Keats, Emily C., B. A. Haider, E. Tam, and Z. A. Bhutta. 2019. "Multiple-Micronutrient Supplementation for Women during Pregnancy." *Cochrane Database of Systematic Reviews* (3).

Keats, Emily C., Christina Oh, Tamara Chau, Dina S. Khalifa, Aamer Imdad, and Zulfiqar A. Bhutta. 2021. "Effects of Vitamin and Mineral Supplementation during Pregnancy on Maternal, Birth, Child Health and Development Outcomes in Low- and Middle-Income Countries: A Systematic Review." *Campbell Systematic Reviews* 17 (2): e1127. https://doi.org/10.1002/cl2.1127.

Kinshella, Mai-Lei Woo, Shazmeen Omar, Kerri Scherbinsky, Marianne Vidler, Laura A. Magee, Peter von Dadelszen, Sophie E. Moore, et al. 2021. "Effects of Maternal Nutritional Supplements and Dietary Interventions on Placental Complications: An Umbrella Review, Meta-Analysis and Evidence Map." *Nutrients* 13 (2): 472. https://doi.org/10.3390/nu13020472.

Kodish, Stephen R., Nancy J. Aburto, Mutina Nseleke Hambayi, Filippo Dibari, and Joel Gittelsohn. 2017. "Patterns and Determinants of Small-Quantity LNS Utilization in Rural Malawi and Mozambique: Considerations for Interventions with Specialized Nutritious Foods." *Maternal & Child Nutrition* 13 (1): 3–6.

Krämer, Marion, Santosh Kumar, and Sebastian Vollmer. 2021. "Improving Child Health and Cognition: Evidence from a School-Based Nutrition Intervention in India." *Review of Economics and Statistics* 103 (5): 818–34.

Kremer, Michael, Stephen P. Luby, Ricardo Maertens, Brandon Tan, and Witold Więcek. 2023. "Water Treatment and Child Mortality: A Meta-Analysis and Cost-Effectiveness Analysis." Working Paper No. 30835, National Bureau of Economic Research, Cambridge, MA.

Kumar, Neha, Samuel Scott, Purnima Menon, Samyuktha Kannan, Kenda Cunningham, Parul Tyagi, Gargi Wable, et al. 2018. "Pathways from Women's Group-Based Programs to Nutrition Change in South Asia: A Conceptual Framework and Literature Review." *Global Food Security* 17: 172–85. https://doi.org/10.1016/j.gfs.2017.11.002.

Kyere, Paul, J. Lennert Veerman, Patricia Lee, and Donald E. Stewart. 2020. "Effectiveness of School-Based Nutrition Interventions in Sub-Saharan Africa: A Systematic Review." *Public Health Nutrition* 23 (14): 2626–36. https://doi.org/10.1017/S1368980020000506.

Larson, Leila M., Shruthi Cyriac, Eric W. Djimeu, Mduduzi N. N. Mbuya, and Lynnette M. Neufeld. 2021. "Can Double Fortification of Salt with Iron and Iodine Reduce Anemia, Iron Deficiency Anemia, Iron Deficiency, Iodine Deficiency, and Functional Outcomes? Evidence of Efficacy, Effectiveness, and Safety." *Journal of Nutrition* 151 (S1): 15S–28S.

Lassi, Zohra S., Sophie E. G. Kedzior, and Zulfiqar A. Bhutta. 2019. "Community-Based Maternal and Newborn Educational Care Packages for Improving Neonatal Health and Survival in Low- and Middle-Income Countries." *Cochrane Database of Systematic Reviews* 2019 (11): CD007647.

Lassi, Zohra S., Jaameeta Kurji, Cristeil Sérgio de Oliveira, Anoosh Moin, and Zulfiqar A. Bhutta. 2020. "Zinc Supplementation for the Promotion of Growth and Prevention of Infections in Infants Less Than Six Months of Age." *Cochrane Database of Systematic Reviews* 4 (4): CD010205. https://doi.org/10.1002/14651858.CD010205.pub2.

Lassi, Zohra S., Zahra A. Padhani, Amna Rabbani, Fahad Rind, Rehana A. Salam, and Zulfiqar A. Bhutta. 2021. "Effects of Nutritional Interventions during Pregnancy on Birth, Child Health and Development Outcomes: A Systematic Review of Evidence from Low- and Middle-Income Countries." *Campbell Systematic Reviews* 17 (2): e1150. https://doi.org/10.1002/cl2.1150.

Lassi, Zohra S., Fahad Rind, Omar Irfan, Rabia Hadi, Jai K. Das, and Zulfiqar A. Bhutta. 2020. "Impact of Infant and Young Child Feeding (IYCF) Nutrition

Interventions on Breastfeeding Practices, Growth and Mortality in Low- and Middle-Income Countries: Systematic Review." *Nutrients* 12 (3): 722. https://doi.org/10.3390/nu12030722.

Lazzerini, Marzia, and Humphrey Wanzira. 2016. "Oral Zinc for Treating Diarrhoea in Children." *Cochrane Database of Systematic Reviews* 12 (12): CD005436.

Leroy, Jef L., Deanna Olney, and Marie Ruel. 2016. "Tubaramure, a Food-Assisted Integrated Health and Nutrition Program in Burundi, Increases Maternal and Child Hemoglobin Concentrations and Reduces Anemia: A Theory-Based Cluster-Randomized Controlled Intervention Trial." *Journal of Nutrition* 146 (8), 1601–08.

Leroy, Jef L., Deanna Olney, and Marie Ruel. 2018. "Tubaramure, a Food-Assisted Integrated Health and Nutrition Program, Reduces Child Stunting in Burundi: A Cluster-Randomized Controlled Intervention Trial." *Journal of Nutrition* 148 (3): 445–52.

Leroy, Jef L., Deanna K. Olney, Lilia Bliznashka, and Marie Ruel. 2020. "Tubaramure, a Food-Assisted Maternal and Child Health and Nutrition Program in Burundi, Increased Household Food Security and Energy and Micronutrient Consumption, and Maternal and Child Dietary Diversity: A Cluster-Randomized Controlled Trial." *Journal of Nutrition* 150 (4): 945–57. https://doi.org/10.1093/jn/nxz295.

Li, Jinrong, Sufei Yang, Fan Yang, Jinhui Wu, and Fei Xiong 2021. "Immediate vs Delayed Cord Clamping in Preterm Infants: A Systematic Review and Meta-Analysis." *International Journal of Clinical Practice* 75 (11): e14709. https://doi.org/10.1111/ijcp.14709.

Lisboa, Cinthia S., Nathalia Sernizon Guimarães, Andrêa Jacqueline Fortes Ferreira, Karine Brito Beck da Silva, Flávia Jôse Oliveira Alves, Aline Dos Santos Rocha, Naiá Ortelan, et al. 2023. "Impact of Cash Transfer Programs on Birth and Child Growth Outcomes: Systematic Review." *Ciência & Saúde Coletiva* 28 (8): 2417–32. https://doi.org/0.1590/1413-81232023288.14082022.

Lowe, Nicola M. 2021. "The Global Challenge of Hidden Hunger: Perspectives from the Field." *Proceedings of the Nutrition Society* 80 (3): 283–289. https://doi.org/10.1017/S0029665121000902.

Mahumud, Rashidul A., Sophiya Uprety, Nidhi Wali, Andre M. N. Renzaho, and Stanley Chitekwe. 2022. "The Effectiveness of Interventions on Nutrition Social Behaviour Change Communication in Improving Child Nutritional Status within the First 1000 Days: Evidence from a Systematic Review and Meta-Analysis." *Maternal & Child Nutrition* 18 (1): e13286. https://doi.org/10.1111/mcn.13286.

Manley, James, Harold Alderman, and Ugo Gentilini. 2022. "More Evidence on Cash Transfers and Child Nutritional Outcomes: A Systematic Review and Meta-Analysis." *BMJ Global Health* 7 (4): e008233.

Margolies, Amy, Christopher G. Kemp, Esther M. Choo, Carol Levin, Deanna Olney, Neha Kumar, Ara Go, et al. 2022. "Nutrition-Sensitive Agriculture Programs Increase Dietary Diversity in Children under 5 Years: A Review and Meta-Analysis." *Journal of Global Health* 12: 08001. https://doi.org/10.7189/jogh .12.08001.

Maternity Benefit for Women in the Informal Economy, S. 148, 19th Congress (2022 Phil.). https://legacy.senate.gov.ph/lis/bill_res.aspx?congress=19&q =SBN-148.

McDonald, Sarah D. 2023. "Deferred Cord Clamping and Cord Milking: Certainty and Quality of the Evidence in Meta-Analyses, and Systematic Reviews of Randomized Control Trials, Guidelines, and Implementation Studies." *Seminars in Perinatology* 47 (5): 151790. https://doi.org/10.1016/j.semperi.2023.151790.

Michaux, Kristina D., Kroeun Hou, Crystal D. Karakochuk, Kyly C. Whitfield, Sokhoing Ly, Vashti Verbowski, Ame Stormer, et al. 2019. "Effect of Enhanced Homestead Food Production on Anaemia among Cambodian Women and Children: A Cluster Randomized Controlled Trial." *Maternal & Child Nutrition* 15 (Supplement 3): e12757. https://doi.org/10.1111/mcn.12757.

Mkambula, Penjani, Mduduzi N. N. Mbuya, Laura A. Rowe, Mawuli Sablah, Valerie M. Friesen, Manpreet Chadha, Akoto K. Osei, et al. 2020. "The Unfinished Agenda for Food Fortification in Low- and Middle-Income Countries: Quantifying Progress, Gaps and Potential Opportunities." *Nutrients* 12 (2): 354. https://doi.org/0.3390/nu12020354.

Moorthy, Denish, Rebecca Merrill, Sorrell Namaste, and Lora Iannotti. 2020. "The Impact of Nutrition-Specific and Nutrition-Sensitive Interventions on Hemoglobin Concentrations and Anemia: A Meta-Review of Systematic Reviews." *Advances in Nutrition* 11 (6): 1631–45. https://doi.org/10.1093 /advances/nmaa070.

Munos, Melinda K., Christa L. Fischer Walker, and Robert E. Black. 2010. "The Effect of Oral Rehydration Solution and Recommended Home Fluids on Diarrhoea Mortality." *International Journal of Epidemiology* 39 (Suppl_1): i75-i87.

Murayama, Nobuko, Mieko Magami, Salima Akter, Israt Ara Hossain, Liaquat Ali, Mahmud Hossain Faruquee, and Sk Akhtar Ahmad. 2018. "A Pilot School Meal Program Using Local Foods with Soybean in Rural Bangladesh: Effects on the Nutritional Status of Children." *Food and Nutrition Sciences* 9 (4): 290–313. https://doi.org/10.4236/fns.2018.94023.

Navarro-Rosenblatt, Deborah, and María-Luisa Garmendia. 2018. "Maternity Leave and Its Impact on Breastfeeding: A Review of the Literature." *Breastfeeding Medicine* 13 (9): 589–97. https://doi.org/10.1089/bfm.2018.0132.

Nguyen, Hoa Thi Mai, Sonia Hernandez-Cordero, Pablo Gaitan-Rossi, Bianca Franco-Lares, Vania Lara-Mejía, Brenda Tapia-Hernandez, Lucía Félix Beltrán. 2024. "Impacts of Nutrition-Sensitive Interventions on Nutrition Outcomes in

Low- and Middle-Income Countries. An Update of the Evidence." PROSPERO 2024 CRD42024552449. https://www.crd.york.ac.uk/prospero/display_record .php?ID=CRD42024552449.

Official Gazette (Philippines). 2019. "Republic Act No. 11210: An Act Increasing the Maternity Leave Period to One Hundred Five (105) Days for Female Workers with an Option to Extend for an Additional Thirty (30) Days Without Pay and Granting an Additional Fifteen (15) Days for Solo Mothers, and for Other Purposes." https://www.officialgazette.gov.ph/downloads/2019/02feb/2019 0220-RA-11210-RRD.pdf.

Ofori, Kelvin F., Sophia Anoniello, Marcia M. English, and Alberta N. A. Aryee. 2022. "Improving Nutrition through Biofortification—A Systematic Review." *Frontiers in Nutrition* 9: 1043655. https://doi.org/10.3389/fnut.2022.1043655.

Oh, Christina, Emily C. Keats, and Zulfiqar A. Bhutta. 2020. "Vitamin and Mineral Supplementation During Pregnancy on Maternal, Birth, Child Health and Development Outcomes in Low- and Middle-Income Countries: A Systematic Review and Meta-Analysis." *Nutrients* 12 (2): 491.

Olney, Deanna K., Abdoulaye Pedehombga, Marie T. Ruel, and Andrew Dillon. 2015. "A 2-Year Integrated Agriculture and Nutrition and Health Behavior Change Communication Program Targeted to Women in Burkina Faso Reduces Anemia, Wasting, and Diarrhea in Children 3–12.9 Months of Age at Baseline: A Cluster-Randomized Controlled Trial." *Journal of Nutrition* 145 (6): 1317–24. https://doi.org/10.3945/jn.114.203539.

Osei, Akoto, Pooja Pandey, Jennifer Nielsen, Alissa Pries, David Spiro, Dale Davis, Victoria Queinn, et al. 2017. "Combining Home Garden, Poultry, and Nutrition Education Program Targeted to Families with Young Children Improved Anemia among Children and Anemia and Underweight among Nonpregnant Women in Nepal." *Food and Nutrition Bulletin* 38 (1): 49–64. https://doi.org/10.1177 /0379572116676427.

Park, Jay J. H., Ellie Siden, Ofir Harari, Louis Dron, Reham Mazoub, Virginia Jeziorska, Noor-E Zannat, et al. 2020. "Interventions to Improve Linear Growth during Exclusive Breastfeeding Life-Stage for Children Aged 0-6 Months Living in Low- and Middle-Income Countries: A Systematic Review with Network and Pairwise Meta-Analyses." *Gates Open Research* 24 (3): 1720. https://doi.org/10.12688/ gatesopenres.13082.2.

Pega, Frank, Roman Pabayo, Claire Benny, Eun-Young Lee, Stefan K. Lhachimi, and Sze Yan Liu. 2022. "Unconditional Cash Transfers for Reducing Poverty and Vulnerabilities: Effect on Use of Health Services and Health Outcomes in Low- and Middle-Income Countries." *Cochrane Database of Systematic Reviews* 3.

Pelletier, David and Saski DePee. 2019. "Micronutrient Powder Programs: New Findings and Future Directions for Implementation Science." *Maternal & Child Nutrition* 15 (Supplement 5): e12802.

Peña-Rosas, Juan Pablo, Prasanna Mithra, Bhaskaran Unnikrishnan, Nihin Kumar, Luz Maria De-Regil, N. Sreekumaran Nair, Maria N. Garcia-Casal, et al. 2019. "Fortification of Rice with Vitamins and Minerals for Addressing Micronutrient Malnutrition." *Cochrane Database of Systematic Reviews* 2019 (10): CD009902. https://doi.org/10.1002/14651858.CD009902.pub2.

Pérez-Escamilla, Rafael, Cecilia Tomori, Sonia Hernández-Cordero, Phillip Baker, Aluisio J. D. Barros, France Bégin, Donna J. Chapman, et al. 2023. "Breastfeeding: Crucially Important, but Increasingly Challenged in a Market-Driven World." *The Lancet* 401 (10375): 472–485. https://doi.org/10.1016/S0140-6736(22)01932-8.

Persad, Emma, Greta Sibrecht, Martin Ringsten, Simon Karlelid, Olga Romantsik, Tommy Ulinder, Israel Júnior Borges do Nascimento, et al. 2021. "Interventions to Minimize Blood Loss in Very Preterm Infants—A Systematic Review and Meta-Analysis." *PLOS ONE* 16 (2): e0246353. https://doi.org/10.1371/journal.pone.0246353.

Premand, Patrick, and Oumar Barry. 2022. "Behavioral Change Promotion, Cash Transfers and Early Childhood Development: Experimental Evidence from a Government Program in a Low-Income Setting." *Journal of Development Economics* 158 (2022): 102921. https://doi.org/10.1016/j.jdeveco.2022.102921.

Rabe, Heike, Gillian M. I. Gyte, José L. Díaz-Rossello, and Lelia Duley. 2019. "Effect of Timing of Umbilical Cord Clamping and Other Strategies to Influence Placental Transfusion at Preterm Birth on Maternal and Infant Outcomes." *Cochrane Database of Systematic Reviews* 9 (9): CD003248. https://doi.org/10.1002/14651858.CD003248.pub4.

Ramírez-Luzuriaga, Maria J., Leila M. Larson, Venkatesh Mannar, and Reynaldo Martorell. 2018. "Impact of Double-Fortified Salt with Iron and Iodine on Hemoglobin, Anemia, and Iron Deficiency Anemia: A Systematic Review and Meta-Analysis." *Advances in Nutrition* 9 (3): 207–18. https://doi.org/10.1093/advances/nmy008.

Ramírez-Luzuriaga, María J., Mishel Unar-Munguía, Sonia Rodríguez-Ramírez, Juan A. Rivera, and Teresa González de Cosío. 2016. "A Food Transfer Program without a Formal Education Component Modifies Complementary Feeding Practices in Poor Rural Mexican Communities." *Journal of Nutrition* 146 (1): 107–13.

Ritchie, Hannah, and Max Roser. 2021. "Clean Water and Sanitation." *Our World in Data*. https://ourworldindata.org/clean-water-sanitation.

Ruel, Marie T., and Harold Alderman. 2013. "Nutrition-Sensitive Interventions and Programmes: How Can They Help to Accelerate Progress in Improving Maternal and Child Nutrition?" *The Lancet* 382 (9891): 536–51.

Ruel, Marie T., Agnes R. Quisumbing, and Mysbah Balagamwala. 2018. "Nutrition-Sensitive Agriculture: What Have We Learned So Far?" *Global Food Security* 17: 128–53. https://doi.org/10.1016/j.gfs.2018.01.002.

Salam, Rehana A., Jai K. Das, and Zulfiqar A. Bhutta. 2021. "Effect of Mass Deworming with Antihelminthics for Soil-Transmitted Helminths during Pregnancy." *Cochrane Database of Systematic Reviews* 2021 (5): CD005547. https://doi.org/10.1002/14651858.CD005547.pub4.

Sarma, Haribondhu, Md Fakhar Uddin, Mohammad Ashraful Islam, Mahfuzur Rahman, Grant J. Aaron, Catherine Harbour, Cathy Banwell, et al. 2021. "Use of Concurrent Evaluation to Improve Implementation of a Home Fortification Programme in Bangladesh: A Methodological Innovation." *Public Health Nutrition* 24 (S1): s37–s47. https://doi.org/10.1017/S1368980020000439.

Schoonees, Anel, Martani J. Lombard, Alfred Musekiwa, Etienne Nel, and Jimmy Volmink. 2019. "Ready-to-Use Therapeutic Food (RUTF) for Home-Based Nutritional Rehabilitation of Severe Acute Malnutrition in Children from Six Months to Five Years of Age." *Cochrane Database of Systematic Reviews* 5 (5): CD009000. https://doi.org/10.1002/14651858.CD009000.pub3.

Scott, Nick, Dominic Delport, Samuel Hainsworth, Ruth Pearson, Christopher Morgan, Sshan Huang, Jonathan K. Akuoku, et al. 2020 "Ending Malnutrition in All Its Forms Requires Scaling Up Proven Nutrition Interventions and Much More: A 129-Country Analysis." *BMC Medicine* 18: 1–19.

Segura-Pérez, Sofia, Rubén Grajeda, and Rafael Pérez-Escamilla, R. 2016. "Conditional Cash Transfer Programs and the Health and Nutrition of Latin American Children." *Revista Panamericana de Salud Pública* 40 (2): 124–37.

Sheoran, Seema, Sandeep Kumar, Vinita Ramtekey, Priyajoy Kar, Ram Swaroop Meena, and Chetan Kumar Jangir. 2022. "Current Status and Potential of Biofortification to Enhance Crop Nutritional Quality: An Overview." *Sustainability* 14 (6): 3301. https://doi.org/10.3390/su14063301.

Sinha, Bireshwar, Ranadip Chowdhury, M. Jeeva Sankar, Jose Martines, Sunita Taneja, Sarmila Mazumder, Nigel Rollins, et al. 2015. "Interventions to Improve Breastfeeding Outcomes: A Systematic Review and Meta-Analysis." *Acta Paediatrica* 104 (S467): 114–34. https://doi.org/10.1111/apa.13127.

Sinha, Bireshwar, Ranadip Chowdhury, Ravi Prakash Upadhyay, Sunita Taneja, Jose Martines, Rajiv Bahl, and Mari Jeeva Sankar. 2017. "Integrated Interventions Delivered in Health Systems, Home, and Community Have the Highest Impact on Breastfeeding Outcomes in Low- and Middle-Income Countries." *Journal of Nutrition* 147 (11): 2179S–87S. https://doi.org/10.3945/jn.116.242321.

Siregar, Adiatma Y. M., Pipit Pitriyan, Donny Hardiawan, Paul Zambrano, Mireya Vilar-Compte, Graciela Ma Teruel Belismelis, Meztli Moncada, et al. 2021. "The Yearly Financing Need of Providing Paid Maternity Leave in the Informal Sector in Indonesia." *International Breastfeeding Journal* 16: 17.

Sivanandan, Sindhu, and Mari Jeeva Sankar. 2023. "Kangaroo Mother Care for Preterm or Low Birth Weight Infants: A Systematic Review and Meta-Analysis." *BMJ Global Health* 8 (6): e010728. https://doi.org/10.1136/bmjgh-2022-010728.

Stewart, Christine P., Charles D. Arnold, Anne M. Williams, Benjamin F. Arnold, Amy J. Pickering, Holly Dentz, Marion Kiprotich, et al. Forthcoming. "Social Desirability Bias in a Randomized Controlled Trial that Included Breastfeeding Promotion in Western Kenya." *Maternal Child Nutrition*.

Stewart, Christine P., K. Ryan Wessells, Charles D. Arnold, Lieven Huybregts, Per Ashorn, Elodie Becquey, Jean H. Humphrey, et al. 2020. "Lipid-Based Nutrient Supplements and All-Cause Mortality in Children 6–24 Months of Age: A Meta-Analysis of Randomized Controlled Trials." *American Journal of Clinical Nutrition* 111 (1): 207–18. https://doi.org/10.1093/ajcn/nqz262.

Suchdev, Parminder S., Maria Elena D. Jefferds, Erika Ota, Katharina da Silva Lopes, and Luz Maria De-Regil. 2020. "Home Fortification of Foods with Multiple Micronutrient Powders for Health and Nutrition in Children under Two Years of Age." *Cochrane Database of Systematic Reviews* 2 (2): CD008959. https://doi .org/10.1002/14651858.CD008959.pub3.

Tam, Emily, Emily C. Keats, Fahad Rind, Jai K. Das, and Zufiqar A. Bhutta. 2020. "Micronutrient Supplementation and Fortification Interventions on Health and Development Outcomes among Children Under-Five in Low- and Middle-Income Countries: A Systematic Review and Meta-Analysis." *Nutrients* 12 (2): 289. https://doi.org/10.3390/nu12020289.

Taneja, Sunita, Ranadip Chowdhury, Neeta Dhabhai, Ravi Prakash Upadhyay, Sarmila Mazumder, Sitanshi Sharma, Kiran Bhatia, et al. for the WINGS Study Group. 2022. "Impact of a Package of Health, Nutrition, Psychosocial Support, and WaSH Interventions Delivered during Preconception, Pregnancy, and Early Childhood Periods on Birth Outcomes and on Linear Growth at 24 Months of Age: Factorial, Individual Randomised Controlled Trial." *BMJ* 379: e072046. https://doi.org/10.1136/bmj-2022-072046.

Taylor-Robinson, David C., Nicola Maayan, Sarah Donegan, Marty Chaplin, and Paul Garner. 2019. "Public Health Deworming Programmes for Soil-Transmitted Helminths in Children Living in Endemic Areas." *Cochrane Database of Systematic Reviews* 9 (9): CD000371. https://doi.org/10.1002/14651858.CD000371.pub7.

The Lancet. 2021. "Maternal and Child Undernutrition Progress." Series from *The Lancet*. https://www.thelancet.com/series/maternal-child-undernutrition -progress.

Ulep, Valerie Gilbert, Paul Zambrano, Janice Datu-Sanguyo, Mireya Vilar-Compte, Graciela Ma Teruel Belismelis, Rafael Pérez-Escamilla, Grace J. Carroll, et al. 2021. "The Financing Need for Expanding Paid Maternity Leave to Support Breastfeeding in the Informal Sector in the Philippines." *Maternal & Child Nutrition* 17 (2): e13098. https://doi.org/10.1111/mcn.13098.

UNICEF (United Nations Children's Fund). 2021. *UNICEF Conceptual Framework on Maternal and Child Nutrition*. New York: UNICEF. https://www.unicef.org /media/113291/file/UNICEF%20Conceptual%20Framework.pdf.

UNICEF (United Nations Children's Fund). 2023. *Small Supplements for the Prevention of Malnutrition in Early Childhood (Small Quantity Lipid-Based Nutrient Supplements).* Brief Guidance Note. Version 1.0. New York: UNICEF. https://www.unicef.org /media/134786/file/SQLNS_Brief_Guidance_Note.pdf.

van Eijk, Anna Maria, David A. Larsen, Kassoum Kayentao, Gibby Koshy, Douglas E. C. Slaughter, Cally Roper, Lucy C. Okell, et al. 2019. "Effect of *Plasmodium falciparum* Sulfadoxine-Pyrimethamine Resistance on the Effectiveness of Intermittent Preventive Therapy for Malaria in Pregnancy in Africa: A Systematic Review and Meta-Analysis." *The Lancet Infectious Diseases* 19 (5): 546–56. https://doi.org/10.1016/S1473-3099(18)30732-1.

van Ginkel, Maarten, and Jeremy Cherfas. 2023. "What Is Wrong with Biofortification." *Global Food Security* 37: 100689.

Vilar-Compte, Mireya, Graciela Teruel, Diana Flores, Grace J. Carroll, Gabriela S. Buccini, and Rafael Pérez-Escamilla. 2019. "Costing a Maternity Leave Cash Transfer to Support Breastfeeding among Informally Employed Mexican Women." *Food and Nutrition Bulletin* 40 (2): 171–81. https://doi.org/10.1177 /0379572119836582.

Vilar-Compte, Mireya, and Hoa Thi Mai Nguyen. 2024. "Nutrition-Specific Interventions That Address Malnutrition in Low- and Middle-Income Countries. An Update of the Evidence." PROSPERO 2024 CRD42024529609. https://www .crd.york.ac.uk/prospero/display_record.php?ID=CRD42024529609.

Wake, Getu Engida, and Yohannes Moges Mittiku. 2021. "Prevalence of Exclusive Breastfeeding Practice and Its Association with Maternal Employment in Ethiopia: A Systematic Review and Meta-Analysis." *International Breastfeeding Journal* 16: 86.

Walker, Christa L. Fischer, and Robert E. Black. 2010. "Zinc for the Treatment of Diarrhoea: Effect on Diarrhoea Morbidity, Mortality and Incidence of Future Episodes." *International Journal of Epidemiology* 39 (Suppl 1): i63.

Wang, Dongqing, and Wafaie W. Fawzi. 2020. "Impacts of School Feeding on Educational and Health Outcomes of School-Age Children and Adolescents in Low- and Middle-Income Countries: Protocol for a Systematic Review and Meta-Analysis." *Systematic Reviews* 9: 55.

Wegmüller, Rita, Kelvin Musau, Lucie Vergari, Emily Custer, Hellen Anyango, William E. S. Donkor, Marion Kiprotich, et al. 2022. "Effectiveness of an Integrated Agriculture, Nutrition-Specific, and Nutrition-Sensitive Program on Child Growth in Western Kenya: A Cluster-Randomized Controlled Trial." *American Journal of Clinical Nutrition* 116 (2): 446–59. https://doi.org/10.1093 /ajcn/nqac098.

Wessells, K. Ryan, Charles D. Arnold, Christine P. Stewart, Elizabeth L. Prado, Souheila Abbeddou, Seth Adu-Afarwuah, Benjamin F. Arnold, et al. 2021. "Characteristics that Modify the Effect of Small-Quantity Lipid-Based Nutrient

Supplementation on Child Anemia and Micronutrient Status: An Individual Participant Data Meta-Analysis of Randomized Controlled Trials." *American Journal of Clinical Nutrition* 114 (Supplement 1): 68S–94S. https://doi.org/10.1093/ajcn/nqab276.

WHO (World Health Organization). 2012. *Guideline: Daily Iron and Folic Acid Supplementation in Pregnant Women*. Geneva: WHO. https://iris.who.int/handle/10665/77770.

WHO (World Health Organization). 2014. *Guideline: Delayed Umbilical Cord Clamping for Improved Maternal and Infant Health and Nutrition Outcomes*. Geneva: WHO. https://iris.who.int/bitstream/handle/10665/148793/9789241508209.

WHO (World Health Organization). 2016. *WHO Recommendations on Antenatal Care for a Positive Pregnancy Experience*. Geneva: WHO. https://iris.who.int/handle/10665/250796.

WHO (World Health Organization). 2020. *WHO Antenatal Care Recommendations for a Positive Pregnancy Experience. Nutritional Interventions Update: Multiple Micronutrient Supplements during Pregnancy*. Geneva: WHO.

WHO (World Health Organization). 2023a. *Burden of Disease Attributable to Unsafe Drinking-Water, Sanitation and Hygiene: 2019 Update*. Geneva: WHO. https://www.who.int/publications/i/item/9789240075610.

WHO (World Health Organization). 2023b. "More Ways, to Save More Lives, for Less Money: World Health Assembly Adopts More Best Buys to Tackle Noncommunicable Diseases." Geneva: WHO. https://www.who.int/news/item/26-05-2023-more-ways--to-save-more-lives--for-less-money----world-health-assembly-adopts-more-best-buys--to-tackle-noncommunicable-diseases.

WHO (World Health Organization). 2023c. *WHO Guidelines for Malaria*. Geneva: WHO. https://reliefweb.int/attachments/bf1186e0-21dc-4a85-ac68-e4faa0a5debf/WHO%20guidelines%20for%20malaria%2C%2016%20October%202023.pdf.

WHO (World Health Organization). 2023d. *Kangaroo Mother Care: Implementation Strategy for Scale-Up Adaptable to Different Country Contexts*. Geneva: WHO. https://iris.who.int/handle/10665/367625.

WHO (World Health Organization). 2023e. *Guideline on the Prevention and Management of Wasting and Nutritional Oedema (Acute Malnutrition) in Infants and Children under 5 years*. Geneva: WHO.

WHO (World Health Organization). 2023f. *Guideline for Complementary Feeding of Infants and Young Children 6–23 Months of Age*. Geneva: WHO.

WHO (World Health Organization), UNICEF (United Nations Children's Fund), and World Bank Group. 2018. *Nurturing Care for Early Childhood Development: A Framework for Helping Children Survive and Thrive to Transform Health and Human Potential*. Geneva: WHO. https://iris.who.int/bitstream/handle/10665/272603/9789241514064-eng.pdf.

Wolf, Jennyfer, Sydney Hubbard, Michael Brauer, Argaw Ambelu, Benjamin F. Arnold, Robert Bain, Valerie Bauza, et al. 2022. "Effectiveness of Interventions to Improve Drinking Water, Sanitation, and Handwashing with Soap on Risk of Diarrhoeal Disease in Children in Low-Income and Middle-Income Settings: A Systematic Review and Meta-Analysis." *The Lancet* 400 (10345): 48–59. https://doi.org/10.1016/S0140-6736(22)00937-0.

Xu, Yvonne Yiru, Talata Sawadogo-Lewis, Shannon E. King, Arlene Mitchell, and Timothy Roberton. 2021. "Integrating Nutrition into the Education Sector in Low- and Middle-Income Countries: A Framework for a Win–Win Collaboration." *Maternal & Child Nutrition* 17 (3): e13156. https://doi.org /10.1111/mcn.13156.

Zhang, Fan, and Christian Borja-Vega. 2024. *Water for Shared Prosperity*. Washington, DC: World Bank.

Zhao, Yang, Rui Hou, Xiu Zhu, Lihua Ren, and Hong Lu. 2019. "Effects of Delayed Cord Clamping on Infants after Neonatal Period: A Systematic Review and Meta-Analysis." *International journal of Nursing Studies* 92: 97–108. https://doi .org/10.1016/j.ijnurstu.2019.01.012.

6

Policies and Fiscal Measures That Address All Forms of Malnutrition

Kyoko Shibata Okamura, Mireya Vilar-Compte, Felipe Dizon, Kate Mandeville, Libby Hattersley, and Meera Shekar

KEY MESSAGES

- Effective and coherent policy actions are critical to support investments in nutrition. A strategically designed package of policy instruments can improve access to nutrition services and influence consumer preferences by modifying social environments, food environments, and commercial determinants of health and dietary behaviors.

- Infant and young child feeding policies support the scale-up of intervention packages that prevent undernutrition and curb the obesity epidemic and related noncommunicable diseases (NCDs). Policy measures such as the Baby Friendly Hospital Initiative and the International Code of Marketing of Breast-milk Substitutes are examples of such policies.

- Fiscal policy measures such as nutrition-targeted health taxation have direct and tangible impacts on prices and purchasing of unhealthy products. They generate domestic resources and yield positive effects on health and nutrition outcomes. To date, these policies have focused on sugar-sweetened beverages that now cover 57 percent of the world's population. Several countries are now expanding them to include ultraprocessed and other unhealthy foods. Ultraprocessed foods (UPFs) are strongly associated with NCDs and have greater climate impacts, including higher carbon footprints.

- To be effective, nutrition-targeted health taxes need to be designed carefully in the context of the broader policy environment, including price-related policies such as production incentives, consumer subsidies, and price controls, as well as complementary policies and interventions that can help shift social norms toward healthier dietary choices such as front-of-package-labeling policies, marketing regulations, and mass media and digital communication approaches.

- Food fortification, a globally recognized high-return development investment, can also be an effective climate adaptation strategy to enhance the nutritional quality of agriculture commodities affected by climate shocks. However, growing evidence on adverse health impacts of UPFs warrants careful, evidence-based selection of food items targeted for fortification.

- Repurposing of public support for agrifood, such as producer subsidies and trade policies, which currently costs $638–$851 billion a year globally, is key to transforming the food system to enable healthier and more sustainable diets.

- The World Bank's new Food and Nutrition Security Global Challenge Program supports many of these policy solutions, along with other high-impact nutrition interventions, to address all forms of malnutrition. Countries are encouraged to develop and implement a coherent package of regulatory and fiscal policies and policy frameworks, accompanied by strong social communications strategies. Scale-up must be carefully calibrated to national contexts, taking into account the economic and political landscape, institutional capacity, and epidemiology of malnutrition and related disease burdens.

- These policies must be designed in each country context to leverage policy coherence and optimize allocation of public resources; maximize economic, health, and climate co-benefits; and minimize negative externalities that affect countries' human capital, economic growth, and sustainable development.

Policy Nexus: Nutrition, Food Systems, and Climate

With rising rates of overweight, obesity, and diet-related noncommunicable diseases (NCDs), low- and middle-income countries (LMICs) face a double burden of malnutrition: the prevalence of both undernutrition and overnutrition in their populations (refer to chapter 2). Furthermore, the syndemic of overweight and obesity, undernutrition, and climate change takes the heaviest toll on the most vulnerable segments of the population, who often lack access to essential health and nutrition services and information, are increasingly exposed to cheap and unhealthy food choices, and are often most adversely affected by climate shocks (Swinburn et al. 2019; also refer to chapter 4). Food price hikes since the onset of the COVID-19 pandemic exemplify such effects, because evidence suggests that lower socioeconomic groups are coping by shifting to cheap ultraprocessed foods (UPFs) that are unhealthy and generate larger carbon footprints (Osendarp et al. 2021).

Effective solutions lie within the nutrition–food system–climate nexus, as highlighted in chapter 4. These require policy shifts and systemic changes beyond traditional program and service boundaries. The nutrition interventions identified in chapter 5 need to be supported with effective policy measures to address all forms of malnutrition and promote healthier and more sustainable diets. Increasing evidence underscores the importance of deploying cohesive policy measures to promote healthier and more sustainable societies while simultaneously pursuing more inclusive economic growth. These policy measures, depicted in figure 6.1, can be grouped into four categories: (1) national nutrition policy frameworks that provide the basis for nutrition strategies, programs, and interventions; (2) technical guidelines, which include normative nutrition recommendations that address specific issues, population groups, or settings; (3) legislative and regulatory frameworks for influencing food consumption, diet, and nutrition; and (4) economic and fiscal measures that use market structures to promote healthier choices.

This chapter highlights how the implementation of these policies, together with the interventions summarized in chapter 5, can improve nutrition outcomes by easing access to quality food and nutrition services and influencing consumer preferences by modifying the social environments, food environments, and commercial determinants of health and dietary behaviors. Hassel and Wegrich (2022) argue that today's complex health and consumer policy problems require policy makers to consider the long-term implications for consumers who have incomplete and sometimes contradictory knowledge and who are often faced with immediate costs to achieve uncertain future benefits. This chapter also sheds light on these considerations, including how countries have used evidence and behavioral economics analyses to design and implement a package of policy measures.

Figure 6.1 Policies and Fiscal Measures to Enable and Promote Better Nutrition

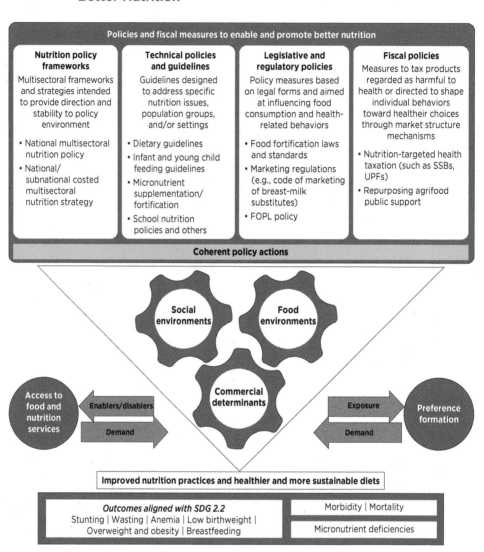

Source: Adapted from Hassel and Wegrich 2022 and Lascoumes and Le Galès 2007.
Note: FOPL = front-of-package labeling; SDG = Sustainable Development Goal; SSBs = sugar-sweetened beverages; UPFs = ultraprocessed foods.

National Nutrition Policy Frameworks and Technical Guidelines

Nutrition Policy Frameworks

As of 2022, all 66 Scaling Up Nutrition (SUN) Movement member countries had developed or were developing a national, multisectoral set of nutrition policies or strategies that serve as a guiding framework for action (SUN 2023).

Such policies need to respond to a country's epidemiological needs through appropriate institutional mechanisms to coordinate, finance, and monitor the intended actions. Countries such as Indonesia and Senegal have a legally binding national nutrition policy and a high-level (often supraministerial) coordination body as well as a stable policy environment to implement a well-financed national multisectoral nutrition strategy. Indonesia has both national and subnational nutrition strategies that are backed up by detailed cost estimates, budget allocation processes even at the district level, and continuous budget monitoring, which provides accountability (Subandoro, Holschneider, and Bergeron 2021). Pakistan has taken a bottom-up approach to formulating nutrition strategies by allowing provincial governments to develop their own strategies first and then consolidating them into a national strategy (Government of Pakistan, Ministry of Planning, Development & Reform, and World Food Programme 2018).

Multisectoral nutrition policy frameworks and their costed strategies need to be anchored in relevant sectoral policies and strategies because sectoral ministries oversee resource allocation and implementation of the relevant nutrition-related activities. The health sector, for example, defines a priority package of services, often referred to as a national essential health care package or benefits package. Nutrition services and interventions delivered in the health sector need to be explicitly prioritized in this package and accompanied by strong policies and financing to strengthen the primary health care (PHC) systems in which most high-impact nutrition services are delivered. Countries such as Peru and Thailand, which are among the few LMICs to have steadily reduced stunting levels over the past few decades to below 15 percent, have a prioritized list of nutrition services in their benefit packages based on a rigorous costing exercise and have historically invested in strengthening PHC (Subandoro et al. 2022). Agriculture sector policies and strategies tend to maximize agricultural productivity and profitability. In recent years, however, climate-related objectives have been incorporated into agriculture strategies with the help of climate-smart agriculture investment plans that maximize the triple wins of increased productivity, enhanced resilience, and reduced emissions (World Bank 2024a). A health and nutrition win could also be added to the equation to further maximize human capital and economic productivity.

Technical Policies and Guidelines

In response to specific nutrition issues, settings, or population groups, the World Health Organization (WHO) has developed a wide range of technical policies that have often been adopted by national governments. These include, among others, dietary guidelines, infant and young child feeding guidelines and strategies, micronutrient supplementation and fortification guidelines, and school nutrition policies and other institutional nutrition service policies. The full range of these policies are available from the WHO's Global Database on the Implementation of Nutrition Action (WHO 2024b).

The evolution of food systems has led to rapid dietary shifts—from unprocessed or minimally processed foods to processed foods and UPFs that are typically high in sugar, sodium, and fat, especially unhealthy saturated and trans fats (Monteiro et al. 2019). These shifts have contributed to concurrent epidemics of overweight and obesity and diet-related NCDs, such as hypertension and diabetes, imposing heavy burdens on health systems and economies. Some high-income countries and organizations such as the WHO and the Food and Agriculture Organization of the United Nations (FAO), which promote normative processes, have consequently developed guidance on healthy diets (such as the US food pyramid) and dietary and nutrient reference intake levels (such as the WHO–FAO human nutrient requirement guidelines (WHO 2024a) and the US Dietary Reference Intakes (USDHHS 2024). These include a focus on nutrients of concern, such as sugar, sodium, and saturated and trans fats. Many of these reference guides have been integrated into national dietary guidelines to inform dietary policies, regulatory frameworks, consumer communication strategies, and assessment and monitoring. In recent decades, many LMICs have also developed food-based dietary guidelines using national food consumption data; FAO (2024) reported that, as of 2020, 85 countries globally had such guidelines.

The Baby-Friendly Hospital Initiative (BFHI) is a type of global technical guideline that can not only address child undernutrition, morbidity, and mortality but also curb the epidemic of obesity and related NCDs by addressing their early determinants (Weng et al. 2012). Launched in 1991 by the WHO and UNICEF, BFHI focuses on adherence to the Ten Steps to Successful Breastfeeding, a set of actions that have been shown to improve breastfeeding outcomes (Pérez-Escamilla, Martinez, and Segura-Pérez 2016). More than 150 countries have since implemented the BFHI (WHO 2023b), but with varying degrees of success. Some key challenges have been to adequately train the health care workforce, finance the structural changes needed at maternity facilities, and ensure adherence to the "International Code of Marketing of Breast-Milk Substitutes" (WHO 1981), which includes regulation on negative industry behaviors such as distribution of free infant formula samples at maternity facilities (refer to the "Marketing Regulations" section). The BFHI also stresses follow-up on breastfeeding actions at the community level, which is often implemented through the infant and young child feeding interventions addressed in chapter 5. Although evidence suggests that investments in BFHI are feasible and can have important long-term social returns (Arslanian et al. 2022; Horton et al. 1996), innovations in financing (that is, infrastructure, monitoring systems, and training), coherence with related policies, and sustained implementation are critical.

Legislative and Regulatory Policies

Legislative and regulatory policies, enshrined within national legal frameworks, are mandatory policy instruments such as norms, laws, or executive orders that are enforced by the state through real or perceived sanctions (Howlett 2019). This section focuses on key policies, such as food fortification laws and standards, front-of-package labeling (FOPL) policies, and marketing regulations, that have been used to influence food consumption and diet.

Food Fortification Laws and Standards

Fortifying foods with micronutrients is known to be one of the smartest development investments because it can deliver specific nutrients to large segments of the population without requiring radical changes in food consumption patterns. Fortification has also proven to have high investment returns through improved health and economic productivity (WHO 2006).[1] Emerging evidence showing the impacts of climate change on reduced nutritional quality of crops further suggests that both commercial food fortification and biofortification can be cost-effective and readily available climate adaptation strategies, as highlighted in chapter 4. This section does not examine specific regulatory measures of biofortified products, which follow a distinctive production, distribution, and sales pathway compared with commercial food fortification. An assessment conducted by the Consortium of International Agricultural Research Centers suggests that biofortified products derived from conventional breeding should be adequately covered by existing food legislation across supply chains, including food labeling, and that specific standards and regulations are unnecessary because they are no more than selected crop varieties (Mitra-Ganguli, Pfeiffer, and Walton 2022).

Food fortification requires a package of legislation, standards, and monitoring guidelines to ensure that fortified foods meet nutrient, quality, and safety standards. As of 2022, 143 countries, of which 112 were LMICs, had mandatory fortification legislation covering at least one of the following foods: wheat flour, maize flour, rice, oil, or salt. Mandatory fortification of wheat flour is in place in 92 countries (2022); maize, in 19 countries (2021); rice, in eight countries (2021); vegetable oil, in 35 countries (2022); and salt, in 126 countries (2019). The content and quality of the policy package also matter to ensure industry compliance with standards. A recent study (Marks et al. 2018) that reviewed 72 mandatory cereal fortification policy packages across the world (covering wheat, maize, and rice) found that only 64 percent required internal monitoring, or quality assurance and control, by industry; and only 64 percent documented the requirement for external monitoring at the production site, of which only half provided detailed protocols and systems. Similarly, just 68 percent described penalties for noncompliance, with only 31 percent publicly documenting the penalties. Very few addressed incentive mechanisms such as reduced taxes for equipment (14 percent) and fortification premix (10 percent).

With increasing consumption of UPFs, a new concern has emerged regarding fortifying food products that are deemed unhealthy. Ultraprocessed food and drinks, such as breakfast cereals and energy drinks, have been fortified and sold as "healthy" options. Some of these products—for example, breakfast cereals and instant noodles—have a large market in LMICs (Baker et al. 2020). A critical appraisal of UPFs as fortification alternatives in Latin America concluded that the packaging of these products carries attractive health and nutrition messages, which makes consumers believe they are healthier than other products or fine to consume (Kroker-Lobos et al. 2022). The authors urged policy makers to carefully regulate voluntary fortification so that UPFs are not used as vehicles for fortification and promoted as so-called healthy products. Chile has adopted regulations that ban the use of the terminology "high in" on packages as a positive attribute of foods, including references to specific micronutrients, for products that have front-of-package (FOP) warnings (Reyes et al. 2019). India has taken a more concrete approach by amending its food fortification regulations to exclude foods that are high in critical nutrients of concern while also considering the inclusion of FOP warning labels (Kroker-Lobos et al. 2022).

FOPL Policies

FOPL aims to visibly indicate the amount of nutrients of concern (and sometimes calories) a product contains so that consumers can make informed choices at the point of purchase or consumption. As of February 2023, 53 countries globally had FOPL policies, of which 16—such as Chile, Mexico, Sri Lanka, and Thailand—have adopted mandatory regulations, and others had enacted policies that encourage voluntary labeling (Global Food Research Program, UNC-Chapel Hill 2023). A systematic review and meta-analysis conducted by Croker et al. in 2020 indicated that FOPL can encourage healthier food purchasing behaviors, including an overall effect of any FOPL compared with no FOPL regarding the sugar and sodium content of purchases and a trend toward energy and saturated content (map 6.1). A recent study in Guatemala found that its FOP warning labels significantly decreased perception of the products' healthfulness and consumers' purchasing intention among adults and children from rural

Map 6.1 Front-of-Package Labels around the World

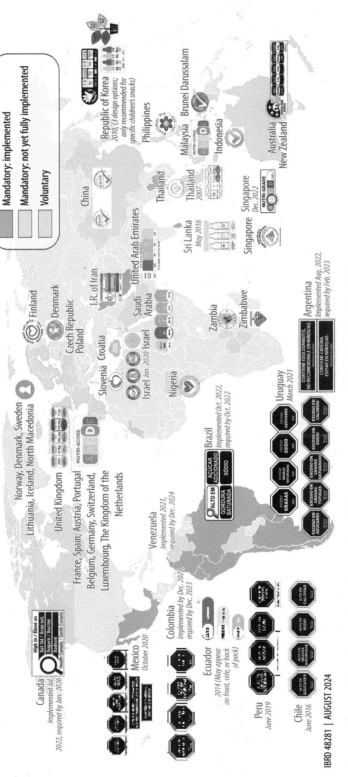

IBRD 48281 | AUGUST 2024

Source: World Bank based on Global Food Research Program, UNC–Chapel Hill 2023.

and urban communities and with less than six years of education (Kroker-Lobos et al. 2023). Labeling approaches and designs (such as "high-in" warnings, Nutri-Score, traffic light icons, Health Star Ratings, and guidelines for daily allowance) matter. Various studies have been conducted to compare the effectiveness of different approaches for different purposes. To help consumers identify unhealthy UPFs and drinks quickly and easily, simple negative warning labels tend to have the strongest evidence for effectiveness (Global Food Research Program, UNC-Chapel Hill 2021).

Marketing Regulations

Food consumption decisions are often considered individual preferences, thereby making individuals—and only individuals—responsible for the consequences. Recent advancements in behavioral economics models, however, have shed new light on how consumer preferences are influenced by a range of food and social environment factors and commercial determinants, such as availability, accessibility, affordability, convenience, and desirability. Foods high in sodium, sugar, and unhealthy fats, as well as UPFs, are increasingly more available and affordable even in rural areas of LMICs. Consequently, lower-income households are more likely than higher-income households to consume these products because their access to proper nutrition knowledge and services is limited, and the products are often cheaper than fresh and healthier choices and aggressively marketed. Marketing to children, often with misleading health messages, is especially detrimental because parents tend to allow children to eat what looks attractive, not recognizing the long-term consequences of such habits. This is called "individual internalities" in economics terms, which refers to the long-term costs to individual health that people do not account for when making consumption decisions. In the case of unhealthy food and beverage products, the aggressive marketing, especially to children and adolescents, distorts individual perceptions of costs and benefits of consumption. Regulating the marketing and promotion of unhealthy foods, especially UPFs, has become a useful policy instrument to address this vulnerability. For example, Chile instituted an advertisement ban on unhealthy "high-in" foods, initially targeting child television programs in 2016, which was further strengthened in 2018 to a comprehensive ban between 6:00 a.m. and 10:00 p.m. A study has shown that the total amount of weekly "high-in" food ads dropped by 64 percent from 2016 (preregulation) levels to 2019. The number of "high-in" food ads dropped by 66 percent and 56 percent in both the 6:00 a.m.–10:00 p.m. and 10:00 p.m.–12:00 a.m. time periods, respectively, although ads were allowed in the latter period (Dillmann Carpentier et al. 2023).

Marketing regulations are also fundamental to protecting optimal infant and young child nutrition. It is widely known that the commercial milk formula industry uses underhanded marketing tactics that have contributed to increasing formula sales, despite the known benefits of breastfeeding, generating revenues of around $55 billion annually (M&C Saatchi World Services 2022). *The Lancet*'s 2023 Series on Breastfeeding calls for policy actions to regulate such marketing (Pérez-Escamilla et al. 2023), including a renewed enforcement of the International Code of Marketing of Breast-Milk Substitutes, which was established to curb these practices. Adherence to and enforcement of the code varies widely across countries (Rollins et al. 2023). As of March 2022, 144 WHO member states have adopted legal measures to implement parts of the code, and 32 countries have measures substantially aligned with it (WHO 2022). In the past five years, 26 countries have updated their laws, with the newer legal instruments more likely to be substantially aligned with the code and to cover children up to age 36 months. However, monitoring and enforcement of the code have remained a key challenge, exemplified by the fact that only 37 countries explicitly address the recent phenomenon of aggressive promotion of breast milk substitutes on digital platforms. Other challenges include the targeted marketing strategies for specialized formulas and growing-up milks (toddler milks), the latter of which is regarded as an ultraprocessed product, with sugar content equivalent to that of SSBs. Some of the recommendations that have been posed include full adoption of the international code as national legislation (in particular, targeting the digital space), development of ongoing monitoring mechanisms at the national level (such as dashboards and other media-based tools), and training of the health care workforce (Lutter et al. 2022). Another suggested policy is to introduce plain packaging for commercial milk formulas and baby products and prohibit the use of images and text suggesting that formulas are equivalent or superior to breast milk and health or nutrition claims, such as endorsement by health professionals or organizations (M&C Saatchi World Services 2022). Such a policy would also reduce exposure to marketing strategies that make the formulas look like branded products recommended throughout the first years of life (that is, pregnancy through toddlerhood), including branding tactics for a variety of baby products targeting different age groups, which can evade the intended impacts of restrictions on advertising (Vilar-Compte et al. 2022).

Mandatory Limits and Bans: Eliminating Trans Fats in the Food Chain

Trans-fatty acids (trans fats) are created when liquid vegetable oils are partially hydrogenated to make them solid at room temperature. They are commonly found in baked and fried foods, snack food products, and cooking oils and spreads (for example, ghee and margarine). The use of trans fats has increased because they have various commercial advantages: they are cheaper than healthier fats, increase the shelf life of food, and are more stable during deep frying. Trans-fat consumption substantially raises the risk of coronary heart disease by raising LDL ("bad") and lowering HDL ("good") cholesterol levels. However, removing trans fats from the production process is straightforward and can make little difference to the taste of products. It can be done through a mandatory national limit of 2 grams of industrially produced trans fat per 100 grams of total fat in all foods, and a mandatory national ban on the production or use of partially hydrogenated oils (a major source of trans fat) as an ingredient in all foods.

As of February 2024, more than half of the world's population (55.5 percent) is currently covered by mandatory trans-fats limits (WHO 2024c). Denmark, one of the earliest adopters, found that deaths from heart disease began falling after it introduced a trans-fats ban in 2001. By 2016, there were 30 fewer deaths from heart disease per 100,000 people than projected if the ban had not been implemented. Significant reductions were also seen in Denmark's rates of adolescent and child obesity (Spruk and Kovač 2020).

Fiscal Policies to Reorient Food Systems to Healthier and More Sustainable Diets

Fiscal policies are increasingly important measures to reorient food systems to promote healthier and more sustainable diets and improve nutrition, and an evidence base for their effectiveness is growing. These policy measures tax products regarded as harmful to health or are directed at shaping the behaviors of individuals to make healthier choices through market structure mechanisms. Nutrition-targeted health taxation also provides modest yet additional revenue sources. Policy and fiscal interventions in agrifood production and trade also provide opportunities. For example, there is increasing attention to repurposing public support for agrifood, including subsidy schemes for unhealthy products, taking into account the negative health and climate externalities that these markets are creating. These policy measures can help maximize a net benefit for healthier, more sustainable, and economically viable food systems if they are designed and implemented as a coherent policy package.

Nutrition-Targeted Health Tax Policies

Nutrition-targeted health taxation, while attracting increasing interest from policy makers worldwide, remains less used than tobacco and alcohol taxes and, to date, has focused mainly on SSBs. SSBs are a key contributor to excess sugar and energy intake around the world and are strongly linked to long-term weight gain, obesity, and multiple NCDs, including type 2 diabetes (World Bank 2020). SSBs are also a discrete, nonessential component of many diets, making them relatively easy to target for taxation. As of 2023, more than 100 economies impose national-level taxes on SSBs, covering more than half (57 percent) of the world's population and more than four in five people (82 percent) in low- and lower-middle-income economies (World Bank 2023; refer to map 6.2). However, many of these are small taxes on nonalcoholic beverages in general, and their design could be optimized to target the health impact of SSBs.

There is strong, consistent evidence that SSB taxes raise prices and reduce sales of taxed beverages (Andreyeva et al. 2022b). Although higher retail prices can be viewed as increasing the tax burden on poorer groups, analysis that considers costs and benefits in the longer term suggests that SSB taxes can have a progressive impact, with lower-income households expected to benefit from a disproportionate share of improved health outcomes, reduced health care costs, extended working lives, and reduced years of life lost (Fuchs Tarlovsky, Mandeville, and Alonso-Soria 2020). Demand for SSBs is highly tax-elastic (more so than demand for tobacco and alcohol), which means consumers, particularly low-income consumers (Venson et al. 2023), tend to shift away from taxed products with even a small increase in the sales price (Andreyeva et al. 2022b; PAHO 2021; Teng et al. 2019). A recent meta-analysis of results from 33 studies of 16 SSB tax policies worldwide found an average estimated price elasticity in demand of −1.59 (95 percent confidence interval [CI], −2.11, −1.08) and a 15 percent mean reduction in sales of taxed products (95 percent CI, −20 percent, −9 percent; Andreyeva et al. 2022b), which aligns with the relatively small size of most evaluated SSB taxes (WHO 2023a).

Map 6.2 Global Coverage of National-Level Taxes on SSBs, August 2023

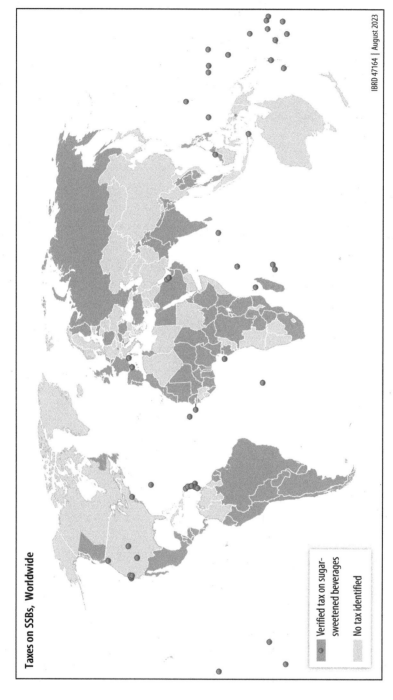

Taxes on SSBs, Worldwide

Verified tax on sugar-sweetened beverages

No tax identified

IBRD 47164 | August 2023

Source: World Bank Global SSB Tax Database, 2023, https://ssbtax.worldbank.org/.

Note: SSBs = sugar-sweetened beverages.

Less evidence is available on changes in consumption in response to SSB taxes, mainly because of the more limited availability of longitudinal consumption data compared with sales data. Similarly, given that systematic evaluation of implemented taxes for health impacts has only recently begun, evidence on the long-term effects of SSB taxes is still limited. However, emerging data from Mexico and the United Kingdom suggests positive impacts on body mass index, particularly among adolescent girls (Gracner, Marquez-Padilla, and Hernandez-Cortes 2022; Rogers, Cummins, et al. 2023), as well as improvements in dental health (Hernández-F, Cantoral, and Colchero 2022; Rogers, Conway, et al. 2023). Beyond demand-side effects, sugar-based and tiered tax designs can also incentivize manufacturers to reduce their tax burden by lowering the sugar content in their products and across their portfolios, amplifying the health benefits of a tax (refer to box 6.1).

As with other health taxes, robust tax design and implementation are crucial to achieving health, equity, and revenue objectives. For example, excise taxes are the instrument most commonly used to tax SSBs (Hattersley et al. 2020), and one-third of LMICs that impose excise taxes on SSBs also tax unsweetened bottled water—a key healthy substitute—at the same or higher rate than SSBs (World Bank 2023). These represent missed opportunities to incentivize healthier diets. These excise taxes could be easily modified to contribute to improving population health and nutrition while also linking them with other important measures to increase access to healthy substitutes, such as the provision of safe drinking water. At the same time, most SSB taxes do not include all SSB categories, which lowers their health and revenue potential. Fewer than half of SSB taxes worldwide cover sweetened milk-based drinks (42 percent), and only 1 in 3 (36 percent) cover 100 percent juices, despite these SSBs carrying health risks similar to those of more easily recognized SSBs, such as carbonated soft drinks. Most existing SSB taxes are ad valorem or volume-based, with fewer than 1 in 5 taxes worldwide targeted at sugar content (and these taxes are concentrated in high-income economies). Finally, tax rates applied to SSBs are generally low, with a global median excise and total tax share of the retail price of an internationally comparable brand of sugar-sweetened carbonated drink of 3.4 percent and 18.4 percent in 2023, respectively (WHO 2023a). Box 6.1 shows an example from Saudi Arabia, where the SSB tax design, which already applied one of the highest rates in the world, has been continuously revised on the basis of rigorous evaluation and implementation research to enhance its effectiveness on population health.

Box 6.1

Saudia Arabia: Moving from a Sugar-Sweetened Beverage Tax Policy to a Comprehensive, Multisectoral Health-Promoting Policy Package

Saudi Arabia's sugar-sweetened beverage (SSB) tax, first implemented in 2017, included a 50 percent ad valorem tax on carbonated beverages and a 100 percent tax on energy drinks, and it continues to be one of the highest SSB tax rates in the world (World Bank 2023). The tax was expanded in 2019 to include a 50 percent tax on all SSBs (World Bank 2023) and designed as an ad valorem uniform-rate excise tax.

One evaluation found that sales of carbonated drinks decreased by 35 percent in Saudi Arabia compared with Gulf Cooperation Council countries without the tax (Alsukait et al. 2020). Another cross-sectional study of 200 adults in Medina pre- and posttax found that soft drink consumption decreased by 19 percent after implementation of the tax (Jalloun and Qurban 2022).

Figure B6.1.1 Saudi Arabia's Front-of-Package Traffic Light Label

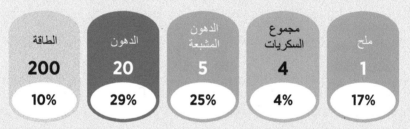

Sources: Saudi Food and Drug Authority 2018. https://sfda.gov.sa/sites/default/files/2019-11/ND6-min.jpg; Informal communications with Reem Alsukait, World Bank.
Note: The labels translate to energy, fat, saturated fat, total sugar, and salt. The traffic-light colors are applied to fat, saturated fat, total sugar and salt on the basis of the percentages of healthy reference intake levels: green = lower levels; amber = medium levels; red = high levels. Energy information should be provided separately in a neutral or no color. The amounts of fat, saturated fat, total sugars, and salt are shown in grams per 100 grams or 100 milliliters. The energy value is expressed in kilocalories per 100 grams or 100 milliliters.

Saudi Food and Drug Authority, "Draft Standard DS—Food Sector, Traffic-Light Labelling," translated by the Translation Bureau of Canada, in "Draft Standard DS: Food Sector, Traffic-Light Labelling." 2018. FOP = front of package labelling.

(continued)

Box 6.1

Saudia Arabia: Moving from a Sugar-Sweetened Beverage Tax Policy to a Comprehensive, Multisectoral Health-Promoting Policy Package *(continued)*

The government of Saudia Arabia is currently considering revising the tax structure even further to enhance its effectiveness. One potential area of improvement is to change the design from a uniform rate to a tiered rate on the basis of sugar content (Alluhidan et al. 2022). It is recognized that one policy instrument, even as successful as an SSB tax, will not be enough to address the alarming burden of diet-related noncommunicable diseases and obesity. Accordingly, since 2017 the government has adopted a comprehensive multisectoral approach to health promotion. Some of the initiatives include the launch of a national healthy food strategy; voluntary traffic-light front-of-package label (FOPL); mandatory menu calorie labeling; food and beverage product reformulations, such as setting upper limits on sodium in baked bread; and a total ban on trans fats (Bin Sunaid et al. 2021).

A recent randomized controlled trial to test the effectiveness of FOPLs in Saudi Arabia, using an online grocery store, found that both a Nutri-Score and a warning label approach positively influenced participants' diet quality (Shin et al. 2023). On the basis of global evidence, further considerations can be made to shift from the current voluntary FOPL policy to a mandatory one to ensure industry uptake and compliance and enhance its intended impacts on population health.

SSBs represent only one subset of unhealthy diets. Yet far fewer jurisdictions apply nutrition health taxes on unhealthy foods (refer to map 6.3). Existing unhealthy food taxes are mostly limited to one or two specified nutrients of concern (such as sugar or salt) and unequivocally unhealthy product categories (such as confectionery, chocolates, biscuits, salty snacks, and high-fat animal products), although some countries are exploring broader taxes (Sassi et al. 2022).

Map 6.3 National-Level Unhealthy Food Taxes, January 2024

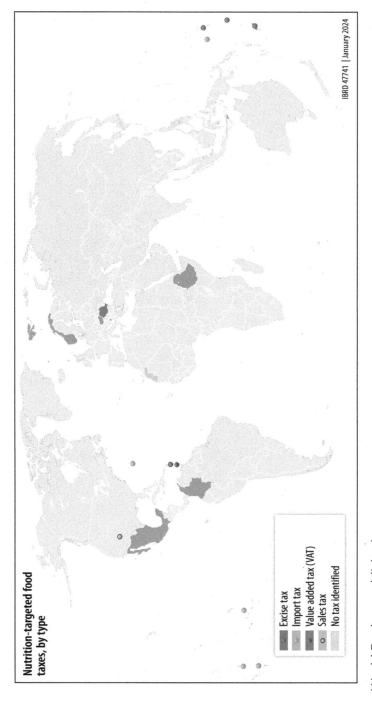

Nutrition-targeted food
taxes, by type

Excise tax
Import tax
Value added tax (VAT)
Sales tax
No tax identified

IBRD 47741 | January 2024

Source: World Bank, unpublished.

Dominica, in the Caribbean, taxes confectionery and chocolate bars, in addition to SSBs. French Polynesia taxes imported confectionery, marmalade, and ice cream. Although narrower food taxes can be simpler to design and administer, they carry a greater risk of encouraging substitution with equally as or more unhealthy products, limiting potential health impacts. Mexico applies a wider 8 percent tax on energy-dense (≥275 kcal/100 g) foods across several product categories, including salty snacks, confectionary, chocolate, desserts, ice cream, and cereal-based products that are high in added sugars. The tax was implemented in January 2014, along with a 1-peso-per-liter tax on SSBs. There were significant reductions in the purchase of taxed foods in the first two years after implementation. However, evidence suggests this may have been compensated for by increases in calories from purchasing untaxed products (Aguilar, Gutierrez, and Seira 2021). Others countries with broader unhealthy food taxes include Ethiopia (which taxes goods "hazardous to health," such as hydrogenated fats and oils with high saturated fat content, and some sugars and sugary products), Tonga (which taxes animal fat products, mayonnaise, and instant noodles), and the Navajo Nation of the United States (which taxes "minimal-to-no nutritional value food items" such as snacks high in salt, saturated fat, and sugar).

Some countries have begun to explore broader unhealthy food taxes across multiple nutrient and product categories (refer to box 6.2). Colombia implemented an excise tax on a wide range of unhealthy foods in November 2023. Although ostensibly the first tax in the world to target UPFs (refer to the "Emerging Evidence and Policy Actions on UPFs" section for more details), it applies a nutrient profiling approach to target products exceeding set thresholds for sugars, sodium, and saturated fat across multiple product categories (defined by tariff headings). Nutrient Profile Models are increasingly being used as a comprehensive and systematic approach to classify and categorize foods for designing various food policies, including FOPL, marketing restrictions, and taxation.

Box 6.2

Design, Approval, and Implementation of Excise Taxes on Sugar-Sweetened Beverages and Ultraprocessed Foods in Colombia

Background

Initial discussions regarding excise taxes on sugar-sweetened beverages (SSBs) in Colombia occurred in 2015 in the context of the country's overall tax reform and was a reaction to rising

(continued)

Box 6.2

Design, Approval, and Implementation of Excise Taxes on Sugar-Sweetened Beverages and Ultraprocessed Foods in Colombia *(continued)*

overweight and obesity rates among both adults and children—from 45.6 percent to 56.5 percent and from 14.4 percent to 24.4 percent, respectively, between 2005 and 2015 (ICBF 2006, 2018), and the increasing burden of noncommunicable diseases. According to the Ministry of Health and Social Protection (MoHSP), 13 percent of deaths from diabetes, 5 percent of deaths from cardiovascular disease, and 1 percent of deaths from cancers were estimated to be attributable to SSB consumption (Government of Colombia, Ministerio de Salud y Protección Social 2016). Despite strong evidence emerging from other countries, such as Mexico, which showed reduced SSB consumption and increased tax revenues, the initial proposal of a 20 percent ad valorem excise tax introduced by the then–Minister of Health and Social Protection was rejected in Congress on the basis of unfounded arguments, including ineffectiveness of the policy, potential job losses and retail business closures, and regressive effects on low-income households. Other healthy diet and SSB tax proposals were presented to Congress in subsequent years, but none of them were discussed and voted upon.

Change in Policy

In 2022, the then–Minister of Finance (MoF) decided to include an excise tax on SSBs and an ad valorem tax on ultraprocessed foods (UPFs) with high sugar content in a tax reform proposal. The initial design included a tiered SSB excise tax based on sugar content (Col$0 for SSBs with less than 4 grams of added sugar per 100 milliliters (ml), Col$18 for those with 4–8 grams, and Col$35 for those with more than 8 grams), and an ad valorem tax of 10 percent of the retail price for UPFs with high added sugar content (Government of Colombia, Ministerio de Hacienda y Crédito Público 2022). The proposal, however, faced active industry lobbying targeted to increasing the threshold values to the level at which most products would fall in the Col$0 category. However, the tax proposal received strong support from civil society, research centers, and the Pan American Health Organization, as well as endorsement by

(continued)

Box 6.2

Design, Approval, and Implementation of Excise Taxes on Sugar-Sweetened Beverages and Ultraprocessed Foods in Colombia *(continued)*

several lawmakers in Congress. As the MoHSP and MoF continued to articulate the design, the policy was finally included in the tax reform package and approved in December 2022, followed by implementation in November 2023. Table B6.2.1 shows the approved SSB excise tax thresholds, which are scheduled to decrease in 2025. A UPF ad valorem tax on the retail price covers products with front-of-package (FOP) warning labels on sodium, added sugars, and saturated fat, with a rate of 10 percent in 2023, 15 percent in 2024, and 20 percent in 2025 (when artisanal products will be excluded). The MoF estimates an expected tax revenue of Col$3 trillion a year (equivalent to US$700 million; Government of Colombia, Ministerio de Hacienda y Crédito Público 2023).

Table B6.2.1 Approved SSB Excise Tax Thresholds

Sugar content of SSBs (grams of added sugar per 100 ml)	Tax rate per 100 ml (Col$)		
	2023	2024	2025
<6	0	0	
≥6 and <10	18	28	
≥10	35	55	
<5			0
≥5 and <9			38
≥9			65

Source: Original table for this publication based on government of Colombia, Ministerio de Hacienda y Crédito Público 2023.
Note: SSBs = sugar-sweetened beverages.

Lessons Learned and the Way Forward

Colombia's experience illuminates important lessons. Approval and implementation of SSB and UPF taxes involve complex processes that require policy champions and continuous technical work to break through opposition and failures. In addition, simultaneous

(continued)

Box 6.2

Design, Approval, and Implementation of Excise Taxes on Sugar-Sweetened Beverages and Ultraprocessed Foods in Colombia *(continued)*

work related to other nutrition-targeted interventions will facilitate synergies; for example, in Colombia, the approval of the FOP warning label policy was crucial to improving the tax design by expanding the tax base to UPFs. Regarding a way forward, Colombia is considering the inclusion of beverages with artificial sweeteners. Furthermore, a package of effective policy actions should be considered that include but are not limited to (1) ensuring availability and affordability of safe drinking water; (2) regulating marketing of unhealthy foods; (3) designing and implementing official dietary guidelines that demote consumption of UPFs; and (4) determining what healthy and sustainable diets constitute in Colombia, their costs, and how to transform the country's food system to make these diets affordable for everyone. Cross-sectoral work, including agriculture, trade, and water, among others, will be fundamental to provide effective access to affordable healthful alternatives and rethink sustainable food systems.

Source: Norman Maldonado and Elisa Cadena, PROESA—Research Center on Health Economics and Social Protection, Universidad Icesi.

Although consistent evidence shows that unhealthy food taxes have increased prices and reduced sales of taxed products, evidence is still limited on their other effects, including substitution with untaxed products, industry reformulation, impacts on consumption and health outcomes, and distributional effects (Andreyeva et al. 2022a). Evaluations of Mexico's tax on nonessential energy-dense foods (Batis et al. 2016) and Hungary's Public Health Product Tax (Biró 2015) found greater reductions in sales of taxed foods to lower-income households.

To be effective, nutrition-targeted health taxes on unhealthy products should be designed on the basis of best practices and scientific evidence. Understanding the context in which these taxes operate can help position them in the broader policy environment, including price-related policies—such as production incentives, consumer subsidies, and price controls—throughout food supply chains as well as complementary policies and other interventions that can help shift social norms toward healthier dietary choices and practices—such as FOPL policies, marketing regulations, and whole-of-society communication approaches.

Repurposing Agrifood Public Support Policies for Healthier and More Sustainable Diets

The global food system today generates $10 trillion in market value each year. However, it also results in $12 trillion worth of hidden costs in health burdens, environmental impacts, and socioeconomic vulnerabilities, including $2.7 trillion from obesity-related NCDs, $1.8 trillion from undernutrition, and $1.5 trillion from greenhouse gas (GHG) emissions, reflecting significant global market failures (FOLU 2019). Globally, public support for the agrifood sector is substantial. A 2022 World Bank report estimated that, between 2016 and 2018, there were net public transfers to the agrifood sector of $638 billion a year on average in 79 countries for which data were available (Gautam et al. 2022). The Organisation for Economic Co-operation and Development's (OECD) estimate for 2020–22 showed $851 billion a year, on average, among 54 OECD members and other major agriculture producers (OECD 2023). Although estimates vary, both analyses consistently found that much of this support contributed to the hidden costs of the food system, driving unsustainable production practices, unhealthy consumption patterns, and inequality. This support is also often distortionary, inefficient, focused on producers, and regressive. An appreciation of the gains from repurposing agricultural policies and support has gained momentum in recent years, and a growing body of literature is emerging to inform charting ways forward for food systems that better benefit people, the planet, and the world's economies (Gautam et al. 2022). A forthcoming World Bank policy note, *Reshaping the Agrifood Sector for Healthier Diets: Exploring the Links between Agrifood Public Support and Diet Quality,* summarizes this ongoing agenda.

Of the total global agrifood public support of $638–$851 billion mentioned earlier, it has been estimated that more than 70 percent was targeted to producers, and most of these measures were market distorting. Much smaller shares of support were allocated to general services support (12 percent), which includes investments in private or public services, such as institutions and infrastructure, and to consumer subsidies (13 percent). Of the support to producers, more than 50 percent was in the form of trade or market policies, which affect market prices of agricultural commodities (OECD 2023). Furthermore, agrifood support measures in LMICs often lead to the most distortionary outcomes, because they tend to prioritize coupled subsidies, unlike high-income countries, where subsidies are commonly uncoupled and have a less distortive impact. In addition, agrifood subsidies in high-income countries focus more on research and infrastructure development than in LMICs, which leads to more market harm in the latter income group (Damania et al. 2023). Between 2020 and 2022, producers received $630 billion on average per year, with 14 percent of gross farm receipts being derived from public support measures. Agrifood subsidies that governments allocate to producers are regressive—they benefit wealthier farmers, because they use more inputs and produce more outputs, and rarely have a positive effect on the efficiency of production.

Public support to the agrifood sector is also imbalanced—higher for commodities with already high consumption and lower for heathier commodities with low consumption. Support for commodities for which consumption already meets or exceeds the recommended amounts far outpaces the support for healthier underconsumed commodities (OECD 2022). The most supported commodities in terms of an absolute amount of support are maize ($57 billion globally), rice ($32 billion), poultry meat ($27 billion), beef and veal ($24 billion), and pork ($31 billion). In 2020–22, sugar was the most supported commodity as a share of farmer income, with about 24 percent of gross farm receipts on sugar coming from agriculture support measures (refer to figure 6.2), which totaled more than $15 billion each year. In contrast, dairy, fruits, and vegetables have very low and negligible levels of public support (and as a share of farmer income).

Global simulation exercises (refer to figure 6.3) suggest that there are opportunities for multiple wins when repurposing agrifood support to target better climate or health outcomes. Modeling shows that repurposing for green innovation, by redirecting public support to research and development and other technological investments, could lead to triple wins for planet, economy, and people. With a baseline year of 2020, one study finds that by 2040, repurposing can lead to a 1.6 percent increase in real national income, a 1 percent reduction in extreme poverty, and an 18 percent reduction in the cost of a healthy diet, compared with a business-as-usual scenario. The modeling in that study also shows agricultural productivity increases: crop production volume is set to rise by 16 percent and livestock production by 11.5 percent. In addition, this repurposing scenario can lead to a 41 percent reduction in emissions from agriculture and land use, which partially derives from a 2.1 percent decrease in agricultural land. However, this scenario might also result in an 8 percent decrease in real farm income per worker, a 10.5 percent reduction in farm employment, and a 27.5 percent increase in the consumption of sugar, an already overconsumed commodity (Gautam et al. 2022).

Figure 6.2 Share of Global Agrifood Support, by Commodity, 2020–22

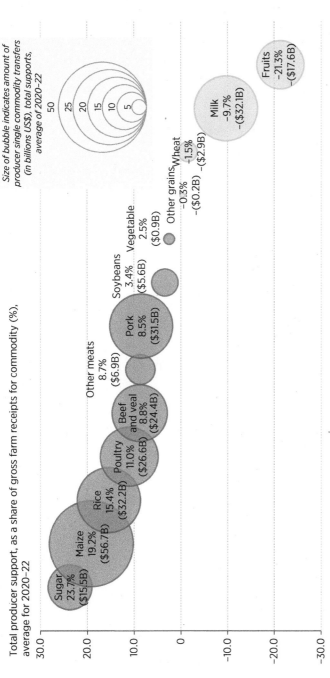

Total producer support, as a share of gross farm receipts for commodity (%), average for 2020–22

Size of bubble indicates amount of producer single commodity transfers (in billions US$), total supports, average of 2020–22

Sugar
23.7%
($15.5B)

Maize
19.2%
($56.7B)

Rice
15.4%
($32.2B)

Poultry
11.0%
($26.6B)

Beef
and veal
8.8%
($24.4B)

Other meats
8.7%
($6.9B)

Pork
8.5%
($31.5B)

Soybeans
3.4%
($5.6B)

Vegetable
2.5%
($0.9B)

Other grains
–0.3%
–($0.2B)

Wheat
–1.5%
–($2.9B)

Milk
–9.7%
–($32.1B)

Fruits
–21.3%
–($17.6B)

Agriculture commodities

Source: World Bank, forthcoming, using data from OECD 2023.

Note: The Organisation for Economic Co-operation and Development (OECD) indicator database includes a total of 60 food groups. A full list of commodities can be found at https://www.oecd.org/agriculture/topics/agricultural-policy-monitoring-and -evaluation/documents/producer-support-estimates-manual.pdf. Data are from 54 countries, including the 38 OECD countries, the 5 non-OECD European Union member states, and 11 emerging economies. Public support is measured by percentage of producer single-commodity transfers of the gross farm receipts for the single commodity and is defined as the total gross transfers from consumers and taxpayers to agricultural producers, measured at the farm gate level, arising from policies linked to the production of a single commodity. "Other meats" includes sheep meat. "Other grains" include alfalfa, oats, sorghum, and barley.

Figure 6.3 Global Modeling Simulations Repurposing Agrifood Support to Improve Climate and Health Outcomes

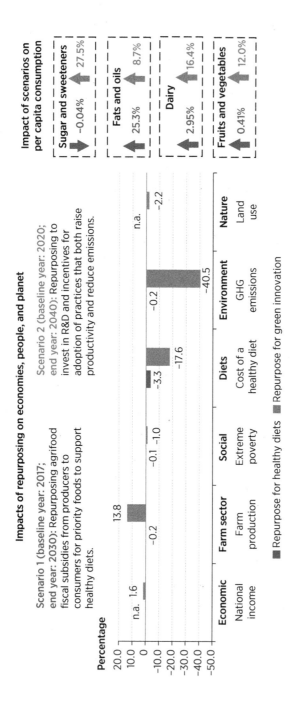

Source: World Bank, forthcoming, using data from Gautam et al. 2022 and FAO et al. 2022.

Note: Scenario 1 is listed as Scenario 6 in the source, shifting fiscal subsidies from producers to consumers in support of healthy diets. In this new scenario, the fiscal subsidies initially allocated to producers no longer stay within the agrifood sector, although they remain within the agrifood system. Scenario 2, listed as Scenario 4 in the source, repurposes a portion of current domestic support for increased spending on green innovations, that is, the development, diffusion, and adoption of new technologies that both reduce emissions and raise productivity. GHG = greenhouse gas; R&D = research and development.

Other global modeling work investigates repurposing for healthy diets—for example, with a scenario of repurposing agrifood support (fiscal subsidies) from producers to consumers for priority foods that support healthy diets (FAO et al. 2022). This scenario targets high-priority foods with a 10-fold increase in consumer subsidies, maintains average consumer subsidies for medium-priority foods, and maintains just one-tenth of the average level of support for low-priority commodities. Using 2017 as a baseline, the study finds that by 2030, this scenario can reduce extreme poverty by 0.06 percent, reduce GHG emissions by 0.18 percent, and decrease the cost of a healthy diet by 3.34 percent. Extreme poverty would fall the most, by 0.22 percent, in low-income countries. Because the repurposing-for-healthy-diets modeling takes into account reducing support for low-priority foods, the consumption of sugar and sweeteners falls by 0.04 percent in this scenario, whereas consumption of dairy, vegetables, and fruits increases. A trade-off in this scenario is the reduction in farm income by 3.74 percent and agricultural production by 0.2 percent. However, this outcome significantly affects high-income countries, and low-income countries experience an increase in farm income by 1.61 percent and in agricultural production by 0.36 percent (FAO et al. 2022).

Although repurposing agrifood policies and support often generates trade-offs across health, environment, and social outcomes, some scenarios indicate that there are opportunities for multiple wins. A careful country-level analytical agenda of the various options in repurposing is fundamental to elaborate on these trade-offs and identify windows of opportunities for multiple wins. Repurposing more explicitly for healthy diets (as opposed to repurposing for other objectives) is more likely to arrive at better diet outcomes, or at least to minimize any negative impacts on healthy diets. Repurposing for more effective nutrition-sensitive agriculture interventions is also more likely to have a positive impact on diets and nutrition (refer to chapter 5, "Food Transfers and Vouchers" section).

Policy Coherence

Emerging Evidence and Policy Actions on UPFs

The evolution of food systems over the past several decades—fueled by the development of food technologies, urbanization, expanded road networks, and cash economies—has led to rapid dietary shifts from unprocessed or minimally processed foods to processed foods and UPFs that tend to be high in sugar, sodium, and unhealthy fats, especially saturated fat, and low in fiber, proteins, and micronutrients. There have been several attempts to define and redefine what constitutes a UPF, such as inclusion of additives, salt, sugars, oils, and unhealthy fats; accessibility; convenience; palatability; and the use of industrial technologies to synthesize food ingredients and enhance sensory qualities (Gibney 2018). Among several different food classification approaches, the NOVA system, developed by researchers at the University of São Paulo in Brazil, is considered the most common in the scientific literature (Moubarac et al. 2014). The NOVA system categorizes foods into four groups: (1) unprocessed and minimally processed foods, (2) processed culinary ingredients, (3) processed foods, and (4) UPFs.

UPFs already make up a significant proportion of people's diet. Available evidence from middle-income and high-income countries (MICs and HICs, respectively) indicates that, although the expansion of UPF consumption started in HICs, MICs, especially in Latin America, are catching up. Studies show that the proportion of dietary energy consumption coming from UPFs has reached 59 percent in the United States (Baraldi et al. 2018), 50 percent in the United Kingdom (Rauber et al. 2019), 30 percent in Mexico (Marrón-Ponce et al. 2018), and 20 percent in Brazil (Louzada et al. 2018). Although evidence is limited for LMICs and low-income countries, an analysis done by Baker et al. (2020) revealed that LMICs had lower per capita UPF sales, by volume, in 2019 compared with most of the upper-middle-income countries (UMICs) and HICs studied. Almost half of the LMICs, such as Cameroon, India, Indonesia, Pakistan, Uzbekistan, and Viet Nam, however, had higher growth rates in per capita UPF sales between 2009 and 2019 (6–11 percent per year, on average) than most of the UMICs and HICs (between −4 and 6 percent; Baker et al. 2020). In Viet Nam, a study found that people in periurban and rural areas had higher average consumption of UPFs than those in urban areas. Consumption of instant noodles, chips, sweets (candies, chocolate, and so forth), and soft drinks was significantly higher in rural areas than in periurban and urban areas; 80 percent of rural households had consumed instant noodles in the past seven days, whereas shares were 70 percent and 64 percent among periurban and urban households, respectively (Nguyen et al. 2021). FAO's analysis of food consumption across the urban–rural continuum in 11 Sub-Saharan African countries suggests that consumption of highly processed foods was more equally dispersed across the urban–rural continuum, even in areas that were one to two or more than two hours away from a city or a town (Dolislager et al. 2023). Children's exposure to UPFs in LMICs poses a particular concern because they are more susceptible to marketing and advertising and because of the consequences of the double burden of malnutrition. A striking study in Nepal revealed that almost 90 percent of children ages 12–23 months in Kathmandu Valley had eaten unhealthy snack foods and beverages (USFBs) within the past 24 hours; such foods and beverages contributed to, on average, almost half of the total energy intake among the highest consumers and one-quarter among all children

(Pries et al. 2019). The study also found an association between USFB consumption and linear growth among these children; the average length-for-age z score was 0.3 standard deviation lower among high USFB consumers than among low consumers. In Mexico, a cross-sectional analysis using National Health and Nutrition Survey data revealed that the consumption of UPFs among children and adolescents increased between 2006 and 2016 and that higher UPF consumption was associated with the double burden of anemia and excess body weight in children of low socioeconomic status (Oviedo-Solís et al. 2022).

How UPF consumption affects population health has drawn enormous attention in recent years, and more evidence continues to emerge. The latest umbrella review of meta-analytic evidence of associations between exposure to UPFs and adverse health outcomes, which involved almost 10 million participants, identified direct associations with 32 (of 45) health parameters, spanning mortality (for example, all-cause and cardiovascular disease–related mortality); cancer (for example, colorectal cancer); and mental (for example, adverse sleep-related and anxiety outcomes), respiratory (for example, wheezing), cardiovascular (combined events and morbidity), gastrointestinal, and metabolic (for example, obesity, abdominal obesity and type 2 diabetes) health outcomes (Lane et al. 2024). Across the 32 parameters, greater exposure to UPFs was consistently associated with a higher risk of adverse health outcomes. The study, as well as other, preceding publications, notes that the adverse health outcomes may not be fully explained by nutrient composition and energy density of UPFs alone, but may also be explained by physical and chemical properties associated with industrial alterations and intensive processing, "cocktail effects" of multiple additives, and potentially harmful by-products linked to possible chronic inflammatory risks (Lane et al. 2024; Tristan Asensi et al. 2023).

UPFs are not only associated with obesity and diet-related NCD burdens, they also have greater environmental impacts, as described in chapter 4. Food supply chains contribute to almost one-third of global GHG emissions. Increasing sales and consumption of UPFs across the world through these supply chains raises serious concerns for both planetary and human health. A systematic review covering 52 studies found that UPFs accounted for 17–39 percent of total diet-related energy use; 36–45 percent of total diet-related biodiversity loss; up to one-third of total diet-related GHG emissions, land use, and food waste; and up to one-quarter of total diet-related water use among adults (Anastasiou et al. 2022). A longitudinal assessment of UPF consumption and its environmental impacts involving more than 5,000 participants in Spain suggests that lower UPF consumption may contribute to reducing GHG emissions and energy use while increasing water use (Garcia et al. 2023).

The challenges associated with the expansion of UPF sales and consumption involve three interrelated aspects: (1) the highly attractive nature of the products, such as affordability, accessibility, convenience, and palatability; (2) the UPF industry's effective and aggressive marketing strategies, which were adapted from the proven tactics of tobacco marketing; and (3) the distorted market price context, which allows the UPF industry to make products cheaply yet energy dense (albeit nutrient poor) compared with heathier options. Given these aspects, a range of policy measures is needed, including marketing regulations; strong behavior science–based interventions, such as FOPL policies; and fiscal incentives to address distortive market pricing structures (Popkin et al. 2021). Policy actions targeting UPFs are slowly emerging. To date, a few countries (for example, Chile and Mexico) have adopted a mandatory FOP warning label carrying a clear message about the added danger of UPFs. Only a handful of countries and territories have expanded SSB taxes to cover unhealthy foods, including UPFs. This includes the most recent comprehensive UPF tax policy approved in Colombia in 2023, which includes edible products formulated from food-derived substances, along with additives that contain added sugars, sodium, and saturated fats and exceed the defined thresholds (Global Food Research Program, UNC-Chapel Hill, n.d.; refer to the "Nutrition-Targeted Health Tax Policies" section for more detailed nutrition-targeted health tax policy designs and box 6.2 for Colombia's UPF taxes). Besides Colombia, other country-based studies to assess the effectiveness of UPF tax policies, for example through their distributive impacts, are emerging. A recent study in Brazil demonstrated that taxes on processed foods and UPFs can have progressive effects in terms of (1) changes in product expenditure, (2) changes in medical expenditure, and (3) changes in years of life lost, especially among households at the lower end of the consumption distribution that are reliant on the public health system (World Bank 2024b). Policy reforms based on repurposing agrifood public support have started to incorporate climate co-benefits, yet more work is needed to also reflect health and nutrition outcomes. Questions that remain unanswered include the following: Are there any specific policies to protect infants and young children from unwarranted UPFs, are there any marketing regulations around UFPs, and (even more fundamentally) have any countries adopted legislation clearly defining what UPFs entail? To date, no country has enacted a comprehensive policy package to systemically halt the growth of UPF consumption.

Additionally, evidence suggests that consumption of UPFs is inversely associated with lower consumption of less processed and healthier food choices that are low in sugar, sodium, and unhealthy fats (Martini et al. 2021). It is important to simultaneously explore effective approaches to improving availability, affordability, and desirability of and actual consumer access to less processed and healthier food choices. A range of policy measures are available, including price incentives in the form of subsidies, rebates, and discounts, as well as consumer-focused incentives such as tax exemption and targeted social assistance to increase the purchasing power of the most vulnerable population groups. Yet, most have only been explored and evaluated in high-income countries. A few other examples from middle-income countries include South Africa's Cash-Back Rebate Program for Healthy Food Purchases, which has demonstrated increases in purchases of healthy foods and decreases in purchases of less-desirable foods (Sturm et al. 2013). Israel has introduced a two-color FOP label that consists of mandatory red warning labels and a voluntary green label on foods in their natural form or those that underwent minimal processing with no food additives. This positive labeling strategy was carefully developed by an independent scientific committee using evidence and built on the positive experience with the "Health Is Possible" labeling strategy, which was applied to bread with a high proportion of whole grains, low sodium, and low calories (Muzzioli et al. 2023).

Policy Coherence on Production and Consumption of Unhealthy Products

Transforming food systems to ensure access to more sustainable and healthier choices requires a comprehensive package of action, supported by multiple and mutually reinforcing policies and accompanying communication measures to enable both supply and demand changes (Adams et al. 2020; Popkin et al. 2021).

Pricing measures targeted to consumers as well as price controls are commonly used in LMICs to address food affordability and security (Asfaw 2007; Ginn and Pourroy 2019; Snowdon et al. 2010). Many LMICs have differentiated value-added tax or sales tax systems, enabling some products to benefit from reduced or zero rates. Reviewing these products to ensure the standard rate is applied to unhealthy products helps ensure policy coherence with nutrition-targeted health taxes and other measures. Subsidies on fruits and vegetables can complement other fiscal policies by encouraging consumers to make healthier choices. A 2022 meta-analysis found that a 10 percent subsidy-induced reduction in the price of fruits and vegetables was associated with a 5.9 percent increase in sales (95 percent CI, −10.4 percent, −1.3 percent; Andreyeva et al. 2022a).

Chile has taken a multipronged approach with a comprehensive set of policy and fiscal measures to curb the consumption of unhealthy foods and promote healthier diets, including mandatory FOP warning labeling, a complete advertisement ban, restrictions on school food sales and marketing, and a SSB tax policy. Evidence of its effectiveness is emerging from the first phase of the comprehensive FOPL and marketing laws, first enacted in 2016: significant decreases in overall purchases of overall calories by 3.5 percent, sugar by 10.2 percent, saturated fat by 3.9 percent, and sodium by 4.7 percent, compared with projected trends if these laws had not been introduced. The study found that these declines were largely driven by reductions in "high-in" food and beverage purchases, with partial compensation from increases in "not-high-in" purchases (Taillie et al. 2021). It should be noted that Chile's initiative has been anchored in its carefully designed nutrient profiling model to align food taxes and other policies with warning label initiatives to create a set of coherent and mutually reinforcing set of fiscal and labeling laws (Colchero, Paraje, and Popkin 2021).

As the various repurposing scenarios outlined in the "Repurposing Agrifood Public Support Policies for Healthier and More Sustainable Diets" section suggest, there are trade-offs when assessing climate, health, and economic benefits, and these need to be further studied to inform coherent policy decisions that can maximize short- and long-term benefits for people, planet, and inclusive growth.

There are certain cases in which agrifood public policy and support might be at odds with public policy in other sectors, such as the health sector. For example, although the production of sugar is one of the most publicly supported, many governments around the world are also taxing the consumption of SSBs in recognition of the harmful effects of a final product with high sugar content. This demonstrates potential inconsistencies in what commodities governments support production of and what commodities they curb consumption of. As figure 6.4 shows, countries such as Costa Rica, India, Mexico, the Philippines, South Africa, and the United States have imposed SSB taxes on their consumers but have also maintained fairly significant support to their sugar producers (whether via fiscal subsidies or trade policy). These countries are close to or have exceeded the WHO recommended maximum threshold of 50 grams per day (g/day) of free sugar consumption.[2] By shifting support to producers, this policy incoherence imposes both short-term and long-term economic burden on people not only as consumers but also as taxpayers. The burden is felt primarily by low-income consumers who would be most affected by long-term consequences, such as reduced productivity and income resulting from overweight and obesity and NCDs, as well as catastrophic medical spending related to these conditions. It is also noteworthy that other countries with high levels of sugar consumption and producer support have not adopted SSB taxes. In Indonesia, for example, the Ministry of Finance has attempted to propose SSB taxes since 2018, using evidence showing their potential to reduce consumption and generate revenue (Widarjono et al. 2023), but to date it has not yet gained sufficient support (Ahsan et al. 2023).

Figure 6.4 Sugar Consumption, SSB Taxes, and Support to Sugar Producers, Selected Countries

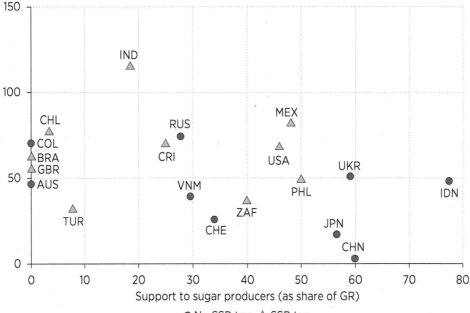

Sugar consumption (grams per day)

Support to sugar producers (as share of GR)

● No SSB tax   △ SSB tax

Source: World Bank, forthcoming, using data from OECD 2023 and "Producer and Consumer Support Estimates," OECD Agriculture Statistics database, https://doi.org/10.1787/agr-pcse-data-en; consumption data come from the Global Dietary Database 2020.

Note: The measure of support to sugar producers, the percentage of Producer Single Commodity Transfers of the gross farm receipts for sugar (GR), is defined as the total gross transfers from consumers and taxpayers to agricultural producers, measured at the farm gate level, arising from policies linked to the production of sugar. For a list of country codes, go to https://www.iso.org/obp/ui/#search. SSB = sugar-sweetened beverage.

Policy Measures and Scale-Up Opportunities, by Income Group

On the basis of the analyses discussed in this chapter, countries are encouraged to develop and implement a coherent package of normative policy frameworks, regulatory policies, and fiscal measures, buttressed by strong social communication strategies. Scale-up must, however, be carefully calibrated to national contexts, taking into account the economic and political landscape, institutional capacities, and epidemiology of malnutrition and related disease burdens. Table 6.1 provides a typology of policy measures and scale-up opportunities for countries with different income statuses. It also summarizes important policy considerations for each policy type based on epidemiological and market conditions.

Table 6.1 Typology of Policy Measures and Scale-Up Opportunities, by Country Income Classification and Epidemiological and Market Conditions

Policy Measure	LICs	MICs	HICs	Epidemiological and market considerations for scale-up	Policy considerations
National Policy Frameworks and Guidelines					
National multisectoral nutrition policy legal framework	**✶ 🌾	**✶ 🌾	**✶ 🌾	Set a scope to reflect the epidemiological status of a country on the basis of evidence. LICs and MICs with a high undernutrition burden should have a policy that can address the double burden of malnutrition and climate challenges.	Multisectorality and legal status matter for effectiveness of the framework as a foundation for a stable policy environment in all countries.
Costed national multisectoral nutrition strategy	**✶ 🌾🌾	**✶ 🌾🌾	**✶ 🌾	Set a scope to reflect the epidemiological status of a country. LICs and MICs with a high undernutrition burden should have a strategy that can address the double burden of malnutrition and climate challenges.	Costing and allocative efficiency considerations across relevant sectors can enhance adequate resource allocation.
Costed subnational multisectoral nutrition strategy	*✶ 🌾🌾🌾	*✶ 🌾🌾🌾	**✶ 🌾	Set a scope to reflect the epidemiological status of each locality. Areas with high undernutrition burden should have a strategy that can address the double burden of malnutrition and climate challenges.	Costing across relevant sectors at the subnational level can further enhance adequate resource allocation for critical community-based nutrition actions.

(continued)

Table 6.1 Typology of Policy Measures and Scale-Up Opportunities, by Country Income Classification and Epidemiological and Market Conditions (continued)

Policy Measure	LICs	MICs	HICs	Epidemiological and market considerations for scale-up	Policy considerations
National dietary guidelines	* 🌾🌾	** 🌾🌾	***	In all epidemiological situations, guidelines on UPF consumption should be included.	It is increasingly more important for LMICs to respond to food system and dietary challenges.
Regulatory Policies					
Food fortification regulations	* 🌾🌾	** 🌾🌾	*** 🌾	Design a legal framework and standards based on evidence of micronutrient deficiencies and food consumption patterns, with a focus on vulnerable women and children. Marketing and FOPL regulations are critical where packaged foods are voluntarily fortified, widely marketed, and consumed.	The strategy is cost-effective and highly relevant, yet accelerated progress is needed, especially in LICs. Consider double burden and health risks of UPFs in selection of food vehicles.
Marketing regulations on unhealthy foods and drinks	* 🌾	* 🌾🌾	** 🌾🌾	This measure is applicable to all epidemiological profiles. It is especially urgent in places where consumption of packaged foods and drinks is high or increasing.	It is important for all MICs and HICs and most of LICs to respond to food system and dietary challenges, including increasing consumption of UPFs.
Marketing regulations on breast milk substitutes	* 🌾🌾	** 🌾🌾	** 🌾	This is applicable to all epidemiological profiles, not only to prevent undernutrition and child mortality, but also to reduce risks of obesity and NCDs later in life. It is crucial in LICs and MICs where more women work as wage laborers, yet access to nutrition services and information is limited. BFHI should be regarded as a paired intervention.	This is a long-standing, globally endorsed strategy, yet progress, especially on strong enforcement measures, is slow in LICs. It must be implemented in all countries and should include stronger enforcement mechanisms such as through digital marketing.

(continued)

Table 6.1 Typology of Policy Measures and Scale-Up Opportunities, by Country Income Classification and Epidemiological and Market Conditions *(continued)*

Policy Measure	LICs	MICs	HICs	Epidemiological and market considerations for scale-up	Policy considerations
FOP warning labels on all "high-in" foods and UPFs	** 🌾	** 🌾🌾	** 🌾🌾	This measure is applicable to all epidemiological profiles, especially in places where consumption of packaged foods and drinks is high or increasing.	This is important in all MICs and HICs, as well as some in LICs where consumption of UPFs is increasing.
FOP positive labels on healthy food choices	*	* 🌾	* 🌾🌾	This measure is applicable in places where healthy packaged alternatives are available and affordable.	It is increasingly more important to inform consumers when there are affordable and accessible alternatives.
Fiscal Policies					
Taxation on SSBs	** 🌾	** 🌾🌾	** 🌾🌾	This measure is applicable to all epidemiological profiles. The SSB market is expanding in many LMICs. Taxes are mostly passed through consumers, who generally respond to price increases by decreasing purchasing. Lower-income households tend to be more responsive to price increases and may benefit more in the long run from health and productivity improvements.	Many LICs and LMICs have existing taxes; however, design and implementation need to be strengthened. This is increasingly important in LICs where SSBs are available at affordable prices.
Taxation on unhealthy foods	*	* 🌾🌾	* 🌾🌾	This measure is applicable to all epidemiological profiles, and it is especially important in places where low-cost UPFs are available and accessible. SBCC is critical for less-educated consumers who may be affected by marketing tactics and still opt for such products to, for example, feed children.	Only a few countries have these policies in place. Need scale-up in MICs and HICs as well as in LMICs as part of a larger policy package for healthier and more sustainable diets.

(continued)

Table 6.1 Typology of Policy Measures and Scale-Up Opportunities, by Country Income Classification and Epidemiological and Market Conditions *(continued)*

Policy Measure	LICs	MICs	HICs	Epidemiological and market considerations for scale-up	Policy considerations
Repurposing	* ⸎	* ⸎	* ⸎	This measure is applicable to all epidemiological profiles. It is especially important in countries with large agrifood sector public support.	It is often politically difficult to shift public support away from producers and against specific commodities because policies and programs are typically long-standing. Robust analytics, high-level multisectoral policy dialogue, and careful transitions are needed.
Others					
Nationwide evidence-led consumer education and communication	* ⸎	** ⸎	*** ⸎	It is critical for all epidemiological profiles to support any combination of policy measures, and it is especially important for less-educated consumers, who may be affected by marketing tactics that make them believe such products are good for health.	Scale-up is needed in all countries, in support of all other policy measures, to shift the social norm. Innovative solutions are needed to increase effectiveness of digital marketing to promote healthier and demote unhealthy dietary choices.

Source: Original table for this publication.

Note: ⸫ = policy largely in place; ⸪ = policy partially in place; * = policy not commonly in place; ⸎⸎ = urgent scale-up needed; ⸎ = scale-up recommended. BFHI = Baby Friendly Hospital Initiative; FOP = front-of-package; FOPL = front-of-package labeling; HICs = high-income countries; LICs = low-income countries; LMICs = lower-middle-income countries; MICs = middle-income countries; NCDs = noncommunicable diseases; SBCC = social and behavioral change communication; SSBs = sugar-sweetened beverages; UPF = ultraprocessed food.

The World Bank's new Food and Nutrition Security Global Challenge Program supports many of these game-changing policy solutions, along with high-impact nutrition interventions, to address all forms of malnutrition.

These policies must be designed to leverage policy coherence to optimize allocation of public resources; maximize economic, health, and climate co-benefits; and minimize negative externalities on countries' human capital, economic growth, and sustainable development.

Notes

1. The Copenhagen Consensus Center, a group of leading economists that advocate for investing in high-return development solutions, identified micronutrient fortification among the top three development priorities in its expert panel ranking in 2008. See Copenhagen Consensus Center (2024).

2. Based on WHO (2015), which recommends reducing intake of free sugars to less than 10 percent of total daily energy intake, an amount which translates to roughly 50 grams of free sugars per day for an average adult consuming 2,000 calories a day.

References

Adams, Jean, Karen Hofman, Jean-Claude Moubarac, and Anne Marie Thow. 2020. "Public Health Response to Ultra-Processed Food and Drinks." *BMJ* 369: m2391.

Aguilar, Arturo, Emilio Gutierrez, and Enrique Seira. 2021. "The Effectiveness of Sin Food Taxes: Evidence from Mexico." *Journal of Health Economics* 77: 102455. https://doi.org/10.1016/j.jhealeco.2021.102455.

Ahsan, Abdillah, Nadira Amalia, Krisna Pudji Rahmayanti, Nadhila Adani, Nur Hadi Wiyona, Althof Endawansa, Maulida Gadis Utami, et al. 2023. "Health Taxes in Indonesia: A Review of Policy Debates on the Tobacco, Alcoholic Beverages and Sugar-Sweetened Beverage Taxes in the Media." *BMJ Global Health* 8 (Suppl 8): e012042. https://doi.org/10.1136/bmjgh-2023-012042.

Alluhidan, Mohammed, Reem F. Alsukait, Taghred Alghaith, Meera Shekar, Nahar Alazemi, and Chrisopher H. Herbst, eds. 2022. *Overweight and Obesity in Saudi Arabia: Consequences and Solutions.* International Development in Focus. Washington, DC: World Bank.

Alsukait, Reem, Parke Wilde, Sara N. Bleich, Gitanjali Singh, and Sara C. Folta. 2020. "Evaluating Saudi Arabia's 50% Carbonated Drink Excise Tax: Changes in Prices and Volume Sales." *Economics & Human Biology* 38: 100868. https://doi.org/10.1016/j.ehb.2020.100868.

Anastasiou, K., P. Baker, M. Hadjikakou, G. A. Hendrie, and M. Lawrence. 2022. "A Conceptual Framework for Understanding the Environmental Impacts of Ultra-Processed Foods and Implications for Sustainable Food Systems." *Journal of Cleaner Production* 368: 133155. https://doi.org/10.1016/j.jclepro.2022.133155.

Andreyeva, Tatiana, Keith Marple, Timothy E. Moore, and Lisa M. Powell. 2022a. "Evaluation of Economic and Health Outcomes Associated with Food Taxes and Subsidies: A Systematic Review and Meta-analysis." *JAMA Network Open* 5 (6): e2214371-e. https://doi.org/10.1001/jamanetworkopen.2022.14371.

Andreyeva, Tatiana, Keith Marple, Samantha Marinello, Timothy E. Moore, and Lisa M. Powell. 2022b. "Outcomes Following Taxation of Sugar-Sweetened Beverages: A Systematic Review and Meta-Analysis." *JAMA Network Open* 5 (6): e2215276-e. https://doi.org/10.1001/jamanetworkopen.2022.15276.

Arslanian, Kendall J., Mireya Vilar-Compte, Graciela Teruel, Annel Lozano-Marrufo, Elizabeth C. Rhodes, Amber Hromi-Fiedler, Erika Garcia, et al. 2022. "How Much Does It Cost to Implement the Baby-Friendly Hospital Initiative Training Step in the United States and Mexico?" *PLOS One* 17 (9): e0273179. https://doi.org/10.1371/journal.pone.0273179.

Asfaw, Abay. 2007. "Do Government Food Price Policies Affect the Prevalence of Obesity? Empirical Evidence from Egypt." *World Development* 35 (4): 687–701.

Baker, Philip, Priscilla Machado, Thiago Santos, Katherine Sievert, Kathryn Backholer, Michalis Hadjikakou, Cherie Russell, et al. 2020. "Ultra-Processed Foods and the Nutrition Transition: Global, Regional and National Trends, Food Systems Transformations and Political Economy Drivers." *Obesity Reviews* 21 (12): e13126.

Baraldi, Larissa Garibaldi, Euridice Steele, Daniela Silva Canella, and Carmelo A. Monteiro. 2018. "Consumption of Ultra-Processed Foods and Associated Sociodemographic Factors in the USA between 2007 and 2012: Evidence from a Nationally Representative Cross-Sectional Study." *BMJ Open* 8 (3).

Batis, Carolina, Juan A. Rivera, Barry M. Popkin, and Lindsey Smith Taillie. 2016. "First-Year Evaluation of Mexico's Tax on Nonessential Energy-Dense Foods: An Observational Study." *PLoS Medicine* 13: e1002057. https://doi.org/10.1371/journal.pmed.1002057.

Bin Sunaid, Faisal Fahad, Ayoub Al-Jawaldeh, Meshal Wasel Almutairi, Rawan Abdulaziz Alobaid, Tagreed Mohammad Alfuraih, Faisal Naser Bensaidan, Atheer Shayea Alragea, et al. 2021. "Saudi Arabia's Healthy Food Strategy: Progress & Hurdles in the 2030 Road." *Nutrients* 13 (7): 2130. https://doi.org/10.3390/nu13072130.

Bíró, Anikó. 2015. "Did the Junk Food Tax Make the Hungarians Eat Healthier?" *Food Policy* 54: 107–15. https://doi.org/10.1016/j.foodpol.2015.05.003.

Colchero, M. Aranxta, Guillermo Paraje, and Barry Popkin. 2021. "The Impacts on Food Purchases and Tax Revenues of a Tax Based on Chile's Nutrient Profiling Model." *PLoS One* 16 (12): e0260693.

Copenhagen Consensus Center. 2024. "Outcomes." Tewksbury, MA: Copenhagen Consensus Center. Accessed February 27, 2024, https://copenhagenconsensus.com/copenhagen-consensus-ii/outcomes.

Croker, H., J. Packer, Simon J. Russell, C. Stansfield, and R. M. Viner. 2020. "Front of Pack Nutritional Labelling Schemes: A Systematic Review and Meta-Analysis of Recent Evidence Relating to Objectively Measured Consumption and Purchasing." *Journal of Human Nutrition and Dietetics* 33 (4): 518–37. https://doi.org/10.1111/jhn.12758.

Damania, Richard, Esteban Balseca, Charlotte de Fontaubert, Joshua Gill, Kichan Kim, Jun Renschler, Jason Russ, and Esha Zaveri. 2023. *Detox Development: Repurposing Environmentally Harmful Subsidies*. Washington, DC: World Bank. http://hdl.handle.net/10986/39423.

Dillman Carpentier, Francis R., Fernanda Mediano Stoltze, Marcela Reyes, Lindsey Smith Taillie, Camila Corvalán, and Teresa Correa. 2023. "Restricting Child-Directed Ads Is Effective, but Adding a Time-Based Ban Is Better: Evaluating a Multi-Phase Regulation to Protect Children from Unhealthy Food Marketing on Television." *International Journal of Behavioral Nutrition and Physical Activity* 20: 62. https://doi.org/10.1186/s12966-023-01454-w.

Dolislager, M. J., C. Holleman, L. S. O. Liverpool-Tasie, and T. Reardon. 2023. "Analysis of Food Demand and Supply across the Rural–Urban Continuum for Selected Countries in Africa." Background paper, *The State of Food Security and Nutrition in the World 2023*. FAO Agricultural Development Economics Working Paper No. 23-09, Food and Agriculture Organization of the United Nations, Rome.

FAO (Food and Agricultural Organization of the United Nations). 2024. "Food-Based Dietary Guidelines: Regions." Rome: FAO. https://www.fao.org/nutrition/education/food-dietary-guidelines/regions/en/.

FAO (Food and Agricultural Organization of the United Nations), IFAD (International Fund for Agricultural Development), UNICEF (United Nations Children's Fund), WFP (World Food Programme), and WHO (World Health Organization). 2022. *The State of Food Security and Nutrition in the World 2022: Repurposing Food and Agricultural Policies to Make Healthy Diets More Affordable*. Rome: FAO. https://openknowledge.fao.org/handle/20.500.14283/cd1254en.

FOLU (Food and Land Use Coalition). 2019. *Growing Better: Ten Critical Transitions to Transform Food and Land Use*. The Global Consultation Report of the Food and Land Use Coalition. London: FOLU. https://www.foodandlandusecoalition.org/wp-content/uploads/2019/09/FOLU-GrowingBetter-GlobalReport.pdf.

Fuchs Tarlovsky, Alan, Kate Mandeville, and Ana Cristina Alonso-Soria. 2020. *Health and Distributional Effects Taxing Sugar-Sweetened Beverages: The Case of Kazakhstan*. Washington, DC: World Bank.

Garcia, Sylvia, Rosario Pastor, Margalida Monserrat-Mesquida, Laura Álvarez-Álvarez, María Rubín-García, Miguel Ángel Martínez-González, Jordi Salas-Salvadó, et al. 2023. "Ultra-Processed Foods Consumption as a Promoting Factor of Greenhouse Gas Emissions, Water, Energy, and Land Use: A Longitudinal Assessment." *Science of the Total Environment* 891: 164417. https://doi.org/10.1016/j.scitotenv.2023.164417.

Gautam, Madhur, David Laborde Debucquet, Abdullah Al-Mamun, Will Martin, Valeria Piñeiro, and Robert Vos. 2022. *Repurposing Agricultural Policies and Support: Options to Transform Agriculture and Food Systems to Better Serve the Health of People, Economies, and the Planet.* Washington, DC: World Bank and International Food Policy Research Institute.

Gibney, Michael J. 2018. "Ultra-Processed Foods: Definitions and Policy Issues." *Current Developments in Nutrition* 3 (2): nzy077.

Ginn, William, and Marc Pourroy. 2019. "Optimal Monetary Policy in the Presence of Food Price Subsidies." *Economic Modelling* 81: 551–75.

Global Food Research Program, UNC-Chapel Hill (University of North Carolina at Chapel Hill). 2021. "Front of Package (FOP) Food Labelling: Empowering Consumers and Promoting Healthy Diets." Global Food Research Program, Chapel Hill, NC.

Global Food Research Program, UNC-Chapel Hill (University of North Carolina at Chapel Hill). 2023. *Front-of-Package Labels around the World.* Chapel Hill, NC: Global Food Research Program. https://www.globalfoodresearchprogram.org /wp-content/uploads/2023/02/GFRP-UNC_FOPL_maps_2023_02.pdf.

Global Food Research Program, UNC-Chapel Hill (University of North Carolina at Chapel Hill). n.d. "Colombia." https://www.globalfoodresearchprogram.org /where-we-work/colombia/.

Government of Colombia, Ministerio de Hacienda y Crédito Público. 2022. *Reforma tributaria para la igualdad y la justicia social. Exposición de motivos.* Bogotá: Government of Colombia. https://www.minhacienda.gov.co/webcenter /ShowProperty?nodeId=/ConexionContent/WCC_CLUSTER-200786.

Government of Colombia, Ministerio de Hacienda y Crédito Público. 2023. *Efectos inflacionarios del impuesto a alimentos ultraprocesados.* Bogotá: Government of Colombia. https://www.minhacienda.gov.co/webcenter/ShowProperty?nodeId =%2FConexionContent%2FWCC_CLUSTER-231553%2F%2FidcPrimaryFile&r evision=latestreleased.

Government of Colombia, Ministerio de Salud y Protección Social. 2016. *Papeles en salud No. 5. Impuestos a las bebidas azucaradas.* Bogotá: Government of Colombia. https://www.minsalud.gov.co/sites/rid/Lists/BibliotecaDigital/RIDE/DE/AS /papeles-salud-n5.pdf.

Government of Pakistan, Ministry of Planning, Development & Reform, and World Food Programme. 2018. *Pakistan Multi-Sectoral Nutrition Strategy (PMNS 2018-25).* Islamabad: Pakistan.

Gracner, Tadeja, Fernanda Marquez-Padilla, and Danae Hernandez-Cortes. 2022. "Changes in Weight-Related Outcomes Among Adolescents Following Consumer Price Increases of Taxed Sugar-Sweetened Beverages." *JAMA Pediatrics* 176 (2): 150–58.

Hassel, Anke, and Kai Wegrich. 2022. "How to Choose and Design Policy Instruments." In *How to Do Public Policy*, edited by Anke Hassel and Kai Wegrich, 93–126. Oxford: Oxford University Press; online edition, Oxford Academic, April 21, 2022, https://doi.org/10.1093/oso/9780198747000 .003.0004.

Hattersley, Libby, Alessia Thiebaud, Alan Fuchs, Alberto Gonima, Lynn Silver, and Kate Mandevill. 2020. *Taxes on Sugar-Sweetened Beverages: International Evidence and Experiences.* World Bank Health Nutrition and Population Global Practice Knowledge Brief. Washington, DC: World Bank. https://thedocs.worldbank.org /en/doc/d9612c480991c5408edca33d54e2028a-0390062021/related /Knowledge-Brief-Taxes-on-Sugar-Sweetened-BeveragesInternational -Evidence-and-Experiences.pdf.

Hernández-F, Mauricio, Alejandra Cantoral, and M. Arantxa Colchero. 2022. "Taxes to Unhealthy Food and Beverages and Oral Health in Mexico: An Observational Study." *Caries Research* 55 (3): 183–92.

Horton, Susan, Tina Sanghvi, Margaret Phillips, John Fiedler, Rafael Perez-Escamilla, Chessa Lutter, Ada Rivera, et al. "Breastfeeding Promotion and Priority Setting in Health." 1996. *Health Policy and Planning* 11 (2): 156–68. https://doi .org/10.1093/heapol/11.2.156.

Howlett, Michael 2019. *Designing Public Policies: Principles and Instruments.* New York: Routledge.

ICBF (Instituto Colombiano de Bienestar Familiar). 2006. Encuesta Nacional de la Situacion Nutricional en Colombia. 2005. Instituto Colombiano de Bienestar Familiar (ICBF), Republica de Colombia. ISBN 958-623-087-2. https://www .minsalud.gov.co/sites/rid/Lists/BibliotecaDigital/RIDE/VS/ED/GCFI/Ensin%20 2005.pdf.

ICBF (Instituto Colombiano de Bienestar Familiar). 2018. Encuesta Nacional de la Situacion Nutricional - ENSIN 2015. Instituto Colombiano de Bienestar Familiar (ICBF), Ministerio de Salud y Proteccion Social, Republica de Colombia. https://www.minsalud.gov.co/sites/rid/Lists/BibliotecaDigital/RIDE/VS/ED /GCFI/documento-metodologico-ensin-2015.pdf.

Jalloun, Rola Adnan, and Moataz Abdulsattar Qurban. 2022. "The Impact of Taxes on Soft Drinks on Adult Consumption and Weight Outcomes in Medina, Saudi Arabia." *Human Nutrition & Metabolism* 27: 200139. https://doi.org/10.1016/j .hnm.2022.200139.

Kroker-Lobos, Maria F., Mónica Mazariegos, Mónica Guamuch, and Manuel Ramirez-Zea. 2022. "Ultraprocessed Products as Food Fortification Alternatives: A Critical Appraisal from Latin America. *Nutrients* 14 (7): 1413.

Kroker-Lobos, Maria Fernanda, Analí Morales-Juárez, Wilton Pérez, Tomo Kanda, Fabio S. Gomes, Manuel Ramírez-Zea, and Carolina Siu-Bermúdez. 2023. "Efficacy of Front-of-Pack Warning Label System versus Guideline for Daily Amount on Healthfulness Perception, Purchase Intention and Objective Understanding of Nutrient Content of Food Products in Guatemala: A Cross-Over Cluster Randomized Controlled Experiment." *Archives of Public Health* 81: 108.

Lane, Melissa M., Elizabeth Gamage, Shutong Du, Deborah N. Ashtree, Amelia J. McGuinness, Sara Gauci, Phillip Baker, et al. 2024. "Ultra-Processed Food Exposure and Adverse Health Outcomes: Umbrella Review of Epidemiological Meta-Analyses." *BMJ* 384: e077310. https://doi.org/10.1136/bmj-2023-077310.

Lascoumes, P., and Le Galès, P. 2007. "Introduction: Understanding Public Policy through Its Instruments—From the Nature of Instruments to the Sociology of Public Policy Instrumentation." *Governance* 20 (1): 1–21.

Louzada, Maria Laura da Costa, Camilla Zancheta Ricardo, Euridice Martinez Steele, Renata Bertazzi Levy, Geoffrey Cannon, and Carlos August Monteio. 2018. "The Share of Ultraprocessed Foods Determines the Overall Nutritional Quality of Diets in Brazil." *Public Health Nutrition* 21 (1): 94–102. https://doi.org/10.1017/S1368980017001434.

Lutter, Chessa K., S. Hernandez-Cordero, L. Grummer-Strawn, V. Lara-Mejía, and A. L. Lozada-Tequeanes. 2022. "Violations of the International Code of Marketing of Breast-Milk Substitutes: A Multi-Country Analysis." *BMC Public Health* 22: 2336.

M&C Saatchi World Services. 2022. *Multi-Country Study Examining the Impact of Marketing of Breast-Milk Substitutes on Infant Feeding Decisions and Practices: Commissioned Report.* Geneva: World Health Organization.

Marks, Kristin J., Corey L. Luthringer, Laird J. Ruth, Laura A. Rowe, Noor A. Khan, Luz María De-Regil, Ximena López, et al. 2018. "Review of Grain Fortification Legislation, Standards, and Monitoring Documents." *Global Health: Science and Practice* 6 (2) 356-71.

Marrón-Ponce, Joaquin A., Tania G. Sánchez-Pimienta, Maria Laura da Costa Louzada, and Carolina Batis. 2018. "Energy Contribution of NOVA Food Groups and Sociodemographic Determinants of Ultra-Processed Food Consumption in the Mexican Population." *Public Health Nutrition* 21 (1): 87–93.

Martini, Daniela, Justyna Godos, Marialaura Bonaccio, Paola Vitaglione, and Giuseppe Grosso. 2021. "Ultra-Processed Foods and Nutritional Dietary Profile: A Meta-Analysis of Nationally Representative Samples." *Nutrients* 13 (10): 3390.

Mitra-Ganguli, Tora, Wolfgang H. Pfeiffer, and Jenny Walton. 2022. "The Global Regulatory Framework for the Commercialization of Nutrient Enriched Biofortified Foods." *Annals of the New York Academy of Sciences* 1517 (1): 154–166.

Monteiro, Carlos Augusto, Geoffrey Cannon, Mark Lawrence, Maria Laura da Costa Louzada, and Priscila Pereira Machado. 2019. *Ultra-Processed Foods, Diet Quality, and Health Using the NOVA Classification System.* Rome: Food and Agriculture Organization of the United Nations.

Moubarac, Jean-Claude, Diana C. Parra, Geoffrey E. Cannon, and Carlos Monteiro. 2014. "Food Classification Systems Based on Food Processing: Significance and Implications for Policies and Actions: A Systematic Literature Review and Assessment and Implications for Policies and Actions: A Systematic Literature Review and Assessment." *Current Obesity Reports* 3 (2): 256–72.

Muzzioli, Luca, Lorenzo Maria Donini, Matteo Mazziotta, Marco Iosa, Francesco Frigerio, Eleonora Poggiogalle, Andrea Lenzi, et al. 2023. "How Much Do Front-Of-Pack Labels Correlate with Food Environmental Impacts?" *Nutrients* 15 (5): 1176.

Nguyen, Trang, Huong Pham Thi Mai, Marrit van den Berg, Tuyen Huynh Thi Thanh, and Christophe Béné. 2021. "Interactions between Food Environment and (Un)healthy Consumption: Evidence along a Rural-Urban Transect in Viet Nam." *Agriculture* 11 (8): 789.

OECD (Organisation for Economic Co-operation and Development). 2022. *Agricultural Policy Monitoring and Evaluation 2022: Reforming Agricultural Policies for Climate Change Mitigation.* Paris: OECD Publishing.

OECD (Organisation for Economic Co-operation and Development). 2023. *Agricultural Policy Monitoring and Evaluation 2023: Adapting Agriculture to Climate Change.* Paris: OECD.

Osendarp, Saskia, Jonathan Kweku Akuoku, Robert E. Black, Derek Headey, Marie Ruel, Nick Scott, Meera Shekar, et al. 2021. "The COVID-19 Crisis Will Exacerbate Maternal and Child Undernutrition and Child Mortality in Low- and Middle-Income Countries." *Nature Food* 2: 476–84.

Oviedo-Solís, Cecilia Isabel, Eric A. Monterrubio-Flores, Gustavo Cediel, Edgar Denova-Gutíerrez, and Simón Barquera. 2022. "Trend of Ultraprocessed Product Intake Is Associated with the Double Burden of Malnutrition in Mexican Children and Adolescents." *Nutrients* 14 (20): 4347. https://doi.org/10.3390/nu14204347.

PAHO (Pan American Health Organization). 2021. *Sugar-Sweetened Beverage Taxation in the Region of the Americas.* Washington, DC: PAHO.

Pérez-Escamilla, Rafael, Josefa L. Martinez, and Sofia Segura-Pérez. 2016. "Impact of the Baby-Friendly Hospital Initiative on Breastfeeding and Child Health Outcomes: A Systematic Review." *Maternal Child Nutrition* 12 (3): 402–17. https://doi.org/10.1111/mcn.12294.

Pérez-Escamilla, Rafael, Cecília Tomori, Sonia Hernández-Cordero, Phillip Baker, Aluisio J. D. Barros, France Bégin, Donna J. Chapman, et al. for the 2023 Lance Breastfeeding Series Group. 2023. "Breastfeeding: Crucially Important, But Increasingly Challenged in a Market-Driven World." *The Lancet* 401 (10375): 472–85. https://doi.org/10.1016/S0140-6736(22)01932-8.

Popkin, Barry M., Simon Barquera, Camila Corvalan, Karen J. Hofman, Carlos Monteiro, Shu Wen Ng, Elizabeth C. Swart, et al. 2021. "Towards Unified and Impactful Policies to Reduce Ultra-Processed Food Consumption and Promote Healthier Eating." *The Lancet Diabetes & Endocrinolology* 9 (7): 462–70. https://doi.org/10.1016/S2213-8587(21)00078-4.

Pries, Alissa M., Nita Sharma, Atul Upadhyay, Andrea M. Rehman, Suzanne Filteau, and Elaine L. Ferguson. 2019. "Energy Intake from Unhealthy Snack Food /Beverage among 12-23-Month-Old Children in Urban Nepal." *Maternal & Child Nutrition* 15 (Supplement 4): e12775. https://doi.org/10.1111/mcn.12775.

Rauber, Fernanda, Maria Laura de Costa Louzada, Euridice Martinez Steele, Leandro F. M. de Rezende, Christopher Millett, Carlos A. Monteiro, and Renata B. Levy. 2019. "Ultra-Processed Foods and Excessive Free Sugar Intake in the UK: A Nationally Representative Cross-Sectional Study." *BMJ Open* 9 (10): e027546.

Reyes, Marcela, Maria-Luisa Garmendia, Sonia Olivares, Claudio Aqueveque, Isabel Zacarías, and Camila Corvalán. 2019. "Development of the Chilean Front-of-Package Food Warning Label." *BMC Public Health* 19: 906.

Rogers, Nina Trivedy, David I. Conway, Oliver Mytton, Chrissy H. Roberts, Harry Rutter, Andrea Sherriff, Martin White, and Jean Adams. 2023. "Estimated Impact of the UK Soft Drinks Industry Levy on Childhood Hospital Admissions for Carious Tooth Extractions: Interrupted Time Series Analysis." *BMJ Nutrition, Prevention & Health* 6 (2): 243–52. https://doi.org/10.1136/bmjnph-2023 -000714.

Rogers, Nina T., Stephen Cummins, Hannah Forde, Catrin P. Jones, Oliver Mytton, Harry Rutter, Stephen J. Sharp, et al. 2023. "Associations between Trajectories of Obesity Prevalence in English Primary School Children and the UK Soft Drinks Industry Levy: An Interrupted Time Series Analysis of Surveillance Data." *PLoS Med* 20 (1): e1004160. https://doi.org/10.1371/journal.pmed.1004160.

Rollins, Nigel, Ellen Piwoz, Phillip Baker, Gillian Kingston, Kopano Matlwa Mabaso, David McCoy, Paulo Augusto Ribeira Neves, et al. for the 2023 Lance Breastfeeding Series Group. 2023. "Marketing of Commercial Milk Formula: A System to Capture Parents, Communities, Science, and Policy." *The Lancet* 401 (10375): 486–502. https://doi.org/10.1016/S0140-6736(22)01931-6.

Sassi, Franco, Maxime Roche, Annalisa Belloni, Elisa Pineda, and Jack Olney. 2022. *Food Taxes for Healthy Eating.* London: Centre for Health Economics and Policy Innovation, Imperial College London.

Shin, S., A. M. Alqunaibet, R. F. Alsukait, A. Alruwaily, Rasha Abdulrahman Alfawaz, Abdullah Algwizani, Christopher H. Herbst, et al. 2023. "A Randomized Controlled Study to Test Front-of-Pack (FOP) Nutrition Labels in the Kingdom of Saudi Arabia." *Nutrients* 15 (13): 2904. https://doi.org/10.3390/nu15132904.

Snowdon, Wendy, Mark Lawrence, Jimaima Schultz, Paula Vivili, and Boyd Swinburn 2010. "Evidence-Informed Process to Identify Policies That Will Promote a Healthy Food Environment in the Pacific Islands." *Public Health Nutrition* 13 (6): 886–92. https://doi.org/10.1017/S136898001000011X.

Spruk, Rok, and Mitja Kovač. 2020. "Does a Ban on Trans Fats Improve Public Health: Synthetic Control Evidence from Denmark." *Swiss Journal of Economics and Statistics* 156: 4.

Sturm, Roland, Ruopeng An, Darren Segal, and Deepak Patel. 2013. "A Cash-Back Rebate Program for Healthy Food Purchases in South Africa: Results from Scanner Data." *American Journal of Preventive Medicine* 44 (6): 567–72.

Subandoro, Ali Winoto, Silvia Holschneider, and Julie Ruel Bergeron. 2021. *Operationalizing Multisectoral Nutrition Programs to Accelerate Progress: A Nutrition Governance Perspective*. Health, Nutrition and Population Discussion Paper. Washington, DC: World Bank.

Subandoro, Ali Winoto, Kyoko Okamura, Michelle Mehta, Huihui Wang, Naina Ahluwalia, Elyssa Finkel, Andrea L. S. Bulungu, et al. 2022. "Positioning Nutrition with Universal Health Coverage: Optimizing Health Financing Levers. Health, Nutrition and Population." Discussion Paper. Washington, DC: World Bank. http://hdl.handle.net/10986/36867.

SUN (Scaling Up Nutrition). 2023. *SUN Movement Stocktake 2022*. Geneva: SUN Movement. https://scalingupnutrition.org/sites/default/files/2023-10/SUN%20Movement%202022%20Annual%20Report.pdf.

Swinburn, Boyd A., Vivica I. Kraak, Steven Allender, Vincent J. Atkins, Phillip I. Baker, Jessica R. Bogard, Hannah Brinsden, et al. 2019. "The Global Syndemic of Obesity, Undernutrition, and Climate Change: *The Lancet* Commission Report." *The Lancet* 393 (10173): 791–846. https://doi.org/10.1016/S0140-6736(18)32822-8.

Taillie, Lindsey Smith, Maxime Bercholz, Barry Popkin, Marcela Reyes, M. Arantxa Colchero, and Camila Corvalán. 2021. "Changes in Food Purchases after the Chilean Policies on Food Labelling, Marketing, and Sales in Schools: A Before and After Study." *The Lancet Planet Health* 5 (8): e526–33. https://doi.org/10.1016/S2542-5196(21)00172-8.

Teng, Andrea M., Amanda C. Jones, Anja Mizdrak, Louise Signal, Murat Genç, and Nick Wilson. 2019. "Impact of Sugar-Sweetened Beverage Taxes on Purchases and Dietary Intake: Systematic Review and Meta-Analysis." *Obesity Reviews* 20 (9): 1187–204. https://doi.org/10.1111/obr.12868.

Tristan Asensi, Marta, Antonia Napoletano, Francesco Sofi, and Monica Dinu. 2023. "Low-Grade Inflammation and Ultra-Processed Foods Consumption: A Review." *Nutrients* 15 (6): 1546.

USDHHS (U.S. Department of Health and Human Services). 2024. *Dietary Reference Intakes*. Washington, DC: USDHHS. https://health.gov/our-work/nutrition -physical-activity/dietary-guidelines/dietary-reference-intakes.

Venson, Auburth Henrik, Larissa Barbosa Cardoso, Flaviane Souza Santiago, Kênia Barreiro de Souza, and Renata Moraes Bielemann. 2023. "Price Elasticity of Demand for Ready-to-Drink Sugar-Sweetened Beverages in Brazil." *PLoS ONE* 18 (11): e0293413. https://doi.org/10.1371/journal.pone.0293413.

Vilar-Compte, Mireya, Sonia Hernández Cordero, Ana C. Castañeda-Márquez, Nigel Rollins, Gillian Kingston, and Rafael Pérez-Escamilla. 2022. "Follow-Up and Growing-Up Formula Promotion among Mexican Pregnant Women and Mothers of Children under 18 Months Old." *Maternal & Child Nutrition* 18 (S3): e13337. https://doi.org/10.1111/mcn.13337.

Weng, Stephen Franklin, Sarah A. Redsell, Julie A. Swift, Min Yang, and Cristine P. Glazebrook. 2012. "Systematic Review and Meta-Analyses of Risk Factors for Childhood Overweight Identifiable during Infancy." *Archives of Disease in Childhood* 97 (12): 1019–26. https://doi.org/10.1136/archdischild-2012-302263.

WHO (World Health Organization). 1981. "International Code of Marketing of Breast-Milk Substitutes." WHO, Geneva.

WHO (World Health Organization). 2006. *Guidelines on Food Fortification with Micronutrients*. Geneva: WHO.

WHO (World Health Organization). 2015. *Guideline: Sugars Intake for Adults and Children*. Geneva: WHO. Accessed April 12, 2024, https://iris.who.int/bitstream /handle/10665/149782/9789241549028_eng.pdf?sequence=1.

WHO (World Health Organization). 2022. *Marketing of Breast-Milk Substitutes: National Implementation of the International Code, Status Report 2022*. Geneva: WHO.

WHO (World Health Organization). 2023a. *Global Report on the Use of Sugar-Sweetened Beverage Taxes*. Geneva: WHO. https://www.who.int/publications/i/item /9789240084995.

WHO (World Health Organization). 2023b. "Implementation of the Baby-Hospital Initiative: Updated August 2023." Geneva: WHO.

WHO (World Health Organization). 2024a. *Establishing Global Nutrient Requirements*. Geneva: WHO. https://www.who.int/activities/establishing-global-nutrient -requirements.

WHO (World Health Organization). 2024b. "The Global Database on the Implementation of Nutrition Action (GINA)." Geneva: WHO. Accessed March 8, 2024, https://extranet.who.int/nutrition/gina/en/home.

WHO (World Health Organization). 2024c. *Trans-Fatty Acid Country Score Card*. Geneva: WHO. Accessed March 19, 2024, https://extranet.who.int/nutrition /gina/en/scorecard/TFA.

Widarjono, Agus, Rifai Afin, Gita Kusnadi, Muhammad Zufiqar Firdaus, and Olivia Herlinda. 2023. "Taxing Sugar Sweetened Beverages in Indonesia: Projections of Demand Change and Fiscal Revenue." *PLoS One* 18 (12): e0293913. https://doi .org10.1371/journal.pone.0293913.

World Bank. 2020. *Taxes on Sugar-Sweetened Beverages: International Evidence and Experiences*. Washington, DC: World Bank.

World Bank. 2023. "Global SSB Tax Database." August 2023 version. Washington, DC: World Bank. https://ssbtax.worldbank.org/.

World Bank. 2024a. "Climate-Smart Agriculture." Washington, DC: World Bank. https://www.worldbank.org/en/topic/climate-smart-agriculture.

World Bank. 2024b. *Distributional Effects of Taxation of Processed Foods in Brazil*. Washington, DC: World Bank.

World Bank. Forthcoming. *Reshaping the Agrifood Sector for Healthier Diets: Exploring the Links between Agrifood Public Support and Diet Quality*.

7

Costs, Benefits, Effectiveness, and Efficiency of Nutrition Interventions

Nick Scott, Meera Shekar, Mireya Vilar-Compte, Chiara Dell'Aira, and Jonathan Kweku Akuoku

KEY MESSAGES

- The additional financing needed to address undernutrition by scaling up a set of evidence-based, high-impact nutrition interventions to 90 percent coverage globally in 2025–34 is $128 billion (approximately $13 billion annually, or $13 per pregnant woman and $17 per child younger than age five years per annum), in addition to the $6.3 billion per annum already being spent to maintain the status quo coverage for addressing undernutrition.

- Financing needs for obesity prevention programs are significantly lower (and harder to quantify), although case studies indicate approximately $3.4–$3.6 purchasing power parity (PPP) per capita annually is required.

- Of the additional financing needs, $52 billion (40 percent) is required for the first five-year period (2025–29), and $76 billion (60 percent) is needed for the subsequent five years (2030–34).

- Some 77 percent ($98 billion) of these needs are for low- and middle-income countries, with $43 billion (34 percent) in South Asia, $34 billion (26 percent) in Sub-Saharan Africa, $19 billion (15 percent) in East Asia and Pacific, and $16 billion (12 percent) in the Middle East and North Africa, reflecting the disproportional burden of poor nutrition outcomes in these regions.

- Scaling up the full set of nutrition interventions could lead to major health and nutrition impacts globally over the 10-year period 2025–34, averting 6.2 million deaths among children under five years old, 27 million stunting cases among children turning age five, 47 million episodes of under-five wasting, 77 million cases of under-five anemia, 6.6 million low birthweight births, 144 million cases of maternal anemia, and 980,000 stillbirths. Such measures could also lead to an additional 85 million exclusively breastfed children.

- The economic benefits of investing in nutrition far outweigh the costs of inaction, highlighting the potential to build human capital and drive global economic development and prosperity. Across the high-burden and high-priority countries assessed, the full scale-up of interventions could generate $2.4 trillion in economic benefits, with a benefit–cost ratio of 23.

- Although the 2017 *Investment Framework for Nutrition* (Shekar et al. 2017) ambitiously estimated financing needs based on the full scale-up of nutrition interventions, this update goes one step further by also optimizing spending to maximize improvements in resource-limited settings. If only 25 percent or 50 percent of total financing needs were met, priority interventions would be as follows:

  - Cash transfers (accompanied with nutrition education or behavior change communication), vitamin A supplementation, preventive zinc supplementation for children, and intermittent preventive treatment of malaria in pregnancy (IPTp) to reduce stunting (and depending on country-specific epidemiological indicators, mixtures of multiple micronutrient supplements [MMS] for pregnant women, small-quantity lipid-based nutrient supplements [SQ-LNS] for children, and infant and young child nutrition counseling)

  - Vitamin A supplementation, preventive zinc supplementation, and SQ-LNS for children to reduce child wasting

  - Delayed cord clamping at birth and micronutrient powders for reducing child anemia

  - Kangaroo mother care and infant and young child nutrition counseling to improve breastfeeding

  - MMS and IPTp for pregnant women to reduce maternal anemia

  - Consideration of prioritizing interventions that affect multiple conditions in countries with a high prevalence of multiple poor nutrition outcomes, such as SQ-LNS for children or MMS for pregnant women.

- Countries can optimize spending by investing in the most cost-effective combination of interventions for their specific context. Each country also has unique contexts and implementation challenges in reprioritizing spending, with varying impacts.

- Financing needs for obesity-reduction interventions are difficult to estimate because they are primarily to support policies. Case studies in Bulgaria, Mexico, and South Africa estimate the relevant costs at approximately $3.5–$3.6 PPP per capita annually; for each $1 PPP invested, approximately $4–$5 PPP, on average, will be returned in economic benefits each year during 2020–50. Mass media campaigns seem to have the largest savings impact associated with reductions in labor market costs, and mass media and food labeling seem to have the largest impacts on health expenditures. Furthermore, some of the policies, such as taxes on unhealthy foods, will generate additional revenue that can offset intervention costs. In Colombia, for example, sugar-sweetened beverage taxes are estimated to generate $700 million annually.

- In Bulgaria, Mexico, and South Africa, the economic costs of overweight and obesity on per capita labor market outputs based on average wages ($ PPP per year), estimated as an average between 2020 and 2050, range from $88 in South Africa to $417 in Bulgaria. If no changes in policy occur, annual costs of treating diseases associated with overweight will amount to, on average, 9 percent of total health spending in Mexico and 8 percent in South Africa and Bulgaria.

Analytic Approaches

This section lays out the overall methodological approaches used in estimating the costs and impacts of scaling up evidence-based interventions to accelerate progress toward achieving the Sustainable Development Goal (SDG) targets for key nutrition outcomes, as well as the approaches to estimating the cost–benefit analyses. The analyses cover the five SDG 2.2 targets of (1) maternal anemia and child stunting, (2) wasting, (3) exclusive breastfeeding, (4) low birthweight (LBW), and (5) child anemia. Proven interventions with quantifiable impacts for all five targets can be modeled. The obesity target is treated differently, focusing primarily on policy approaches, as outlined in chapter 6. Overall, this methodology draws heavily from the approaches adopted in the 2017 *Investment Framework for Nutrition* (Shekar et al. 2017), and any changes to the assumptions and approaches (for example, for obesity prevention) are noted accordingly.

Selection of Outcomes and Interventions

The 2017 *Investment Framework* focused on addressing four of the six World Health Assembly (WHA) and SDG 2.2 targets: stunting, wasting, exclusive breastfeeding, and anemia among women. The targets for LBW and overweight were excluded at the time because of the lack of proven interventions or unavailability of prevalence data. Since then, the data and evidence landscape has evolved. Modeled estimates of LBW data have been developed jointly by the WHO and UNICEF, with the first series released in 2019 (UNICEF and WHO 2019) and updated in 2023. In addition, there is growing consensus on meaningful interventions to address LBW; many of these interventions also have impacts on other nutrition outcomes and have yielded quantifiable data that can be modeled using available tools. For overweight and obesity, the evidence base continues to develop, and current intervention approaches largely focus on sectoral policies to disincentivize poor food and nutrition choices, promote the availability and accessibility of healthier options, reduce consumption of unhealthy foods, and promote increased physical activity (Shekar and Popkin 2020). Although promising, the available evidence cannot be modeled using existing tools. Therefore, these policies are presented as a narrative rather than included in the impact model.

Child anemia was excluded from the previous analysis because, at the time, the focus was strictly on WHA target outcomes. Yet, SDG 2.2 sets an ambitious aim of ending all forms of hunger, including anemia among children. Furthermore, there is a strong evidence base for interventions that demonstrate significant impacts on reducing the prevalence of child anemia.

The Lancet's Series on Maternal and Child Nutrition, first published in 2008 (Bhutta et al. 2008) and updated in 2013 (Bhutta et al. 2013) and 2021 (Keats et al. 2021), identified a set of high-impact, evidence-based interventions for addressing the nutrition outcomes of interest. This evidence base was amplified through a series of additional rigorous reviews, examining the latest evidence across multiple sectors, as discussed in chapter 5. The interventions considered can influence the outcomes of interest through both direct and indirect pathways, as outlined in figure 7A.2 in annex 7A, depicting the relationships among interventions, risk factors, and mortality. For example, randomized trials of vitamin A and zinc supplementation for children have shown direct impacts on reducing diarrhea incidence, and these effects on diarrhea are then assumed (based on other studies) to influence the risk of stunting and wasting, whereas randomized trials of small-quantity lipid-based nutrient supplements (SQ-LNS) for children have shown direct effects on reducing stunting and wasting.

Country Sample Selection

Low- and middle-income countries (LMICs) tend to have the greatest burden of malnutrition; this is reflected in the selection of countries for the analysis presented in this chapter, which focuses on a sample of countries with the greatest absolute burden and greatest prevalence of each of the key malnutrition outcomes. For each outcome, the 20 countries with the greatest burden were selected for inclusion.[1] In addition, countries with prevalence values above a certain threshold of programmatic and policy significance were also included. For example, countries not in the top 20 stunting and wasting burden countries were included if they had stunting prevalence above 30 percent or wasting prevalence above 15 percent, both of which are levels of very high public health significance (de Onis et al. 2019). Countries selected according to these criteria are listed in annex 7B (refer to table 7B.1). This approach ensures representation of both large countries, which contribute disproportionately to the global burden, and smaller countries with high prevalence rates, which would have significant implications for human capital development and economic growth.

Although analysis of each nutrition outcome relies on data from the set of sample countries, the overall aim of the financing analysis is to estimate the total global financing need to accelerate progress toward achieving the nutrition SDG 2.2 targets. Following the approach of the 2017 *Investment Framework*, a multiplier (displayed and described in table 7B.2 and the "Subanalyses by Condition" section of annex 7B, respectively) is used to extrapolate the estimated costs and impacts from the sample countries to all countries. For each target, the multiplier is simply the inverse of the proportion of the global burden represented by the countries in the sample. In the case of the wasting target, a multiplier of 1/0.841, or 1.19, is applied to the sample estimates to approximate the total cost in all LMICs. This approach, although imperfect, is consistent with the 2017 *Investment Framework* and previous costing studies (Horton et al. 2010) and assumes that, on average, the cost of delivering interventions in LMICs outside the sample is similar to the estimates produced for the LMICs that are part of the sample.

Intervention Costing

Unit costs from existing sources are used for the analysis and are sourced from previous analytical studies conducted by the World Bank (for example, investment cases, Optima Nutrition), a review of recent literature, and the global costs taken from the 2017 *Investment Framework*.

These sources used both program experience and "ingredients-based," bottom-up costing to estimate the unit costs of interventions. A program experience approach to costing uses empirical expenditure and beneficiary coverage data to estimate the total and unit costs for delivering an intervention, incorporating the various direct costs and inefficiencies associated with that delivery. In some instances, intervention-level expenditure data are not readily available, and an alternative approach is required to derive intervention cost estimates. An ingredients-based approach itemizes and costs every component necessary for delivering an intervention to one beneficiary. These include the cost of commodities, equipment, personnel time, logistics, and other program administration costs. This approach assumes that the intervention is delivered as efficiently as possible, without inefficiencies, such as wastage or the wrong staff mix. When both types of costing data are available for an intervention in a country, preference is given to estimates derived from the program experience approach.

The unit cost for each intervention is estimated for each country in the sample. When this cost is not available for a particular country, the average unit cost for other countries in the same region is used. In cases in which there are no unit cost data for any country in a region, the average unit cost from other regions is used, and a regional adjustment factor is applied, which is consistent with the 2017 *Investment Framework* and Horton et al. (2010). Unit costs are summarized in annex 7C.

Intervention Scale-Up

The total financing need for each intervention is estimated as the incremental cost of scaling up from baseline coverage to 90 percent, as follows:

$$FN_y = UC \times IC_y \times Pop_y,$$

where FN_y represents the annual financing required for a specific intervention in year y, UC denotes the unit cost, IC_y refers to the incremental coverage expected for year y, and Pop_y indicates the target population for that year. This is done for each country in the sample, and the total financing need per nutrition target is the sum of the total financing need over the 10-year analytic horizon for all interventions included in the target.

Unit costs were assumed to be constant for each intervention, because limited evidence is available to inform how unit costs may vary with scale (which may lead to underestimating costs at high coverage) or efficiencies when interventions are delivered as a package (which may lead to overestimation of costs). Country-specific assessments will be required to disaggregate costs by sector or delivery platform.

It is assumed that interventions are scaled up to 90 percent coverage over a five-year period and maintained at full coverage for a subsequent five years. This is the same approach used in the 2017 *Investment Framework* and allows for children to benefit from the interventions over the critical first five years of life. The impacts of the interventions are modeled using the Optima Nutrition tool (Pearson et al. 2018), which replicates the cohort-based impact modeling of the Lives Saved Tool. By modeling an additional five years after interventions reach 90 percent coverage, the analysis captures the downstream benefits that some interventions can have over the five years they are tracked in the model. For example, it accounts for the benefits that interventions given to pregnant women can provide in reducing small for gestational age (SGA) births, a key risk factor for stunting among children.

Estimating Intervention Impacts

The impacts of interventions were modeled using the aforementioned Optima Nutrition tool, an allocative efficiency modeling tool that includes a component to model the scale-up of one or multiple interventions. The Optima Nutrition tool can estimate the impact of changing coverage of interventions on nutrition, mortality, and morbidity outcomes for children younger than age five years and women of reproductive age. Interventions were classified according to which nutrition outcomes they affect (child stunting, wasting, anemia, breastfeeding, LBW, or maternal anemia, with multiple impacts possible). For each nutrition outcome, the package of interventions was scaled up in the corresponding high-burden and high-priority countries. The estimated impact in these sample countries was then extrapolated to a global estimate using the multipliers mentioned in the "Country Sample Selection" section (and listed in table 7B.2 of annex 7B).

Benefit–Cost Analysis

The improved health and nutrition outcomes gained from scaling up interventions were translated into economic benefits in the form of increased potential income, from either increased workforce size (from deaths averted) or increased workforce productivity (from improved child development or reduced maternal anemia).

The economic benefits included in this analysis were as follows: for stunting interventions, child deaths averted and increased future productivity (based on Hoddinott et al. 2013); for wasting interventions, deaths averted (Horton and Ross 2003); for child anemia interventions, maternal and child deaths averted and increased future productivity (based on Horton and Ross 2003);

for breastfeeding interventions, deaths averted and increased future productivity (based on Hanushek and Woessman 2008, and Wigg et al. 1998); for LBW interventions, deaths averted and increased future productivity (based on Alderman and Behrman 2006); and for maternal anemia interventions, maternal deaths averted, child deaths averted, and improved productivity among women in some occupations (based on Horton and Ross 2003). In addition, multiple micronutrient supplements (MMS) for pregnant women have been shown to reduce stillbirths, and these benefits were considered where this intervention was scaled up. Sensitivity analyses were conducted considering only mortality benefits.

For all components of these benefits, working life was assumed to be ages 18–65 years, with potential earnings based on per capita GDP, adjusted for annual GDP growth, labor share of GDP, and percentage of lifetime earnings that could be realized. Not all children who receive the interventions will survive until age 18 or for the entire age 18–65 working life to fully accrue these benefits; thus, adjustments were made for country- and age-specific all-cause mortality across the life of the cohorts who receive the interventions.

Although intervention costs are incurred in the present, economic benefits will only accrue sometime in the future. Following the approach in the 2017 *Investment Framework*, costs and benefits are discounted to present value. The discount rate to apply has been continually debated. For this analysis, we follow the most recent guidance from the World Health Organization's Choosing Interventions that are Cost-Effective project and apply a base discount rate of 3 percent to both costs and benefits (Bertram et al. 2021). Sensitivity analyses are included with a 5 percent discount rate applied to both costs and benefits and with no benefits discounting.

Economic benefit estimates may be underestimated for a number of reasons: first, we have calculated economic benefits as increased potential income, which is a more conservative approach than using Value of Statistical Life methods; second, long-term benefits of improved undernutrition on noncommunicable diseases (NCDs) are not estimated; and third, a static model is used to capture the increased size of the productive labor force, which does not include any second-order benefits from increased human capital accumulation. However, the economic benefits may be overestimated because secular improvements may reduce rates of disease and malnutrition in the absence of interventions. Additional details on the benefit calculations are in annex 7D.

Allocative Efficiency Analysis

The 2017 *Investment Framework* proposed an ambitious level of investment from country governments and development partners to accelerate progress toward achieving the SDG targets for nutrition. In most contexts, significant resource constraints and competing health and development priorities result in less-than-ideal levels of funding for nutrition programs. To maximize the impact of the available resources for nutrition, an allocative efficiency analysis was undertaken for each country in the sample using the Optima Nutrition modeling tool to identify sets of interventions that can achieve the greatest impact for a fixed budget. The scenarios considered optimizing resources if 0 percent, 25 percent, and 50 percent of additional financing needs are met. For stunting, the objective was to maximize alive and nonstunted children, whereas for wasting, child anemia, and maternal anemia, the objective was to minimize the prevalence of these conditions. Optimizations for breastfeeding (for which only two interventions are available and included in the analysis) or LBW (full-impact pathways are not currently available in the model) were not considered in this example. Similarly, no optimizations are feasible for obesity prevention.

Results

Although the estimation of financing needs was performed for each SDG 2.2 target (except obesity, which is summarized later in this chapter), in real-world scenarios policy makers generally do not focus solely on improving one specific nutrition outcome. A comprehensive nutrition policy and programming approach is essential to address multiple interrelated nutrition goals simultaneously and achieve the SDG 2.2 targets. Recognizing this, the following section presents a comprehensive package that integrates various nutrition interventions as well as the total financing needs to implement them, using an evidence-based approach. Detailed analyses for each individual SDG target are presented in annex 7D,which outline the interventions included, unit costs, and assumptions used for the intervention coverage (baseline and scale-up).

Estimated Total Financing Need

Scaling up the set of evidence-based nutrition interventions to 90 percent coverage was estimated to require an additional $128 billion (discounted) for the 10-year period 2025–34 (refer to figure 7.1). This average additional $13 billion per year is approximately $13 per pregnant woman and $17 per child younger than age five years per annum, and it is on top of the

Figure 7.1 Total Global Financing Needs, Undiscounted, for Full Scale-Up of Undernutrition Interventions

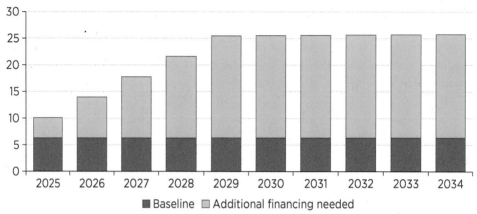

Annual costs 2023 (US$, billions, undiscounted)

■ Baseline ■ Additional financing needed

Source: Original figure for this publication.
Note: Dark blue bars = costs of maintaining existing intervention coverage, light blue bars = the annual additional financing requirements to increase the coverage of interventions to 90 percent over a five-year period (2025–29) and maintain coverage for an additional five years.

estimated $6.3 billion per annum that is already being spent to maintain the status quo coverage (refer to chapter 9).

Of the additional financing needs, $52 billion (40 percent) is required for the five-year intervention scale-up period (2025–29), and $76 billion (60 percent) is required for the subsequent five years (2030–34) to maintain coverage.

A large proportion of the financing needed to scale up interventions is for South Asia ($43 billion; 34 percent) and Sub-Saharan Africa ($34 billion; 26 percent), with an additional $19 billion (15 percent) for East Asia and Pacific and $16 billion (12 percent) for the Middle East and North Africa (refer to figure 7.2, panel a), reflecting the disproportional burden of poor nutrition outcomes in these regions, and 77 percent ($98 billion) of financing needs are for LMICs (refer to figure 7.2, panel b).

Most of the costs of the full scale-up scenario are for treatment of severe acute malnutrition (SAM) ($39 billion; 30 percent), micronutrient powders for children ($20 billion; 16 percent), SQ-LNS for children ($17 billion; 13 percent), and MMS for pregnant women ($16 billion; 13 percent) (refer to figure 7.2, panel c).

Figure 7.2 Global Financing Needs to Scale Up Undernutrition Interventions, by World Bank Region, Country Income Level, and Intervention

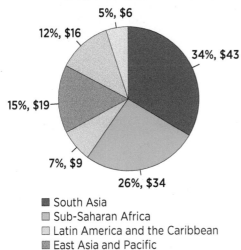

a. Financing needs by region
(US$, billions, discounted)

- ■ South Asia
- ▨ Sub-Saharan Africa
- ☐ Latin America and the Caribbean
- ▨ East Asia and Pacific
- ▨ Middle East and North Africa
- ☐ Europe and Central Asia

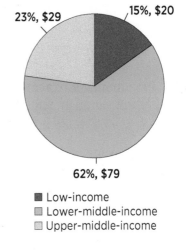

b. Financing needs by country income status (US$, billions, discounted)

- ■ Low-income
- ☐ Lower-middle-income
- ☐ Upper-middle-income

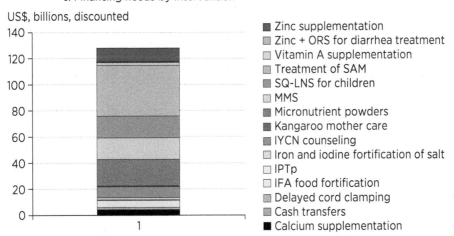

c. Financing needs by intervention

US$, billions, discounted

- ■ Zinc supplementation
- ▨ Zinc + ORS for diarrhea treatment
- ☐ Vitamin A supplementation
- ▨ Treatment of SAM
- ■ SQ-LNS for children
- ☐ MMS
- ▨ Micronutrient powders
- ■ Kangaroo mother care
- ▨ IYCN counseling
- ☐ Iron and iodine fortification of salt
- ☐ IPTp
- ☐ IFA food fortification
- ▨ Delayed cord clamping
- ▨ Cash transfers
- ■ Calcium supplementation

Source: Original figure for this publication, based on Optima Nutrition model outputs.

Note: Estimated cost to increase the coverage of interventions from their current levels to 90 percent over a five-year period (2025–29) and then maintain coverage for an additional five years. IFA = iron–folic acid; IPTp = intermittent preventive treatment of malaria in pregnancy; IYCN = infant and young child nutrition; MMS = multiple micronutrient supplements; ORS = oral rehydrating solution; SAM = severe acute malnutrition; SQ-LNS = small-quantity lipid-based nutrient supplement.

Anticipated Impacts of the Investments

Outcomes by Condition

The full scale-up of nutrition interventions could avert 6.2 million deaths among children younger than age five years and 980,000 stillbirths between 2025–34 and have positive impacts on other nutrition outcomes.

When considering specific interventions for each nutrition outcome of interest, in 2025–34,

- Stunting interventions would require an additional $53 billion (discounted), which could avert an additional 27 million stunting cases among children turning age five

- Wasting interventions would require an additional $80 billion (discounted), which could avert an additional 47 million wasting episodes among children younger than age five

- Child anemia interventions would require an additional $41 billion (discounted), which could avert an additional 77 million cases of anemia among children younger than age five

- Early breastfeeding interventions would require an additional $7 billion (discounted), which could lead to an additional 85 million exclusively breastfed children

- LBW interventions would require an additional $14 billion (discounted), which could avert an additional 6.6 million LBW births

- Maternal anemia interventions would require an additional $20 billion (discounted), which could avert an additional 144 million cases of anemia among pregnant women.

Note that, because some interventions affect multiple conditions, the total costs by nutrition outcome presented in table 7.1 do not add up to the total costs of the full scale-up scenario.

Note also that in the 2017 *Investment Framework*, the projected reductions in child stunting cases averted include the estimated impact of scaling up the high-impact investments, as well as an estimated decline associated with improvements in women's education, women's health, dietary diversity, and food availability. Given the recent polycrises over the past five years, similar improvements in these indicators are not expected. Furthermore, a recent WHO discussion paper (WHO and UNICEF 2024) suggests that if current trajectories in stunting continue, there could be 17.5 million fewer stunted children in 2034 compared with 2025 (138.2 million in 2025 versus

Table 7.1 Total Additional Financing Needs for Maternal Anemia, Low Birthweight, Breastfeeding, Child Stunting, Wasting, and Child Anemia, US$, Millions, 2025–34

Intervention	Maternal anemia	LBW	Breastfeeding	Stunting	Wasting	Child anemia	Full scale-up
Calcium supplementation				4,279			4,279
Cash transfers				1,715			1,718
Delayed cord clamping						56	56
IFA food fortification	4,710	4,048		4,395		4,299	5,371
IPTp	268	170		240			361
Iron and iodine fortification of salt	1,635					1,536	1,735
IYCN counseling			6,621	4,239	5,269		8,221
KMC			619				619
Micronutrient powders						20,378	20,429
MMS	13,836	9,402		12,891	12,280		16,399
SQ-LNS				13,930	12,263	14,856	16,673
Treatment of SAM					38,710		38,763
Vitamin A supplementation				1,879	2,139		2,256
Zinc + ORS for treatment of diarrhea					416		420
Zinc supplementation				9,292	9,236		10,576
Total	**20,449**	**13,620**	**7,240**	**52,861**	**80,313**	**41,126**	**127,876**

Source: Original table for this publication.
Note: Intervention costs are slightly different in the full scale-up scenario compared to when subsets of interventions are scaled up, due to population changes (such as fewer deaths resulting in different needs). IFA = iron–folic acid; IPTp = intermittent preventive treatment of malaria in pregnancy; IYCN = infant and young child nutrition; KMC = kangaroo mother care; LBW = low birthweight; MMS = multiple micronutrient supplements; ORS = oral rehydration solution; SAM = severe acute malnutrition; SQ-LNS = small-quantity lipid-based nutrient supplements.

120.7 million in 2034 [linearly extrapolated from WHA 2025–30 estimates without adjustments]). These would be over and above the estimated 27 million child stunting cases averted because of the scale-up of the proposed interventions.

Table 7.2 shows the impact and cost-effectiveness of individual interventions on different outcomes, estimated by comparing the scale-up scenario with and without the individual intervention. Many interventions, such as MMS for pregnant women and SQ-LNS for children, have benefits for multiple conditions at different degrees of cost-effectiveness. When combined, the full scale-up scenario was estimated to deliver impacts, with the following costs associated with each outcome:

- $20,700 per child death averted

- $4,800 per stunting case averted

- $2,700 per child wasting episode averted

- $1,700 per child anemia case averted

- $890 per maternal anemia case averted

- $1,500 per additional exclusively breastfed child.

These cost-effectiveness estimates relate to the total cost of the full package of interventions; however, some interventions stand out as having particularly favorable cost-per-case averted results (refer to table 7.2). This includes cash transfers in concert with behavior change communication or nutrition education and vitamin A supplementation for stunting; vitamin A supplementation, zinc supplementation, and SQ-LNS for wasting; delayed cord clamping at birth and micronutrient powders for child anemia; infant and young child nutrition counseling and kangaroo mother care (KMC) for breastfeeding; and intermittent preventive treatment of malaria in pregnancy (IPTp) and MMS for maternal anemia. For the cash transfers intervention, cost-effectiveness needs to be interpreted with significant caution because the unit cost used for this analysis does not factor in the cash itself, only the cost of combining the transfers with nutrition advice and messages to produce an impact on child stunting. This is because these transfers are usually implemented with the primary objective of poverty reduction rather than nutritional improvement. Yet, it does highlight how critical a multisectoral approach is to achieve the SDG targets and how different delivery platforms outside of health can be used to deliver nutrition services.

Table 7.2 Impact and Cost-Effectiveness of Interventions on Different Undernutrition Outcomes, US$

Intervention	Child deaths averted	Stunted children turning age five averted	Child wasting episodes averted*	Child anemia averted	Maternal anemia averted	Maternal deaths averted	Additional exclusively breastfed children
Full package of interventions							
Cost per case ($)	20,700	4,800	2,700	1,700	890	702,900	1,500
Impact (thousand cases)	6,192	26,682	47,093	76,798	144,201	182	85,060
Calcium supplementation							
Cost per case ($)	8,400	22,900					
Impact (thousand cases)	510	187	—	—	—	—	—
Cash transfers†							
Cost per case ($)	22,700	377					
Impact (thousand cases)	76	4,559	—	—	—	—	—
Delayed cord clamping							
Cost per case ($)				17			
Impact (thousand cases)	—	—	—	3,199	—	—	—
IFA food fortification							
Cost per case ($)	39,900			3,200	1,500	1,193,000	
Impact (thousand cases)	135	—	—	1,663	3,473	5	—
IPTp							
Cost per case ($)	2,700	1,800			124	58,700	
Impact (thousand cases)	133	200	—	—	2,911	6	—
Iron and iodine fortification of salt							
Cost per case ($)				721	300	247,700	
Impact (thousand cases)	—	—	—	2,407	5,008	7	—

(continued)

Table 7.2 Impact and Cost-Effectiveness of Interventions on Different Undernutrition Outcomes, US$ (continued)

Intervention	Child deaths averted	Stunted children turning age five averted	Child wasting episodes averted*	Child anemia averted	Maternal anemia averted	Maternal deaths averted	Additional exclusively breastfed children
IYCN counseling							
Cost per case ($)	16,700	7,300	3,400				97
Impact (thousand cases)	493	1,131	2,394	—	—	—	84,334
KMC							
Cost per case ($)	349						716
Impact (thousand cases)	1,775	—	—	—	—	—	864
Micronutrient powders							
Cost per case ($)				375			
Impact (thousand cases)	—	—	—	54,537	—	—	—
MMS							
Cost per case ($)	8,300	3,500	8,400		125	101,200	
Impact (thousand cases)	1,974	4,715	1,944	—	131,238	162	—
SQ-LNS							
Cost per case ($)	68,600	4,300	921	3,000			
Impact (thousand cases)	243	3,916	18,100	5,470			
Treatment of SAM							
Cost per case ($)	123,100						
Impact (thousand cases)	315	—	—	—	—	—	—
Vitamin A supplementation							
Cost per case ($)	13,800	508	204				
Impact (thousand cases)	163	4,444	11,064	—	—	—	—

(continued)

Table 7.2 Impact and Cost-Effectiveness of Interventions on Different Undernutrition Outcomes, US$ (continued)

Intervention	Child deaths averted	Stunted children turning age five averted	Child wasting episodes averted*	Child anemia averted	Maternal anemia averted	Maternal deaths averted	Additional exclusively breastfed children
Zinc + ORS for treatment of diarrhea							
Cost per case ($)	4,000						
Impact (thousand cases)	106	—	—	—	—	—	—
Zinc supplementation							
Cost per case ($)	89,500	1,700	690				
Impact (thousand cases)	118	6,348	15,331	—	—	—	—

Source: Original table for this publication.

Note: Attributable impacts were estimated by comparing the scale-up scenario with and without the intervention. This table is a simplified version of a more detailed cost-effectiveness table, with total costs per intervention, available in table 7E.1 of annex 7E. Cost per case values are presented in full numerical amounts. Dashes indicate that the intervention does not affect the corresponding outcome or the impact was not assessed as part of this analysis. KMC = kangaroo mother care; IFA = iron-folic acid; IPTp = intermittent preventive treatment of malaria in pregnancy; IYCN = infant and young child nutrition; MMS = multiple micronutrient supplements; ORS = oral rehydration solution; SAM = severe acute malnutrition; SQ-LNS = small-quantity lipid-based nutrient supplements.

* The Optima Nutrition model tracks the prevalence of wasting and anemia among children each year rather than by incidence; person-years of wasting and anemia averted from model outputs were converted to episodes and cases averted, respectively, by assuming a wasting relapse rate of 2.6 times per year and that anemia in children persists for the entire younger-than-age-five period.

† Cash transfers have a relatively high cost-effectiveness because the only costs included here are the additional requirements for IYCN communication campaigns to make cash transfers conditional or accompany cash transfers with nutrition messaging, with the assumption that cash transfers are instituted primarily for poverty reduction and therefore financed from other budgets.

Economic Benefits of the Investments

The full scale-up of nutrition interventions results not only in health and nutrition impacts, but also in substantial economic benefits. Economic returns associated with investing in stunting, wasting, child anemia, breastfeeding, LBW, and maternal anemia were estimated for each country in the corresponding high-burden and high-priority analytical sample. Country-level tables with net benefits and benefit–cost ratios are presented in annex 7E.

Across the high-burden and high-priority country sample considered, the full scale-up of interventions was estimated to generate $2.4 trillion in economic benefits, with a benefit–cost ratio of 23. Return on investment varied by country, related to country-specific epidemiological, demographic, and economic indicators (refer to annex 7E).

Overall, this underscores the substantial economic returns from scaling up the full package of interventions, although substantial economic and health gains can be achieved with less than the full amount required over the 10-year period.

Optimizing Investments for Maximum Impact

Optimization of Limited Budgets

Where resources are limited, decisions need to be made about how to prioritize efforts for maximal impact. Optima Nutrition was used to assess how resources could be optimally allocated across interventions if 0 percent, 25 percent, or 50 percent of total financing need was obtained (refer to figure 7.3).

The model demonstrates that improved nutrition outcomes could be achieved without additional resources by simply optimizing current spending (refer to table 7.3). If total financing needs could not be met and only limited resources were available, the following examples of cost-effective interventions were identified:

- *Stunting.* Cash transfers (accompanied with nutrition education or behavior change communication), vitamin A supplementation, preventive zinc supplementation for children, IPTp for pregnant women, and, depending on country-specific epidemiological indicators, mixtures of MMS for pregnant women, SQ-LNS for children, and infant and young child nutrition counseling

**Figure 7.3 Optimized Budget Allocations: Potential Scenarios If
0 percent, 25 percent, or 50 Percent of Additional
Financing Needs Are Met**

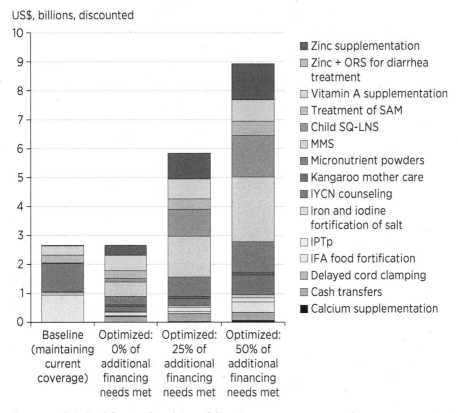

US$, billions, discounted

Legend:
- Zinc supplementation
- Zinc + ORS for diarrhea treatment
- Vitamin A supplementation
- Treatment of SAM
- Child SQ-LNS
- MMS
- Micronutrient powders
- Kangaroo mother care
- IYCN counseling
- Iron and iodine fortification of salt
- IPTp
- IFA food fortification
- Delayed cord clamping
- Cash transfers
- Calcium supplementation

x-axis categories:
- Baseline (maintaining current coverage)
- Optimized: 0% of additional financing needs met
- Optimized: 25% of additional financing needs met
- Optimized: 50% of additional financing needs met

Source: Original figure for this publication.
Note: Outcomes represent the aggregate of individual optimizations for each country and condition-specific intervention sets. Stunting interventions were optimized to maximize alive and nonstunted children turning age five in 2025–34; wasting, child anemia, and maternal anemia interventions were optimized to minimize the corresponding prevalence in 2034. Optimizations do not include the objective of breastfeeding (affected by only two interventions in the model, IYCN counseling and KMC) or LBW. Spending allocations are assumed to change in 2025 and remain fixed up to 2034. Baseline spending does not add up to the estimated $6.3 billion because not all spending is included in this optimization example. Spending on interventions does not necessarily reflect coverage because they each have different unit costs. IFA = iron–folic acid; IPTp = intermittent preventive treatment of malaria in pregnancy; IYCN = infant and young child nutrition; KMC = kangaroo mother care; LBW = low birthweight; MMS = multiple micronutrient supplements; ORS = oral rehydrating solutions; SAM = severe acute malnutrition; SQ-LNS = small-quantity lipid-based nutrient supplement.

Table 7.3 Impact of Optimization Scenarios versus Baseline Outcomes and Full Scale-Up Scenario, 2025–34

Modeled scenario	Additional alive, nonstunted children turning age five	Episodes of child wasting averted	Cases of child anemia averted	Cases of maternal anemia averted
Baseline	613,884,555	1,408,217,151	310,068,104	385,102,927
Optimized: 0% of additional financing needs met	13,068,053	13,452,354	11,554,583	33,939,774
Optimized: 25% of additional financing needs met	21,285,467	28,016,715	25,555,191	72,225,766
Optimized: 50% of additional financing needs met	25,792,475	32,342,632	37,847,748	93,957,472

Source: Original table for this publication.

Note: Breastfeeding and low birthweight outcomes are not included in this example. Regarding wasting optimizations, some optimized budgets achieve more impact on wasting episodes averted than the full scale-up scenario. This is because the full scale-up scenario includes significant investment in treatment of SAM, and although this prevents a lot of mortality among children suffering from wasting, it means wasting prevalence increases.

- *Wasting.* Vitamin A supplementation, preventive zinc supplementation, and SQ-LNS for children

- *Child anemia.* Delayed cord clamping and micronutrient powders

- *Maternal anemia.* MMS and IPTp for pregnant women.

For example, if only 25 percent of total financing need was obtained but new and current investments were optimized, compared with the full scale-up scenario, it may be possible to achieve 75 percent of the impact on stunting, 59 percent of the impact on wasting, 33 percent of the impact on child anemia, and 50 percent of the impact on maternal anemia.

Exclusive breastfeeding was not included in the optimizations because only two interventions affect these outcomes, KMC and infant and young child nutrition (IYCN) counseling (impacts and cost-effectiveness data for these interventions are shown in table 7.2). Although preventive zinc supplementation is prioritized in this optimization modeling on the basis of its impacts on reducing diarrhea incidence, in fact the platforms in place to support scale-up of stand-alone zinc supplementation are limited for both cost and logistical reasons.

This analysis considered high-burden and high-priority countries according to single nutrition outcomes. However, countries with high prevalence of multiple poor nutrition outcomes may consider prioritizing interventions that affect multiple conditions, such as SQ-LNS for children or MMS for pregnant women.

Each country will have unique contexts and practical barriers to shifting nutrition intervention spending and will need to undertake more detailed and localized analyses accounting for these constraints. However, the results presented here demonstrate the importance of allocative efficiency in nutrition programming.

Costs and Benefits of Implementing Policies to Tackle Overweight and Obesity

Because there are no meaningful global data available on this issue, this section summarizes evidence from three upper-middle-income countries in different world regions—Bulgaria, Mexico, and South Africa—on the costs associated with implementing obesity-related policies. The aim is to showcase how public health interventions addressing overweight and obesity are sound social investments. Data are based on the 2019 Organisation for Economic Co-operation and Development (OECD) estimations of the Strategic Public Health Planning for noncommunicable diseases (SPHeP-NCDs) model, which is an advanced modeling tool for public health policy. The model simulates the impact of major risk factors, including obesity, disease incidence, health expenditures, and the labor market.[2]

Costs of Inaction

Overweight and obesity are associated with chronic diseases that worsen health and decrease life expectancy. According to OECD estimates, from 2020 to 2050, overweight and its related diseases will reduce life expectancy by about 3.5 years in Bulgaria, 4.2 years in Mexico, and 1.7 years in South Africa. As shown in figure 7.4, if no policy changes occur, treating the diseases associated with overweight will cost, on average per year, 9 percent of total health expenditure in Mexico and approximately 8 percent of total health expenditure in Bulgaria and South Africa (net of spending for long-term care).

Overweight and obesity have also been linked to economic costs such as labor force participation and productivity. For example, absenteeism and

Figure 7.4 Annual Health Expenditures Associated with Overweight (Preobesity + Obesity) in Mexico, South Africa, and Bulgaria, 2020–50 Average

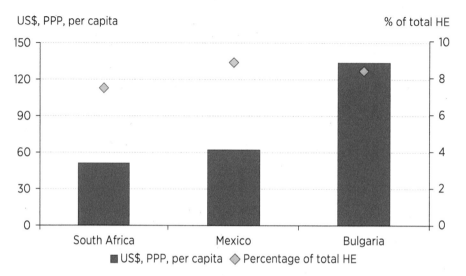

Source: OECD 2019.

Note: HE = health expenditure; PPP = purchasing power parity.

presenteeism can lead to wage payment without a return in productivity. Unemployment and early retirement affect the workforce through the loss of productive workers. Figure 7.5 summarizes such economic impacts as annual averages for 2020–50. Overweight will cost the economy $88 purchasing power parity (PPP) per year per person in South Africa, $210 PPP in Mexico, and $417 PPP in Bulgaria. Variation across countries is driven by differences in overweight and disease prevalence and is mainly due to wage differentials.

When combined, the impact of overweight and obesity on life expectancy, health expenditures, and labor market productivity has overall impacts on macroeconomic indicators. The OECD SPHeP-NCDs model projects that in 2020–50, overweight and obesity will reduce GDP by 5.3 percent in Mexico and 3.8 percent in South Africa (no estimates are available for Bulgaria).

Other models have also estimated the economic impacts associated with overweight and obesity. For example, the Global Obesity Observatory includes medical and nonmedical costs (such as travel costs to treatment), as well as indirect costs, including absenteeism, presenteeism, and premature mortality (World Obesity Federation 2024). Table 7.4 presents the economic costs of the selected countries as a percentage of GDP by 2050. Differences arise from methodological issues (such as assumptions and costs considered), but the estimated effects are within close ranges.

Figure 7.5 Economic Costs of Overweight (Preobesity + Obesity) on Per Capita Labor Market Output in Bulgaria, Mexico, and South Africa and Average Annual Wages, 2020–50

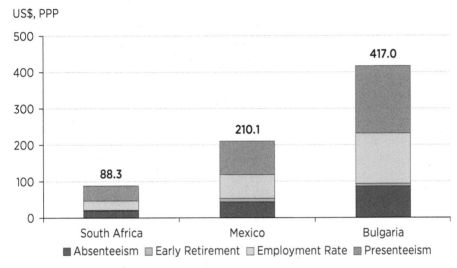

Source: OECD 2019.
Note: PPP = purchasing power parity.

Table 7.4 Economic Costs of Obesity, Estimated as Percentage Reduction in Gross Domestic Product by 2050, by Model

Model	Mexico	South Africa	Bulgaria
OECD SPHeP-NCDs, estimated reduction in 2020–50	5.3	3.8	NA
WOF Global Obesity Observatory, predicted by 2050	4.15	4.16	6.42

Source: Original table for this publication.
Note: NA = not available; OECD SPHeP-NCDs = Organisation for Economic Co-operation and Development Strategic Public Health Planning for noncommunicable diseases; WOF = World Obesity Federation.

Rationale for Action and Policy Options

There is a strong rationale for government intervention to tackle overweight and obesity, and there are a wide range of policies potentially available (see chapter 6). This section assesses four policies—food labeling, mass media campaigns, mobile apps, and advertising regulations—for Bulgaria, Mexico, and South Africa.

This section builds heavily on a recent OECD report (OECD 2019) and analyzes actions to tackle obesity in different regions in the three LMICs. Although the modeled costs are averages mainly used for high-income countries (HICs) and the model assumptions are based on literature applicable to HICs, they do provide some information on costs and benefits that countries can draw on to develop their own strategies.

Benefits and Costs of Implementing Obesity-Prevention Policies

The assumptions underlying the SPHeP-NCDs model are summarized in annex 7F. Based on such considerations, the model estimates the policies' impacts on morbidity and mortality, reduction in health expenditures, and labor market gains; implementation costs are computed for each country (see note 2). The interventions' implementation costs per country are presented in figure 7.6. Per capita annual costs per intervention are similar across countries. Food labeling and mass media campaigns carry higher costs (around $1.2 PPP per capita, annually) compared with food advertisement regulations and mobile apps (approximately $0.5 PPP per capita annually).

Figure 7.6 Costs of Implementing Selected Policies in Bulgaria, Mexico, and South Africa, Per Capita Annual Average, 2020–50

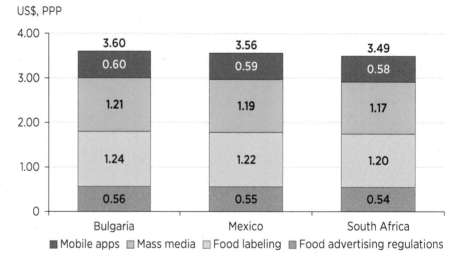

Source: OECD 2019.
Note: PPP = purchasing power parity.

The model predicts positive impacts on population health in Bulgaria, Mexico, and South Africa for all four interventions, which are estimated to improve life years (LYs) and disability-adjusted life years (DALYs). In all three assessed countries, the largest gains in LYs and DALYs are estimated for food labeling and mass media campaigns (see figure 7.7). Differences in the estimated magnitude across countries are due to differences in aspects such as the relative prevalence of overweight and the projected burden of premature mortality.

Findings from the model further estimate the reduction in health expenditures linked to the public health policies assessed annually, as well as cumulatively by 2050. Examining both estimates is critical: even in the short run, preexisting obesity cases may still be driving the expenses even if interventions are working. Hence, cumulative effects—estimated at health expenditure savings of $51.1 PPP in Bulgaria, $11.7 PPP in Mexico, and $8.5 PPP in South Africa (OECD 2019)[3]—may be more illustrative of the impact of these policies. Mass media campaigns and food labeling are estimated to generate the largest savings in health expenditures. Advertising regulations have a smaller relative effect on health expenditures, mostly because of the relatively short time horizon imputed into the model (that is, no life course impacts are imputed

Figure 7.7 Population-Standardized Effects of Selected Policies on Life Years Gained in Bulgaria, Mexico, and South Africa, 2020–50 Average

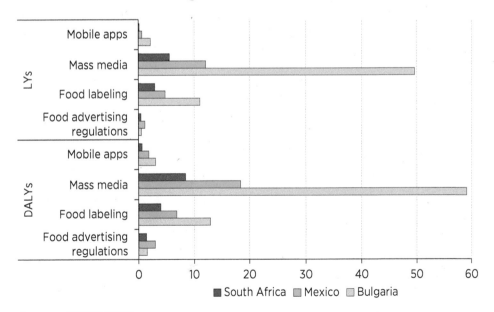

Source: OECD 2019.
Note: Data are LYs and DALYs gained per 100,000 population annually.
DALYs = disability-adjusted life years; LYs = life years.

into the model). Differences across countries result mainly from differentials in cost of medical care and life expectancy.

These health expenditure savings are compounded by additional positive impacts, including the combined labor productivity cost avoided by the interventions, as well as the overall macroeconomic impacts. As shown in figure 7.8, the public health interventions considered have important impacts on labor market outputs. When looking at the effect on total employment, the collective effect of the four policies would add an average of 1,796 workers annually to the workforce in Bulgaria, 29,795 in Mexico, and 5,521 in South Africa. In terms of specific policies, mass media campaigns have the largest impact—adding around 1,290 workers annually to the workforce in Bulgaria, 13,010 in Mexico, and 2,513 in South Africa, followed by food labeling in Bulgaria and regulations on advertising in Mexico and South Africa. When expressed in monetary terms (that is, converting missed work time into wages), estimates suggest important savings associated with reductions in labor market costs brought about by the interventions. Aggregating the impacts of the four interventions standardized by population size would lead to average annual savings (costs avoided) of $7.16 PPP in Bulgaria, $2.70 PPP in Mexico, and $0.88 PPP in South Africa. Mass media yields the largest savings, with up to $4.70 PPP per capita saved in Bulgaria, $1.20 PPP saved in Mexico, and $0.40 PPP saved in South Africa. The second-largest savings result from advertising regulations.

Figure 7.8 Effects of Selected Policies on Health in Bulgaria, Mexico, and South Africa, by Labor Market Impact

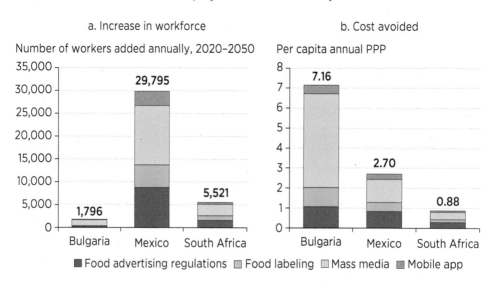

Source: OECD 2019.

Note: PPP= purchasing power parity.

The OECD (2019) estimates an average annual increase in GDP of 0.009 percent for food labelling, 0.021 percent for mass media campaigns, 0.006 percent for mobile apps, and 0.010 percent for advertising regulation for 2020–50. Combining the GDP increase with the cost of implementing the policies suggests good value for the money, because implementing food labeling and mobile apps is about 40 percent of the benefit in terms of GDP, whereas for mass media campaigns and advertising regulations, the cost is around 20 percent of the predicted benefit to the economy. This implies that, annually, for each $1 PPP invested, approximately $4–$5 PPP will be returned in economic benefit on average from 2020 to 2050.

Although the results presented here are based on a limited number of countries, they can provide guidance for policy makers in other countries who are considering implementing such policies and may need to adapt models such as the SPHeP-NCDs to their individual country contexts by taking into consideration costs (refer to box 7.1 for a country-based example), assumptions, and the types of interventions modeled.

Box 7.1

Cost Considerations for Implementing the Chilean Food Labeling and Marketing Law

In 2016, after a long legislative discussion, Chile implemented the Food Labeling and Marketing Law. Precise costs of the design, implementation, and evaluation of this policy have not been estimated. Such estimations are valuable for two potential reasons: (1) assessing the cost-effectiveness of food labeling and marketing regulations and (2) providing financial estimates that can shed light on the budgetary needs for countries considering the implementation of food labeling and marketing regulations. Chile's case provides a systematized listing of the actions that need to be considered for such costing and for successful resource allocation when designing, implementing, and monitoring such policy (see table B7.1.1). It is important to underscore that this listing needs to be contextualized within each country's capacity and structure.

(continued)

Box 7.1

Cost Considerations for Implementing the Chilean Food Labeling and Marketing Law *(continued)*

Table B7.1.1 Systematized Listing of Actions That Need to Be Costed for Design, Implementation, and Monitoring of Food Labeling and Marketing Regulation Interventions

Type of activity	Specifics
Design	
***Research and development.* Costs associated with expert-level work on the definition of norms, implementation and monitoring protocols, and communication strategies**	• Definition of the norms of the regulation (labeling and marketing) and the nutrient profiling • Definition of implementation protocols and resources • Definition of monitoring protocols and resources • Design of communication campaigns and documents for policy dissemination with key stakeholders • Drafting of final legal text
***Administrative.* Costs associated with the coordination, interaction, and consultation processes with key stakeholders**	• Coordination with other governmental institutions: ministries (education, agriculture, finance, and so forth) and other agencies (school feeding program, national TV council, national institute of industrial property, and so forth)* • Coordination with other key stakeholders (regular meetings)* • Interactions with civil society: participatory research with civil society and other health promotion activities, including articulation with consumers organizations • Open consultation process: definition, review, results, responses*

(continued)

Box 7.1

Cost Considerations for Implementing the Chilean Food Labeling and Marketing Law *(continued)*

Table B7.1.1 Systematized Listing of Actions That Need to Be Costed for Design, Implementation, and Monitoring of Food Labeling and Marketing Regulation Interventions *(continued)*

Type of activity	Specifics
Implementation	
Material resources. **Costs associated with the publication and dissemination of the guidelines and tool box linked to the regulation and monitoring**	• Material resources linked to implementation guidelines and implementation tool box with a special focus on small vendors from schools and food entrepreneurs and monitoring guidelines, including human and material resource allocation*
Training. **Costs associated with training of vendors and food producers**	• Short training courses for school kiosk vendors • Workshops for small and medium food producers*
Administrative. **Costs associated with coordination with other governmental stakeholders and national agencies involved in the actual implementation of the regulations and related actions**	• Coordination with other governmental institutions: ministries (education, agriculture, finance, and so forth) and other agencies (school feeding program, national TV council, national institute of industrial property, and so forth)*
Communication campaigns. **Costs associated with expert consultancy for the campaign development and media and school communication campaigns**	• Communication expert in charge of defining key dissemination messages • TV, radio, and billboards (2 months) • Special focus on school campaigns (12 months)
Legal specialized services: **costs associated with legal demands or claims, and actions with the international World Trade Organization***	• Response to legal demands and claims • Consultations with the international World Trade Organization

(continued)

Box 7.1

Cost Considerations for Implementing the Chilean Food Labeling and Marketing Law *(continued)*

Table B7.1.1 Systematized Listing of Actions That Need to Be Costed for Design, Implementation, and Monitoring of Food Labeling and Marketing Regulation Interventions *(continued)*

Type of activity	Specifics
Monitoring and Evaluation	
Resources. **Costs associated with human and technological resources needed for monitoring compliance**	• Hiring of human resources for monitoring compliance of implementation • Technological resources, development of monitoring software, and purchase of marketing databases
Training. **Costs associated with the training of monitoring inspectors and other governmental actors responsible for monitoring**	• Training of monitoring inspectors, including trips and other operational costs associated with the training
Research and development. **Costs associated with internal and external process evaluations needed to calibrate the implementation**	• Internal process evaluation at 6 months based on monitoring reports* • External process evaluation at 6 and 18 months • Consumers' attitudes and perceptions evaluation • Small studies on specific aspects of the law: school environments, consumers, and so forth • Biochemical laboratory testing of labeling compliance in selected food groups* • Implementation of a monitoring system for assessing the compliance of marketing restrictions

Source: Original table for this publication.

*This aspect corresponds to costs that, in Chile's case, have importantly been covered by existing governmental infrastructure.

(continued)

Box 7.1

Cost Considerations for Implementing the Chilean Food Labeling and Marketing Law *(continued)*

It is relevant to highlight that Chile is a country whose government is well-structured, and several of the activities described here relied on the interministerial and interagency coordination that might not be as easy to achieve in other country settings. For Chile, this implied that several activities incurred only marginal additional expenses. For example, the monitoring of the implementation was done by the existing health monitoring system's adding one inspector per region. More generally, this suggests that costing the implementation of such policies may need to account for the coordination efforts in both planning and execution, as noted in table B7.1.1. It is also important to note that these cost lines include only the governmental expenses. Other costs incurred by the private sector are not considered in the proposed listing.

Although this case study does not provide actual costs of the food labeling and marketing intervention in Chile, it provides an explicit list of inputs and resources that are needed to implement such types of policies. Estimating the actual costs and generating a methodology for doing so in other countries would be an invaluable implementation tool box for country governments.

Conclusion

Overall, an estimated $12.8 billion is required each year in the developing world, over and above the $6.3 billion that is currently being spent annually. A large proportion of these financing needs are concentrated in South Asia ($43 billion; 34 percent) and Sub-Saharan Africa ($34 billion; 26 percent), reflecting the disproportionate burden of poor nutrition outcomes in these regions. If this financing is made available, it would help the world move closer to the SDG 2.2 targets by averting an additional 6.2 million child deaths, 980,000 stillbirths, 27 million child stunting cases, 47 million under-five wasting episodes, 77 million cases of under-five anemia cases, 6.6 million LBW births, and 144 million cases of maternal anemia and leading to 85 million additional children exclusively breastfed. The economic benefits associated with investment in nutrition far outweigh the costs of inaction, with an overall benefit–cost ratio from the full package estimated to be 23.

Although these investments are critical to achieving the nutrition targets, it is also possible to improve nutrition outcomes simply by optimizing current spending. If only 25 percent or 50 percent of the financing needs could be met in low-resource contexts, countries would be able to scale up important priority interventions, achieving significant nutrition improvements.

For obesity prevention policies, the costs are significantly lower, albeit harder to quantify with available evidence. Case studies in Bulgaria, Mexico, and South Africa estimate the costs of food labeling, mass media campaigns, mobile apps, and health advertising regulations at approximately $3.4–$3.6 PPP per capita annually. These studies also show that for every $1 PPP invested, approximately $4–$5 PPP, on average, will be returned in economic benefits each year for 2020–50, with large impacts on labor market productivity.

Collectively, increased investments in reducing undernutrition and obesity are crucial to meeting the SDG 2.2 nutrition targets. These investments have unparalleled potential to build human capital and drive economic growth and prosperity—and, as described in chapter 4, when carefully designed with environmental considerations, they also provide climate co-benefits.

Notes

1. That is, the countries selected had the highest number of children younger than age five with stunting, of children younger than age five with wasting, of LBW children, of children younger than age six months who were not exclusively breastfed, of children ages 6 months to 59 months with anemia, and of women of reproductive age with anemia.

2. For SPHeP-NCDs documentation, see http://oecdpublichealthexplorer.org /ncd-doc.

3. For data source, see https://doi.org/10.1787/67450d67-en.

References

Alderman, Harold, and Jere R. Behrman. 2006. "Reducing the Incidence of Low Birth Weight in Low-Income Countries Has Substantial Economic Benefits." *World Bank Research Observer* 21 (1): 25–48. https://doi.org/10.1093/wbro /lkj001.

Bertram, Melanie Y., Jeremy A. Lauer, Karin Stenberg, and Tessa Tan Torres Edejer. 2021. "Methods for the Economic Evaluation of Health Care Interventions for Priority Setting in the Health System: An Update from WHO CHOICE."

International Journal of Health Policy and Management 10 (Special Issue on WHO-CHOICE Update): 673–77. https://doi.org/10.34172/ijhpm.2020.244.

Bhutta, Zulfiqar A., Tahmeed Ahmed, Robert E. Black, Simon Cousens, Kathryn Dewey, Elsa Giugliani, Batool A. Haider, et al.; Maternal and Child Undernutrition Study Group. 2008. "What Works? Interventions for Maternal and Child Undernutrition and Survival." *The Lancet* 371 (9610): 417–40. https://doi.org/10.1016/S0140-6736(07)61693-6.

Bhutta, Zulfiqar A., Jai K. Das, Arjuman Rizvi, Michelle F. Gaffey, Neff Walker, Susan Horton, Patrick Webb, et al.; Lancet Nutrition Interventions Review Group, Maternal and Child Nutrition Study Group. 2013. "Evidence-Based Interventions for Improvement of Maternal and Child Nutrition: What Can Be Done and at What Cost?" *The Lancet* 382 (9890): 452–77. https://doi.org/10.1016/S0140-6736(13)60996-4.

de Onis, Mercedes, Elaine Borghi, Mary Arimond, Patrick Webb, Trevor Croft, Kuntal Saha, Luz Maria De-Regil, et al. 2019. "Prevalence Thresholds for Wasting, Overweight and Stunting in Children under 5 Years." *Public Health Nutrition* 22 (1): 175–79. https://doi.org/10.1017/S1368980018002434.

Hanushek, Eric A., and Ludger Woessmann. 2008. "The Role of Cognitive Skills in Economic Development." *Journal of Economic Literature* 46 (3): 607–68.

Hoddinott, John, Harold Alderman, Jere R. Behrman, Lawrence Haddad, and Susan Horton. 2013. "The Economic Rationale for Investing in Stunting Reduction." *Maternal & Child Nutrition* 9 (Supplement 2): 69–82. https://doi.org/10.1111/mcn.12080.

Horton, Susan E., Jana Krystene Brooks, Ajay S. Mahal, Christine Mcdonald, and Meera Shekar. 2010. *Scaling Up Nutrition: What Will It Cost?* Directions in Development Series. Washington, DC: World Bank. http://documents.worldbank.org/curated/en/655431468163481083/Scaling-up-nutrition-what-will-it-cost.

Horton, S., and J. Ross. 2003. "The Economics of Iron Deficiency." *Food Policy* 28 (1): 51–75. https://doi.org/10.1016/S0306-9192(02)00070-2.

Keats, Emily C., Jai K. Das, Rehana A. Salam, Zohra S. Lassi, Aamer Imdad, Robert E. Black, and Zulfiqar A. Bhutta. 2021. "Effective Interventions to Address Maternal and Child Malnutrition: An Update of the Evidence." *Lancet Child & Adolescent Health* 5 (5): 367–84. https://doi.org/10.1016/S2352-4642(20)30274-1.

OECD (Organisation of Economic Co-operation and Development). 2019. *The Heavy Burden of Obesity: The Economics of Prevention*. OECD Health Policy Studies. Paris: OECD Publishing.

Pearson, Ruth, Madhura Killedar, Janka Petravic, Jakub J. Kakietek, Nick Scott, Kelsey L. Grantham, Robyn M. Stuart, et al. 2018. "Optima Nutrition: An Allocative Efficiency Tool to Reduce Childhood Stunting by Better Targeting of Nutrition-Related Interventions." *BMC Public Health* 18 (1): 384. https://doi.org/10.1186/s12889-018-5294-z.

Shekar, Meera, Jakub Kakietek, Julia Dayton Eberwein, and Dylan Walters. 2017. *An Investment Framework for Nutrition: Reaching the Global Targets for Stunting, Anemia, Breastfeeding, and Wasting*. Washington, DC: World Bank. https://doi.org/10.1596/978-1-4648-1010-7.

Shekar, Meera, and Barry Popkin, eds. 2020. *Obesity: Health and Economic Consequences of an Impending Global Challenge*. Human Development Perspectives series. Washington, DC: World Bank. https://doi.org/10.1596/978-1-4648-1491-4.

UNICEF (United Nations Children's Fund) and WHO (World Health Organization). 2019. *UNICEF-WHO Low Birthweight Estimates: Levels and Trends 2000–2015*. Geneva: WHO.

WHO (World Health Organization) and UNICEF (United Nations Children's Fund). 2024. "The Extension of the 2025 Maternal, Infant and Young Child Nutrition Targets to 2030." WHO/UNICEF Discussion Paper, WHO, Geneva. https://data.unicef.org/resources/who-unicef-discussion-paper-nutrition-targets/.

Wigg, N. R., S. Tong, A. J. McMichael, P. A. Baghurst, G. Vimpani, and R. Roberts. 1998. "Does Breastfeeding at Six Months Predict Cognitive Development?" *Australian and New Zealand Journal of Public Health* 22 (2): 232–36. https://doi.org/10.1111/j.1467-842x.1998.tb01179.x.

World Obesity Federation. 2024. "Economic Impact of Overweight and Obesity." *Global Obesity Observatory*. Accessed May 12, 2024. https://data.worldobesity.org/economic-impact-new/methodology/.

8

Scaling Up Nutrition Actions: Operational Considerations

Michelle Mehta, Kyoko Shibata Okamura, Ali Winoto Subandoro, and Lisa Shireen Saldanha

KEY MESSAGES

- The rationale for investing in nutrition is compelling. However, in environments of constrained resources, the prioritization of evidence-based nutrition interventions is essential to maximize impacts across sectors. Prioritizing and scaling up evidence-based nutrition interventions involves policy dialogue, advocacy, and leadership at all levels of administration, as well as subnational targeting of vulnerable groups to improve equity.

- Tools are available to maximize nutrition investments, including Optima Nutrition allocative efficiency analyses, nutrition-responsive budgeting and public financial management reforms, and health financing arrangements such as revenue raising, pooling, and strategic purchasing to include nutrition in universal health coverage programs. There are also digital solutions for improved data-driven decision-making, and many countries are starting to use these tools.

- Improvements in nutrition outcomes require strong institutional and governance arrangements that facilitate cross-sectoral actions that converge with nutrition interventions delivered across multiple sectors. Holding key sectors accountable at both national and subnational levels is key to addressing direct and underlying drivers of malnutrition.

• Scaling up cross-sectoral solutions is vital for meeting global food and nutrition security challenges through continued investment in high-impact nutrition interventions, including new and innovative approaches as exemplified by country examples provided in this chapter, as well as putting into place budget tracking tools that enhance accountability, as has been done in Indonesia, Pakistan, Rwanda, and several other countries.

Introduction

The previous chapters provided a compendium of best-buy nutrition interventions delivered across platforms in multiple sectors as well as the rationale and evidence for investing in nutrition. This chapter and the following chapter discuss operational considerations in scaling up nutrition actions and the opportunities and trends in financing these investments. Many ministries of finance and planning in low- and middle-income countries (LMICs) have recognized that accelerated investments in people are needed for greater equity and economic growth and that improving nutrition is a critical input in improving human capital. Correspondingly, the World Bank portfolio of nutrition investments across sectors has more than doubled in the past eight years, from $876 million per year in FY2017 to $2,077 million per year in FY2023. High-level advocacy efforts to push the nutrition agenda forward, such as the Nutrition Accountability Framework (Global Nutrition Report 2024), which tracks Nutrition for Growth (N4G) country commitments, continue to promote key policy messages to maximize nutrition investment. Yet, despite this progress, the additional financing need of $12.8 billion annually required to scale the recommended interventions to 90 percent coverage underscores the persistent challenges with political economy and the need to ensure efficient targeting and design of nutrition investments—including leveraging untapped resources such as adaptive safety-net programs, agrifood sector investments, and climate financing—that can also improve nutrition (refer to chapter 7). This process often starts with analytics and dialogue to build understanding of the links among malnutrition, human capital, and economic productivity losses, which can generate stronger demand for investments in nutrition. The sections that follow discuss selected country experiences and operational tools that can support this process at national and subnational levels, followed by strategic opportunities in which further engagement and investment are urgently needed to accelerate scaling up of innovative cross-sectoral solutions to improve nutrition.

Key Considerations in Scaling Nutrition Investment and Prioritizing Evidence-Based Interventions

Scaling up nutrition investments involves strengthening policy dialogue, advocacy, leadership, and governance at all levels of administration. The 2017 *Investment Framework for Nutrition* (Shekar et al. 2017) laid the groundwork of providing evidence on why investing in nutrition makes sense and what investment returns can be achieved, and chapter 5 further elaborates on the latest evidence. This section outlines how to scale up nutrition interventions and realize additional gains from various resources (refer to annex 8A for a full list of tools for prioritizing and maximizing nutrition investments).

Investment Starts with Analytics and Policy Dialogue to Foster Commitments

Beginning in 2012 and culminating in the 2017 *Investment Framework for Nutrition*, the World Bank undertook a series of country- and regional-level costing advisory services and analytics with national governments and local partners to estimate the financing needs for scaling up high-impact interventions to meet global nutrition targets.[1] This work informed focused policy dialogue and advocacy for new nutrition investments to set ambitious targets to reduce stunting, anemia, and wasting, as well as to improve breastfeeding outcomes. Similar analyses and investment case exercises have informed national prioritization processes and helped secure domestic development assistance and innovative nutrition financing in Côte d'Ivoire, the Democratic Republic of Congo, and Madagascar, among other countries. Equally as important, these country analyses were collaborative exercises that engaged local governments, partners, and other stakeholders to better plan and harmonize nutrition investments.

Furthermore, an increased understanding of the human capital and economic productivity losses associated with malnutrition (which encompasses undernutrition, overweight, and obesity) is critical for government authorities, particularly ministries of finance and planning, to cultivate long-term investments to improve nutrition. Recently, the World Bank developed a human development diagnostic tool, Human Capital Review (HCR), that presents a comprehensive view of the state of human capital in a country; assesses endowments and constraints to human capital development across a broad range of areas, including nutrition as one of the key ingredients of human capital (refer to chapter 2); and identifies priority human capital outcomes that need improvement. HCR results are discussed in countries to inform high-level policy dialogue on strengthening national investments for inclusive growth and shared prosperity. Nutrition is often highlighted in HCRs as an important investment area when analyses reveal its burden on people's well-being and the economy. Several countries have completed the dissemination of HCRs, and high-level commitments to nutrition have already been seen to emerge from follow-up policy dialogues, and many more countries are currently conducting similar analyses.

- Timor-Leste's HCR concluded that malnutrition, especially high child-stunting rates, drives its Human Capital Index (Andrews et al. 2023) and that decisive investment could mark a turning point to help unlock the next generation's potential. This dialogue led to formation of the high-level Inter-Ministerial Task Force for Social Affairs to make the most of available resources and improve service delivery with a focus on nutrition and food security, early childhood development, and youth empowerment (World Bank 2023b).

- Pakistan's HCR highlighted the need to shift resources and improve efficiency in the existing allocations to human development sectors. This was linked to a specific recommendation to make nutrition a national priority as well as mobilizing financing and tracking spending and progress on nutrition investments. The HCR also presented an estimation that full utilization of increased human capital investments would grow its gross domestic product eight times more than a business-as-usual scenario in the coming two decades. To make this a reality, it recommends a long-term commitment that goes beyond any political cycle (Ersado et al. 2023).

Broader social equity and social justice agendas may also be part of policy dialogue and can be leveraged to generate nutrition wins. For example, India's Supreme Court ruled that certain government programs providing nutritional programs were legal entitlements that should be provided universally under the constitutional right to food, which led the way to universal coverage of the Integrated Child Development Services program (Chakrabarti et al. 2019). This was a result of explicit political dialogue and advocacy on the importance of nutrition in the growth and development of young children.

Prioritization and Allocative Efficiency

Seminal publications, such as *The Lancet Series on Maternal and Child Nutrition* (*The Lancet* 2008, 2013) and *Scaling Up Nutrition: What Will It Cost?* (Horton et al. 2009), established the evidence base for what to invest in to improve nutrition. However, in environments of constrained resources, priority setting is essential to maximize nutrition investment and impact across sectors. Key considerations for priority setting include types of malnutrition and their epidemiological burdens, geographical distribution of malnutrition, cost-effectiveness of potential interventions within the available service delivery platforms, and scale-up capacity.

Prioritization and allocative efficiency tools ensure that nutrition investments are used in a manner that is likely to achieve the best outcomes and targeted to reach scale. In the context of limited resources and even more constrained fiscal space now faced by many LMICs, it is not possible to implement the full suite of recommended interventions. However, one tool warrants highlighting. The Optima Nutrition modeling tool assists governments in decision-making processes by proposing scenarios for optimal allocation of resources based on the most recent evidence on high-impact nutrition interventions, as presented in chapters 5 and 7, and country-specific costing, coverage, and demographic data. On the basis of a country's national priorities for nutrition, the tool optimizes a package of high-impact interventions within a given budgetary profile, for subnational contexts, and to meet country-specific nutrition objectives. The tool is designed to be highly participatory, with inputs coming primarily from a government-led technical working group (refer to box 8.1).

Box 8.1

Embedding Evidence-Based Decision-Making Analyses into Budget Planning: Nigeria Optima Nutrition Case Study

Nigeria, like many other countries in the region and across the world, is facing a fiscal crisis that is putting unprecedented constraints on public sector financing for critical programs, such as those covering nutrition, that are designed to boost human capital. To address this, the World Bank and partners supported the Nigerian Federal and State Ministries of Budget and National Planning to undertake an Optima Nutrition analysis in four pilot states. A government-selected expert working group guided and informed the Optima Nutrition analyses, which first estimated the impact of each of the four pilot states' current spending on largely direct nutrition interventions delivered through the health system and then determined the best

(continued)

Box 8.1

Embedding Evidence-Based Decision-Making Analyses into Budget Planning: Nigeria Optima Nutrition Case Study *(continued)*

mix of interventions to achieve greater impacts on reducing stunting, wasting, and anemia among children and pregnant women.

In Kano State, the analyses provided a decision-making tool to prioritize investment in a set of direct nutrition interventions and set nutrition targets for the state's Multi-Sectoral Nutrition Action Plan (MSPAN).[a] Through engagement and advocacy, the Optima Nutrition analyses provided the evidence base needed to prioritize and efficiently allocate resources in annual nutrition budgeting cycles. The analyses were subsequently embedded into the state MSPAN, as well as the budget circular for the 2024 budget cycle. This process has enabled Kano State to make credible progress, in a fiscally constrained environment, toward achieving nutrition outcomes and longer-term impact, and it provides a prioritized and evidence-based package of interventions around which the government of Nigeria and donors can align.

a. High-impact interventions included iron and folic acid (IFA) supplementation of pregnant women in health facilities and in the community, providing micronutrient powder supplementation to children, treatment of severe acute malnutrition, education on infant and young child feeding in health facilities in the community and via mass media, and treatment of childhood diarrhea with zinc and oral rehydration solutions.

Strengthening Governance and Accountability for Nutrition at All Levels

Improve Subnational Targeting to Improve Equity

Despite improvements in global malnutrition rates (refer to chapter 2), progress remains slow and inequitable. Even impressive reductions in national stunting prevalence may mask important subnational disparities. For example, Côte d'Ivoire reduced stunting to 23 percent in 2021, yet some regions face alarmingly high rates of stunting at near to or more than 30 percent, which is considered very high prevalence, according to World Health Organization (WHO) international standards (de Onis et al. 2019). Ghana has also shown exemplary success in reducing stunting from

28 percent to 17 percent between 2008 and 2022, yet the prevalence of anemia among pregnant women is still above the WHO's public health significance level of 40 percent (World Bank 2024), and the country's rising overweight and obesity burdens are affecting more women than men. These regional and gender disparities often persist where supply- or demand-side barriers, or both, reduce access to services among vulnerable groups or displaced populations. These barriers need to be identified and addressed through evidence-based investments. In Ghana, subnational assessments identified important regional variations in the contributions of the health and non–health sectors (for example, water and education) in driving changes in stunting, underscoring the need for context-specific planning to improve targeting (Aryeetey et al. 2022). The Philippines is currently undertaking comprehensive subnational analyses of malnutrition burdens—looking at convergence and quality of service delivery, equity, and access; enabling environment; and impacts of recent crises on the delivery of nutrition-related services—to provide operational guidance to the ongoing large-scale Philippines Multisectoral Nutrition Project and further inform investment opportunities to alleviate the burden of malnutrition and promote healthy diets.

Strengthen Governance and Accountability

In some countries, the establishment of an institutional home for nutrition linked to a high-level office increased the visibility of the nutrition agenda and fostered greater coordination and collaboration among relevant sectors. For example, in Senegal, high-level leadership and champions have promoted an understanding that nutrition is essential to the development of human capital. The Nutrition Coordination Unit (Cellule de Lutte Contre la Malnutrition, or CLM) was created in 2001 in the prime minister's office and was responsible for implementation of the World Bank–financed Nutrition Enhancement Program (Programme de Renforcement de la Nutrition). The CLM ensured cross-sectoral collaboration, coordination, and accountability at national and subnational levels (Spray 2018).

Leadership at the highest levels of government is essential, but this commitment must be reinforced at subnational levels to achieve the most impact. It is of particular importance for nutrition investments to be well managed at subnational levels through subnational leadership, capacity building, and systematic targeting of vulnerable groups. In Nigeria, costing analyses (World Bank 2014) were embedded into the National Strategic Plan of Action for Nutrition and subsequently provided the basis for the country's largest ever nutrition investment of $232 million, cofinanced by the International Development Association and the Global Financing Facility, which was designed to scale up a basic package of nutrition interventions in 12 states through the Accelerating Nutrition Results in Nigeria project. This effort has also resulted in growing federal and state recognition of the importance of investing in nutrition to achieve human capital goals.

In Uganda, ministries responsible for agriculture, education, health, and local government jointly implemented the Multisectoral Food Security and Nutrition Project (2015–24) to improve child and maternal nutrition.[2] The project's institutional and governance arrangements were aligned to the national nutrition governance arrangements in the Uganda Nutrition Action Plan. Overall leadership by the Office of the Prime Minister, a supraministerial mechanism, was critical in mobilizing and ensuring the participation of all the participating ministries. District Nutrition Coordination Committees met quarterly to develop and monitor the implementation of District Nutrition Action Plans. The project design ensured alignment of activities and resources with the mandates of the participating ministries. At the community level, primary schools were the center for nutrition demonstrations and distribution of input packages, which included planting materials and biofortified crops. Nutrition-supporting activities were delivered through different community resource persons, with technical support from each sector: education (school management committees and parent groups), health (health unit management committees, village health teams, and lead mothers), and agriculture (lead farmers).

In Indonesia, political buy-in at the presidential level starting in 2017 was achieved through advocacy that linked evidence on scaling up high-impact nutrition interventions, as well as the need for convergence across sectors, to the country's development agenda. A coordination mechanism was subsequently instituted to connect the central government with provincial and district stunting task forces to manage implementation using a clear accountability framework for achieving results at all levels. Implementation of District Convergence Action Plans was further supported by mobile multisectoral technical assistance teams at the provincial level that could respond to local requests for support. These elements have culminated in Indonesia's success in creating a whole-of-government approach to reducing stunting, which has led directly to an unprecedented decline in the national stunting rate from 30.8 percent to 21.6 percent between 2018 and 2022 (Murthi 2022; Subandoro, Holschneider, and Bergeron 2021).

Cross-Sectoral Actions to Improve Nutrition

The evidence presented in earlier chapters shows that gains in human capital and nutrition outcomes are achieved when high-impact nutrition interventions delivered through different sectors effectively reach women, adolescent girls, and young children. Skoufias, Vinha, and Sato (2019) also found that children who had simultaneous access to two or more nutrition-relevant services that address key drivers of stunting (such as food and care; health; and water, sanitation, and hygiene [WASH]) had lower stunting rates compared with those who had access to only one or none of these services. However, reaching these target groups with the full suite of interventions requires strong coordination across key sectors, including health, social protection, water and sanitation, education, and agriculture. Several countries have shown the value of establishing operational platforms and processes to support careful program design, monitoring, and accountability. An evaluation of World Bank support for reducing child undernutrition highlighted the importance of institutional strengthening to enable sustained support of nutrition, including developing leadership, systems, policies, and evidence across multiple actors and sectors (World Bank 2021).

Operational Convergence Approach to Driving Nutrition Outcomes across Sectors

Convergence at an operational level has been a key contributing factor to success (Subandoro, Holschneider, and Bergeron 2021). Many countries, such as Indonesia, the Lao People's Democratic Republic, the Philippines, Papua New Guinea, and Rwanda, have operationalized their multisectoral approaches through a convergence approach, which includes some or all of the following important features. First, select direct nutrition interventions, typically delivered through the health system, are colocated in the same geographical areas with context-appropriate, indirect nutrition actions delivered by actors across sectors. This often includes coordination in the design and delivery of nutrition-related messaging through multiple sectors, including health, social protection, agriculture, WASH, and others. Second, priority groups, such as "1,000-day households" with pregnant women and children younger than age two years, are targeted to receive key interventions from different sectors simultaneously. Finally, an integrated monitoring and evaluation (M&E) system, including a shared results framework and convergence scorecard, tracks commitments and achievements from each sector. Ideally, a mechanism is put in place to track convergence of services at the household level. These integrated tools are essential to increase accountability of sectoral service providers and local government authorities that are expected to monitor and improve nutrition results and to ensure that the target populations are being reached with the full range of interventions needed to address the multifactorial causes of malnutrition.

- In Uganda, reaching households through multiple pathways through the Multisectoral Food Security and Nutrition Project (2015–24) increased adoption of micronutrient-rich crops, improved household dietary diversity, reduced food insecurity, and improved caregivers' knowledge of nutrition practices. These achievements have, in turn, improved child feeding practices and reduced childhood stunting, wasting, and anemia among the households that directly participated in the project activities. This strengthened platform will now be expanded to scale up multiple micronutrient supplements (MMS) to reach pregnant women, including through coordination of nutrition messaging.

- In Cambodia, local governments are being assessed on their ability to plan, finance, implement, and monitor community-based health and nutrition activities, including community outreach in collaboration with health workers and social mobilization.

- The government of Lao PDR, with support from the World Bank, is implementing a Nutrition Convergence Program (NCP) to address maternal and child nutrition through a convergence approach. Interventions from key sectors, such as health, education, water, social protection, and rural livelihoods, are geographically colocated to target the same beneficiaries, using a common M&E framework and coordination of their respective social and behavior change (SBC) activities and community delivery platforms. Robust impact evaluation shows that NCP has already proven to be an effective program to mitigate the adverse impacts of COVID-19 and high inflation on child nutrition.

- The government of the Philippines is implementing the Philippine Multisectoral Nutrition Program, a large-scale and innovative project that uses a multisectoral nutrition approach to deliver a coordinated package of nutrition interventions in 235 municipalities with the highest poverty rates and stunting prevalence. The program helps local governments mainstreaming nutrition as part of their larger efforts to strengthen primary care and incorporates innovative financing mechanisms, such as performance-based grants, which link financing with the achievement of nutrition targets at the local level.

- The governments of Indonesia and Rwanda have operationalized a convergence approach by institutionalizing the use of the Village Convergence Scorecard, or Community Scorecard tool, which tracks simultaneous utilization of key nutrition interventions across sectors at the individual level and visualizes coverages and gaps. This approach has allowed local authorities, service providers, and community members to monitor delivery of these critical services and hold themselves collectively accountable for established nutrition results. Both Indonesia and Rwanda have digitalized the scorecard tool used by human development workers in Indonesia and community health workers in Rwanda at the community level to record their activities, diagnose situations, report progress and challenges, and receive support from supervisors. Lao PDR, Papua New Guinea, and the Philippines have also recently introduced convergence scorecards.

Scaling Up Innovative Cross-Sectoral Solutions for Nutrition and Healthy Diets

Promoting high-impact cross-sectoral solutions for nutrition and healthy diets is one of the three new action areas in the World Bank's Food and Nutrition Security (FNS) Global Challenge Program, along with enhancing FNS crisis prevention, preparedness, and response and supporting the development of a more productive, low-emissions, and climate-resilient food system. Several priority areas have been identified where further investment is urgently needed, including scaling up small-quantity lipid-based nutrient supplements (SQ-LNSs; refer to box 8.2), MMS (refer to box 8.3), reaching target groups during the first 1,000 days with SBC messages, and enhancing use of digital technology and data for evidence-based decision-making (refer to box 8.4). Additional priority areas include expanding large-scale food fortification wherever possible and implementing policy and fiscal measures to promote healthy and sustainable diets—all through concerted multisectoral and multistakeholder efforts to achieve scale, speed, and impact.

Some of these new high-impact nutrition solutions, namely SQ-LNS and MMS, may be delivered through strengthened nutrition-sensitive platforms, such as social protection programs, in coordination with health operations. However, as pointed out in chapter 5, some reviews of multisectoral nutrition interventions have found that integration of these interventions into existing platforms is achieved with varying degrees of success, because issues of workload, supervision, and competing priorities can affect the fidelity of implementation. Well-designed implementation, research, and contextualized implementation strategies are needed to minimize the gap between evidence-based interventions and actual implementation outcomes. Contextual factors, stakeholder dynamics, and system-level barriers should be key considerations (Proctor, Powell, and McMillen 2013). After scale-up, implementation monitoring is needed for continuous improvement.

Box 8.2

Scaling Up Small-Quantity Lipid-Based Nutrient Supplements to Vulnerable Populations Using Existing Health Platforms

In response to an increasingly fragile and conflict-affected environment, the government of Burkina Faso contracted the World Food Program (WFP) in 2022 to deliver small-quantity lipid-based nutrient supplements (SQ-LNS) in two regions where government facilities were becoming increasingly difficult for the population to access. Using WFP's existing supplementary feeding program platform and the government's database on internally displaced and host populations, community health workers identified children eligible for SQ-LNS and provided social and behavior change communication to caregivers in group and household settings. An assessment of the intervention showed that community involvement and reestablishment of community nutrition groups increased access to and uptake of SQ-LNS.

In Madagascar, initial operational research in a highly food-insecure area found that preventive nutritional supplementation among children ages 6 months to 18 months was linked to a 9 percent reduction in stunting (Galasso et al. 2019). The government is now scaling up this intervention to preventively cover all children ages 6 months to 23 months in new regions affected by multiple climate change stressors, such as drought and flooding. Distribution builds on the existing community-based nutrition and health platform through which children receive a package of other services focused on stunting reduction. Production capacity for SQ-LNS has been expanded through a partnership with a local manufacturer.

Box 8.3

Implementation Research Supports Scale-Up of Multiple Micronutrient Supplements

In Indonesia (Anggondowat et al. 2023) and Pakistan (Busch-Hallen et al. 2023), implementation research is being used to understand barriers to and enablers of supply, demand, and delivery of multiple micronutrient supplements (MMS). According to the research, enabling factors included commitment of authorities, trust in health care providers, access to antenatal care (ANC) during the first trimester, and potential use of digital technology to promote MMS adherence. Barriers included limited counseling during ANC visits, stock shortages, and limited knowledge among health care providers about MMS. MMS, which includes iron and folic acid (IFA) in its standard formulation, is expected to replace the existing IFA supplements that are already in the delivery system. However, IFA supplementation itself has not achieved optimal coverage and adherence in many countries because of supply, service quality, and demand challenges. For example, IFA may not be available at health centers or included as part of free ANC, service providers may not be trained in counseling on IFA, and pregnant women often do not adhere to the recommended regimen. Understanding these nuances is an essential step in designing contextual-based strategies to deliver MMS effectively and achieve intended results. In Bangladesh, a results-based approach is being designed to scale up MMS as part of the government's regular ANC package delivered through community clinics in selected rural areas. The program will first incentivize the institutionalization of relevant policies and supply chains to deliver the MMS, followed by incentives to reach annual targets for MMS distribution.

Chapter 6 highlighted examples of potentially powerful policy measures around food systems and healthy diets. Institutionalization and implementation of such policy actions, especially regulatory and fiscal policy measures on unhealthy diets, often face political economy challenges. For example, Slater et al. (2024) conducted detailed mapping and analyses of the ultraprocessed food (UPF) industry's corporate interest groups and their relationships. The study suggests that UPF manufacturing corporations strategically engage and expand these groups into weblike networks that influence various components of the food systems, including consumer behaviors (for example, branding and advertising) and even policy and governance (for example, sustainability, corporate social responsibilities), which were until recently predominantly controlled and led by the public sector (Slater et al. 2024). These policy measures are not free from the complex political economy that undermines its intended benefits to the population. However, as examples from Colombia and other countries illustrate, challenges can be overcome with the existence of strong policy champions; persistent efforts to generate and use evidence; whole-of-society approaches to setting strong social norms, including engagement of the civil society; and careful implementation of a package of interventions that can collectively make impacts.

Technological Innovations to Address Nutrition Service Delivery Challenges

Technological innovations offer an opportunity to address key bottlenecks in service delivery, monitoring, supervision, and SBC at both family and community levels. Technology-based job aids and digital tools have been developed to support frontline workers with assessing and responding to malnutrition cases, improving referral and follow-up and providing peer support. Digital technologies can also improve the reach and the targeting of SBC messages, such as providing age-tailored counseling to improve infant and young child feeding programs. For example, the World Bank's support for India's POSHAN Abhiyaan (or the National Nutrition Mission) led to the development of the Poshan Tracker, an easy-to-use mobile-based nutrition tracking service and decision-making tool for frontline workers (World Bank Group 2023a; refer to box 8.4).

Box 8.4

Poshan Tracker: India's Innovative Mobile App to Transform Community-Based Nutrition Service Delivery and Monitoring

Launched in March 2018, India's Poshan Abhiyaan (or the National Nutrition Mission) aims at achieving improvement in the nutritional status of children, adolescents, and women. The program leveraged transformational technology to improve community-level services delivered by Anganwadi workers (AWWs)—frontline nutrition workers who deliver six key nutrition and health services under the Integrated Child Development Services (ICDS) scheme. It introduced an innovative mobile phone–based application, initially called ICDS

(continued)

Box 8.4

Poshan Tracker: India's Innovative Mobile App to Transform Community-Based Nutrition Service Delivery and Monitoring *(continued)*

Common Application Software (ICDS-CAS), which was changed to Poshan Tracker in 2021 and uses a more comprehensive information technology system. The applications were designed to support the program with multiple functions, including beneficiary registration, daily service tracking and home visit records by AWWs, SMS alerts to trigger beneficiaries' service uptake at critical times, and real-time monitoring by supervisors and officials, which allowed informed decisions on supportive supervision. Additionally, the previous ICDS-CAS version had a job aid for use during counseling. Currently, the Poshan Tracker is being actively used by almost all the AWWs (1.35 million of 1.39 million AWWs) in the country. The Poshan Knowledge and Behavior Survey conducted in 2021 found that the data on key indicators for iron and folic acid consumption, diet during pregnancy, and receipt of key services were higher in CAS districts than in non-CAS districts at an aggregate level. Breastfeeding within the first hour of birth and exclusive breastfeeding among children younger than age six months were significantly higher in CAS districts than in non-CAS districts (70 percent versus 64 percent and 84 percent versus 76 percent, respectively).

Institutional Strengthening to Maximize and Sustain Nutrition Investment and Returns

As described in previous sections, improvements in nutrition outcomes require strong institutional and governance arrangements that facilitate cross-sectoral nutrition actions at national and subnational levels, maximize the delivery platforms from each sector, and hold key sectors accountable for addressing direct and underlying drivers of malnutrition.

Although initiatives related to governance and institutional strengthening for nutrition have been extensively assessed and discussed elsewhere (Scaling Up Nutrition 2024; Subandoro, Holschneider, and Bergeron 2021),[3] this section focuses on how public financial management (PFM) reform processes and health financing levers, including subnational applications, have helped to strengthen the political economy and institutional capacities for nutrition financing and accountability in countries.

Nutrition-Responsive Public Financial Management Reforms to Drive Nutrition Investments across Sectors

How well public resources are managed matters to how effective governments can be in investing their resources to achieve the intended results. However, country PFM systems are often not set up to serve the multisectoral needs that are required for an effective nutrition response. Strengthening institutional setup and PFM processes with a nutrition lens is critical to secure adequate domestic resources for nutrition-contributing activities and make them visible in government planning, budgeting, budget-execution monitoring, feedback reporting, and course correction across all relevant sectors. Unless they are visible in usual government PFM processes, financiers and implementers will not be held accountable for the spending and its results. Although more details are provided in chapter 9, this section summarizes examples of a few countries that have undertaken nutrition-responsive PFM reform initiatives that allow their financial management information systems to continuously track and monitor nutrition budget allocations and expenditures to facilitate informed decision-making by financing authorities (Piatti-Fünfkirchen et al. 2023):

- In Indonesia, key reforms to achieving reductions in stunting include setting and monitoring budget disbursement targets for nutrition initiatives for all ministries, budget tagging and tracking to monitor budget trends, and fiscal transfers to ensure that national priorities are implemented at subnational levels. Indonesia's tracking system has helped make the entire nutrition spending visible to decision-makers for the first time, which led to a commitment, announced at the Tokyo N4G Summit in 2021, to maintain more than $2 billion in annual budget allocation to nutrition up to 2024.

- The government of Rwanda introduced reforms on budget tagging and tracking in 2021 in a collaboration between the Ministry of Finance and the National Child Development Agency. National budgets across sectors were linked through a single action plan to facilitate tracking of finances and a full overview of nutrition spending in the country's Integrated Financial Management Information System (IFMIS). The data generated from this system contributed to a substantial increase in the nutrition budget allocation between 2021 and 2022, even though the total domestic resource envelope did not grow at a similar rate.

- The government of Pakistan institutionalized a nutrition lens approach in annual and medium-term planning and budgeting through its IFMIS with an aim of strengthening coordination across different ministries and agencies in the country and accountability for nutrition budgeting processes. The nutrition expenditure reporting guideline developed by the controller general accounts has been used across the federal and provincial governments. Further work is envisioned to expand the system to the district level and to link the financial performance information with programmatic output and outcome indicators to enhance stakeholder accountability for program results.

• In Nigeria, nutrition-responsive public financing mechanisms, budget tagging and tracking, and sustainable financing frameworks have laid the groundwork for a strong advocacy effort, whereby state-level officials are voicing their support for and urgency regarding a whole-of-government nutrition agenda.

Optimizing Health Financing Levers for Improved Nutrition Service Delivery

Health financing arrangements—such as revenue raising, pooling, and strategic purchasing—can be leveraged to improve the quality and coverage of nutrition services. For example, to increase coverage of nutrition interventions such as MMS in pregnancy, health service purchasers could explicitly include this intervention in output-based payment schemes. Another approach through results-based financing is being implemented in the Democratic Republic of Congo, where a set of nutrition services was added to the facility-level performance-based financing system to incentivize delivery of high-priority nutrition interventions. Much of Peru's success story in reducing stunting was built on a performance-based budgeting system that calculated and secured financing for nutrition and created incentives for government actors to be transparent with spending. As a result, program managers made budget prioritizations based on nutrition outcomes and impacts rather than inputs (Subandoro et al. 2022).

Notes

1. The countries were Afghanistan, Arab Republic of Egypt, Bangladesh, Burkina Faso, Democratic Republic of Congo, Guinea-Bissau, India, Kenya, Madagascar, Mali, Myanmar, Nigeria, Uganda, and Zambia, plus the regional Stunting Reduction in Sub-Saharan Africa (World Bank 2017) that included analyses for Benin, Côte d'Ivoire, Ethiopia, Niger, and Rwanda.

2. The Global Agriculture and Food Security Program financed the operation with grant financing through the World Bank, which also provided technical support.

3. The Scaling Up Nutrition Movement's online resource library includes a list of reports and briefs under the search topic "multistakeholder/multisectoral approach."

References

Andrews, Kathryn, Lander Bosch, Janssen Teixeira, Ilsa Meidina, and Somil Nagpal. 2023. *Seizing Opportunities of a Lifetime: The Timor-Leste Human Capital Review*. Washington, DC: World Bank. https://doi.org/10.1596/40623.

Anggondowat, Trisari, Evi Martha, Tika Rianty, Tiara Amelia, Basuki Imanhadi, Nancy Kosasih, Akhir Riyanti, et al. 2023. "Formative Research: Barriers and Enablers for Successful Implementation of Antenatal MMS in Indonesia." In *Focusing on Multiple Micronutrient Supplements in Pregnancy: Second Edition*, edited by Klaus Kraemer and Rebecca Olson, 79–82. Basel: Sight and Life. https://cms .sightandlife.org/wp-content/uploads/2023/05/202305-MMS-2-sightandlife.pdf.

Aryeetey, Richmond, Afua Atuobi-Yeboah, Lucy Billings, Nicholas Nisbett, Mara van den Bold, and Mariama Toure. 2022. "Stories of Change in Nutrition in Ghana: A Focus on Stunting and Anemia Among Children under Five Years (2009–2018)." *Food Security* 14: 355–79.

Busch-Hallen, Jennifer, Sarah Rowe, Mandana Arabi, and Shabina Raza. 2023. "Implementation Research in Pakistan: Paving the Way for a Successful Transition to Multiple Micronutrient Supplementation." In *Focusing on Multiple Micronutrient Supplements in Pregnancy: Second Edition*, edited by Klaus Kraemer and Rebecca Olson, 50–54. Basel: Sight and Life. https://cms.sightandlife.org /wp-content/uploads/2023/05/202305-MMS-2-sightandlife.pdf.

Chakrabarti, Suman, Kalyani Raghunathan, Harold Alderman, Purnima Menon, and Phuong Nguyen. 2019. "India's Integrated Child Development Services Programme; Equity and Extent of Coverage in 2006 and 2016." *Bulletin of the World Health Organization* 97(4): 270–82.

de Onis, Mercedes, Elaine Borghi, Mary Arimond, Patrick Webb, Trevor Crot, Kuntal Saha, Luz Maria De-Regil, et al. 2019. "Prevalence Thresholds for Wasting, Overweight and Stunting in Children under 5 Years." *Public Health Nutrition* 22 (1): 175–79. https://doi.org/10.1017/S1368980018002434.

Ersado, Lire, Amer Hasan, Koen Martijn Geven, Ashi Kohli Kathuria, Juan Baron, May Bend, and S. Amer Ahmed. 2023. *Pakistan Human Capital Review: Building Capabilities throughout Life*. Washington, DC: World Bank.

Galasso, Emanuela, Anne M. Weber, Christine P. Stewart, Lisy Ratsifandrihamanana, and Lia C. H. Fernald. 2019. "Effects of Nutritional Supplementation and Home Visiting on Growth and Development in Young Children in Madagascar:

A Cluster-Randomised Controlled Trial." *The Lancet Global Health* 7 (9): e1257–e1268. https://doi.org/10.1016/S2214-109X(19)30317-1.

Global Nutrition Report. 2024. "The Nutrition Accountability Framework." Accessed April 8, 2024. https://globalnutritionreport.org/resources/naf/.

Horton, Susan E., Jana Krystene Brooks, Ajay S. Mahal, Christine Mcdonald, and Meera Shekar. 2009. *Scaling Up Nutrition: What Will It Cost (English).* Directions in Development; Human Development. Washington, DC: World Bank. http://documents.worldbank.org/curated/en/655431468163481083/Scaling-up-nutrition-what-will-it-cost.

The Lancet. 2008. *Series on Maternal and Child Undernutrition.* Accessed April 8, 2024. https://www.thelancet.com/series/maternal-and-child-undernutrition.

The Lancet. 2013. *Series on Maternal and Child Nutrition.* Accessed April 8, 2024. https://www.thelancet.com/series/maternal-and-child-nutrition.

Murthi, Mamta. 2022. "Reducing Child Stunting: An Investment in the Future of Indonesia." *Investing in Health Blog,* December 12, 2022. https://blogs.worldbank.org/en/health/reducing-child-stunting-investment-future-indonesia.

Piatti-Fünfkirchen, Moritz, Ali Winoto Subandoro, Timothy Williamson, and Kyoko Shibata Okamura. 2023. *Driving Nutrition Action through the Budget. A Guide to Nutrition-Responsive Budgeting.* Washington, DC: World Bank. https://www.worldbank.org/en/topic/nutrition/publication/nutrition-action-through-budget.

Proctor, Enola K., Byron J. Powell, and J. Curtis McMillen. 2013. "Implementation Strategies: Recommendations for Specifying and Reporting." *Implementation Science* 8: 139.

Scaling Up Nutrition. 2024. "Resource Library." Accessed May 21, 2024. https://scalingupnutrition.org/resources/resource-library?f%5B0%5D=document_library_resource_topics%3A1022.

Shekar, Meera, Jakub Kakietek, Julia Dayton Eberwein, and Dylan Walters. 2017. *An Investment Framework for Nutrition: Reaching the Global Targets for Stunting, Anemia, Breastfeeding, and Wasting.* Washington, DC: World Bank. https://doi.org/10.1596/978-1-4648-1010-7.

Skoufias, Emmanuel, Katja Vinha, and Ryoko Sato. 2019. *All Hands on Deck: Reducing Stunting through Multisectoral Efforts in Sub-Saharan Africa.* Africa Development Forum series. Washington, DC: World Bank.

Slater, Scott, Mark Lawrence, Benjamin Wood, Paulo Serodio, and Phillip Baker. 2024. "Corporate Interest Groups and Their Implications for Global Food Governance: Mapping and Analysing the Global Corporate Influence Network of the Transnational Ultra-Processed Food Industry." *Global Health* 20: 16.

Spray, Andrea L. 2018. "Evolution of Nutrition Policy in Senegal." *Analysis & Perspective: 15 Years of Experience in the Development of Nutrition Policy in Senegal.* Washington, DC: World Bank; Dakar: Senegal. https://documents1.worldbank .org/curated/en/244341537165468896/pdf/Evolution-of-Nutrition-Policy-in -Senegal.pdf.

Subandoro, Ali Winoto, Silvia Holschneider, and Julie Ruel Bergeron. 2021. "Operationalizing Multisectoral Nutrition Programs to Accelerate Progress: A Nutrition Governance Perspective." Health, Nutrition and Population Discussion Paper, World Bank, Washington, DC. http://documents.worldbank .org/curated/en/716431640257867136/Operationalizing-Multisectoral -Nutrition-Programs-to-Accelerate-Progress-A-Nutrition-Governance -Perspective.

Subandoro, Ali Winoto, Kyoko Shibata Okamura, Michelle Mehta, Huihui Wang, Naina Ahluwalia, Elyssa Finkel, Andrea L. S. Bulungu, et al. 2022. *Positioning Nutrition within Universal Health Coverage: Optimizing Health Financing Levers.* Washington, DC: World Bank.

World Bank. 2014. "Costed Plan for Scaling Up Nutrition: Nigeria." Health, Nutrition and Population Discussion Paper. World Bank, Washington, DC.

World Bank. 2017. "Stunting Reduction in Sub-Saharan Africa." Health, Nutrition and Population Discussion Paper, World Bank, Washington, DC.

World Bank. 2021. *World Bank Support to Reducing Child Undernutrition: An Independent Evaluation.* Washington, DC: World Bank.

World Bank. 2023a. *Digital-in-Health: Unlocking the Value for Everyone.* Washington, DC: World Bank.

World Bank. 2023b. "World Bank Stresses Human Capital as Key to Timor-Leste's Growth and Development." Press release, November 14, 2023. https://www .worldbank.org/en/news/press-release/2023/11/14/world-bank-stresses -human-capital-as-key-to-timor-leste-growth-and-development.

World Bank. 2024. "Prevalence of Anemia among Pregnant Women (%)—Ghana." World Development Indicators database. Accessed April 11, 2024, https://data .worldbank.org/indicator/SH.PRG.ANEM?locations=GH.

9

Financing the Global Nutrition Targets: Progress to Date

Meera Shekar, Kyoko Shibata Okamura, Mary D'Alimonte, and Chiara Dell'Aira

KEY MESSAGES

- Estimates of additional financing needed to address the global undernutrition challenge are about $13 billion annually. Over and above this, additional financing is also needed to implement obesity reduction policies, although the costs for such policy efforts have not yet been estimated, as discussed in chapter 7. These resources need to be leveraged from domestic, development assistance, and innovative financing options. Although these financing needs seem substantial, the returns to investment are very high at $23 for every $1 invested, and the costs of inaction are significantly higher. The cost of malnutrition to the global economy is estimated to be $4.1 trillion per year—$2.1 trillion from undernutrition and micronutrient deficiencies and an estimated $2 trillion per year from the economic and social burden of overweight and obesity.

- Overall domestic financing for nutrition in the health sector has increased since 2015. Domestic nutrition-specific expenditures as a share of health expenditures increased from 2.6 percent to 3.3 percent on average between 2015 and 2021. In 2025, it is estimated that countries will spend $4.5 billion on nutrition interventions in the health sector, albeit mainly in upper-middle-income countries, and if trends continue, this amount will increase to $6 billion by 2034. The increases may be a result of global initiatives such as the Human Capital Project and the Nutrition for Growth (N4G) summits. However, nutrition spending still comprises a very small share of overall domestic health expenditures—at just 3 percent, on average. Among lower- and middle-income countries, which include several highly populated countries with the highest malnutrition burdens, the share is even smaller, at less than 2 percent.

Even when domestic health resource envelopes increased (for example, during the COVID-19 pandemic), the share for nutrition remained small, suggesting that domestic health resource expansion does not trickle down to domestic nutrition spending. Data are not yet available for other sectors, although some countries are undertaking public financial management reforms that include the establishment of a nutrition expenditure tracking system across sectors.

- Annual development assistance disbursements from the Organisation for Economic Co-operation and Development Creditor Reporting System to evidence-based high-impact nutrition interventions, including through humanitarian assistance, increased steadily, from $1.14 billion in 2015 to $1.60 billion in 2020, with a two-year average increase of 11 percent per annum. However, these disbursements plateaued between 2020 and 2022, increasing by a mere 0.4 percent per annum. This aligns with the likely impacts of the COVID-19 pandemic on development assistance flows for nutrition that forecast a slow recovery to prepandemic trends only by 2028, without accounting for the potential impacts of the Ukraine conflict on development assistance financing. Across the four major nutrition targets of stunting, wasting, anemia, and breastfeeding, only the treatment of wasting received increased development assistance disbursements during this period.

- Between 2024 and 2034, traditional financing from development assistance and domestic sources is likely to increase only marginally if the trajectory is unchanged, from an overall $6.3 billion annually in 2024 to $7.9 billion annually by 2034. This amount will fall far short of the needed financing. Given these constraints, exploring innovative financing is critical, yet nutrition lags other sectors in catalyzing it.

- Only 4.3 percent of climate financing is currently directed to the agrifood sector, despite the fact that this sector contributes nearly 30 percent of greenhouse gas emissions, and investments in this sector could yield a 16-fold return by 2030, benefiting both nutrition and climate. Large agrifood emitters could put in place sustainable transition plans to help them access climate financing. Opportunities for nutrition-smart adaptation financing also exist, especially for gender-responsive intersectoral activities as well as options such as redirecting public investments toward breastfeeding, which will not only support nutrition but also offer valuable carbon offsets. To date, however, none of these opportunities have been maximized.

- The financing needs highlighted in chapter 7 suggest that much more money is needed for nutrition than was estimated in 2017. However, efforts to increase nutrition financing must be accompanied by measures to enhance the efficiency of existing financing to maximize results, such as institutionalization of nutrition-responsive public financial management, allocative efficiency analytics (for example, Optima Nutrition), repurposing agrifood public support for healthier diets, and leveraging financing from universal health coverage (UHC) and nutrition-responsive safety-net programs.

- Given this scenario, it is imperative for the nutrition community to step up to renew financial commitments at the Paris N4G Summit and at the same time explore new and innovative sources of financing to support countries to scale up evidence-based nutrition actions. There are untapped opportunities, such as prioritizing nutrition in UHC financing and leveraging adaptive safety-net programs, repurposing agrifood subsidies for healthier diets, and accessing climate funds. Nontraditional and innovative sources, including sovereign wealth funds and private sector environmental, social, and governance (ESG) investing, offer other new opportunities. Nutrition lags other sectors in catalyzing these sources, even though food systems hold some of the most powerful opportunities to improve human and planetary health while increasing productivity; the private sector has a key role to play in this.

- In mobilizing private capital, the nutrition sector has much to learn from the climate movement, which has benefited from public capital investing in new technologies to the point at which renewable energy can now be generated more cheaply than fossil fuel energy. To catalyze significant ESG investing for food and nutrition security from the private sector, the nutrition community needs to bring together metrics, advocacy, catalytic capital (leveraging the balance sheets of development finance institutions and multilateral development bank communities), and strategic capital by incentivizing and encouraging companies and investors to invest in the food systems of tomorrow. With these four elements in place, private sector investment groups will pivot toward nutrition-positive investments, just as they did with climate investments and initiatives.

Domestic Financing for Nutrition

Domestic budget allocation is critical for sustainable financing for nutrition. Yet most countries do not have visibility on how much of their domestic budgets are allocated and spent on nutrition across sectors. A handful of countries have conducted nutrition-focused public expenditure reviews,[1] but in most cases, they have faced both data limitations in generating sufficiently granular analyses and human resource challenges in repeating the exercise periodically to analyze trends over time. Some attempts have been made to analyze available data from the System of Health Accounts (SHA), with the caveat that SHA data are limited in the health sector. It is also of concern that, among all disease categories covered by the SHA, the nutritional deficiencies (hereinafter, domestic nutrition expenditure) category receives the smallest share of government budgets, at less than 3 percent, on average. The nutritional deficiencies category is also the one that is most dependent on external aid (WHO 2021).

Analyses of available SHA data from WHO's Global Health Expenditure Database (GHED) show that domestic health expenditures (as a percentage of general government expenditure) increase as country income levels rise from low- and lower-middle- to upper-middle-income classification. However, domestic nutrition expenditures (as a percentage of government health expenditures) do not follow the same pattern; they are lowest among lower-middle-income countries (LMICs; below 2 percent), whereas those of low-income countries (LICs) and upper-middle-income countries (UMICs) are slightly higher (between 2 and 5 percent; refer to figure 9.1). Furthermore, the percentages for the LMIC group showed a downward trend between 2015 and 2021, even as their domestic health expenditures steadily increased (note that 2021 had a very small sample size). This confirms that there is no evidence suggesting a trickle-down of domestic health resource expansion to domestic nutrition spending.

Looking at average domestic nutrition expenditure levels in absolute terms, expenditures in the LIC and LMIC groups remained low at very similar levels, whereas expenditures in UMICs were much higher. It is of concern that domestic nutrition expenditure is particularly limited in LMICs, because this group includes highly populated, high-malnutrition-burden countries, such as Nigeria, Pakistan, and the Philippines. This warrants further assessment and consideration that the epidemiological burden of malnutrition, and its related risk factors, be included when prioritizing health resource allocation, especially in LMICs with high malnutrition burdens.

Figure 9.1   Trends in Domestic Expenditures for Health and Nutrition, 2015–21

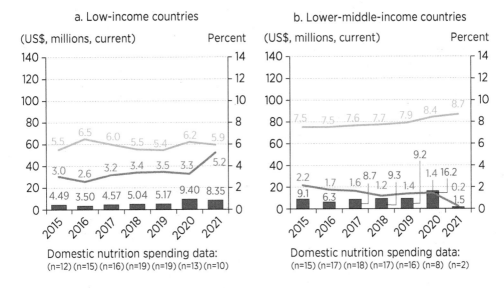

a. Low-income countries

Domestic nutrition spending data:
(n=12) (n=15) (n=16) (n=19) (n=19) (n=13) (n=10)

b. Lower-middle-income countries

Domestic nutrition spending data:
(n=15) (n=17) (n=18) (n=17) (n=16) (n=8) (n=2)

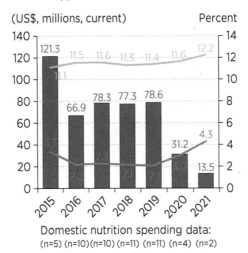

c. Upper-middle-income countries

Domestic nutrition spending data:
(n=5) (n=10)(n=10) (n=11) (n=11) (n=4) (n=2)

■ Average domestic nutrition spending (US$, millions, current)
── Average domestic health spending as % of general government expenditure
── Average domestic nutrition spending as % of domestic health spending

Source: Original figure for this publication, based on data extracted from the World Health Organization Global Health Expenditure Database (https://apps.who.int/nha/database), accessed April 8, 2024.

An in-depth analysis of country-level SHA data shows that several countries did not increase domestic nutrition expenditures at all between 2016 and 2019 (importantly, prepandemic years), even when their domestic health expenditures increased (refer to figure 9.2). These countries include Guinea, Niger, São Tomé and Príncipe, and many others (they are clustered around the *x*-axis in figure 9.2). However, some countries, such as Malawi and Uganda, increased domestic nutrition expenditures when their domestic health expenditures stagnated or even decreased. This indicates that, although the relative importance of nutrition in health sector spending varies across countries, a majority of countries do not allocate increased domestic health resources to nutrition.

Figure 9.2 When Domestic Health Expenditures Increase, Domestic Nutrition Expenditures Do Not Increase Proportionately in the Majority of Low- and Middle-Income Countries, 2016–19

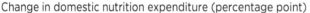

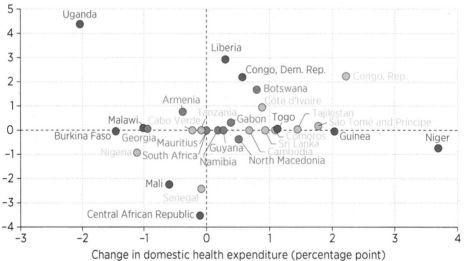

Source: Original figure for this publication, based on data extracted from the World Health Organization Global Health Expenditure Database (https://apps .who.int/nha/database), accessed April 8, 2024.

Figure 9.3 illustrates the relationship between domestic nutrition expenditures, as a share of overall domestic health expenditures, and the prevalence of stunting. In general, the higher the stunting burden, the more domestic health expenditures tend to be allocated to nutrition. However, the level of domestic resource prioritization for nutrition differs by country even when stunting prevalence is similar. For example, among countries that had stunting rates of around 35 percent in 2019, domestic nutrition expenditures as a share of domestic health expenditures ranged from 10 percent in Malawi to less than 2 percent in the Central African Republic, Ethiopia, Nigeria, and Sudan, although the percentages differ by year.

Figure 9.3   Domestic Nutrition Expenditures Relative to Stunting Burden, by Country, 2019

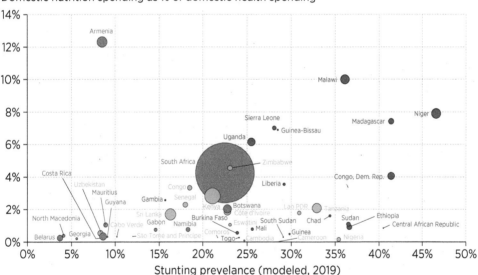

Source: Original figure for this publication, based on data extracted from the WHO Global Health Expenditure Database (https://apps.who.int/nha /database), accessed April 8, 2024, and the World Bank–UNICEF–WHO Joint Child Malnutrition Estimates 2023 (https://datatopics.worldbank.org /child-malnutrition/), accessed May 22, 2024.

Note: Bubble size represents actual domestic nutrition expenditures: the larger the bubble, the greater the expenditures. WHO = World Health Organization.

The 2025 domestic nutrition financing levels for the 73 countries included in this analysis were estimated (refer to annex 9A for details on the methodology). Data were taken from the GHED, and originally from SHA, and the Global Expected Health Spending database (modeled estimates; IHME 2022, 2023). For countries with large budget sizes, other data sources, such as country budget analysis data or public expenditure review results, were also assessed to triangulate the estimates wherever possible. Although data availability has improved, information on total cross-sectoral nutrition spending is limited. These projections, therefore, focus on a package of priority nutrition interventions that were costed in chapter 7 and for which information is available.

The total 2025 projected domestic nutrition expenditure for the countries analyzed was estimated to be $4.5 billion, with $2.8 billion, $1.5 billion, and $0.16 billion for 24 UMICs, 32 LMICs, and 17 LICs, respectively. This seems to reflect an increasing trend in domestic nutrition expenditures in the health sector, compared with the 2015 expenditure of $2.9 billion estimated at the time of the 2017 Investment Framework for Nutrition analysis. It is noteworthy that several LICs and LMICs (such as Côte d'Ivoire, Ethiopia, Madagascar, Niger, Uganda, and Sierra Leone) increased domestic allocations, albeit some high-burden LICs and LMICs (for example, Haiti, Nigeria, and even Senegal) saw a decline in domestic allocations for the past few years. It is likely that global initiatives such as the Human Capital Project and the Nutrition for Growth (N4G) summits, which raised the profile of nutrition with many heads of state, may have contributed to the additional domestic allocations.

Development Assistance for Nutrition

On the basis of data available in the Organisation for Economic Co-operation and Development Creditor Reporting System (OECD-CRS), annual development assistance disbursements to a set of evidence-based, high-impact nutrition interventions that were included in the costing analyses in chapter 7 were analyzed, including those provided through humanitarian assistance. The analysis revealed that the total disbursement increased steadily from $1.14 billion in 2015 (OECD 2024),[2] two years after the first N4G summit, to $1.60 billion in 2020, and especially in 2018–20, which had a two-year average increase of 11 percent per annum (Andridge et al. 2024). However, the latest analysis also shows that development assistance financing to this set of nutrition interventions began to plateau between 2020 and 2022, at around $1.6 billion per year, which represents a mere 0.4 percent increase per annum (refer to figure 9.4). Figure 9.5 shows that among the top six development assistance providers, only the World Bank, the Bill and Melinda Gates Foundation (BMGF), and Germany had a sizable increase in disbursements between 2020 and 2022, whereas bilateral contributions from the United

States, the European Union institutions, and the United Kingdom stagnated or declined by as much as 27 percent (Andridge et al. 2024; refer to figure 9.5). The analyses also show that development assistance financing was much more focused on wasting than on the wider nutrition agenda that would build future resilience (Andridge et al. 2024; refer to figure 9.8).

Analyses of major development assistance funding sources—namely, bilateral donors, multilateral organizations, and private donors—indicate that, although bilateral donor financing for nutrition-specific interventions increased between 2019 and 2020, it has been declining ever since. Multilateral organizations' financing (including multilateral development banks, multilateral financing facilities, and United Nations agencies, among others) peaked in 2019 and shrank in both 2020 and 2021, presumably as an immediate reaction to the COVID-19 pandemic. Private donors (philanthropic foundations that report to OECD-CRS) have steadily increased their total nutrition-specific disbursements since 2019 (refer to figure 9.6). France (2024) announced a €742 million budget cut in its development assistance for 2024; in 2021, the United Kingdom (2024) decided to reduce development assistance spending from 0.7 percent of gross national income to 0.5 percent; and for many major donors, such as the United States, nutrition funding has also been on the decline in recent years.

Figure 9.4 OECD-CRS Development Assistance Disbursements to Evidence-Based High-Impact Nutrition Interventions, 2015–22

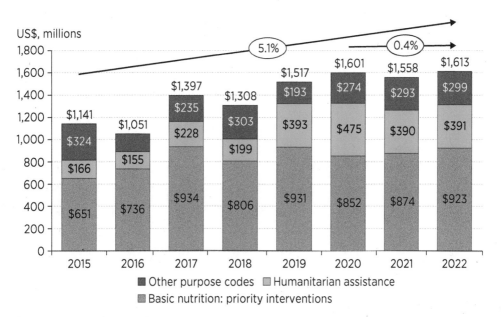

Source: Andridge et al. 2024.
Note: OECD-CRS = Organisation for Economic Co-operation and Development Creditor Reporting System.

Figure 9.5   OECD-CRS Development Assistance Disbursements to Evidence-Based High-Impact Nutrition Interventions from the Top Six Providers as of 2022, Annualized Percent Change, 2015–22

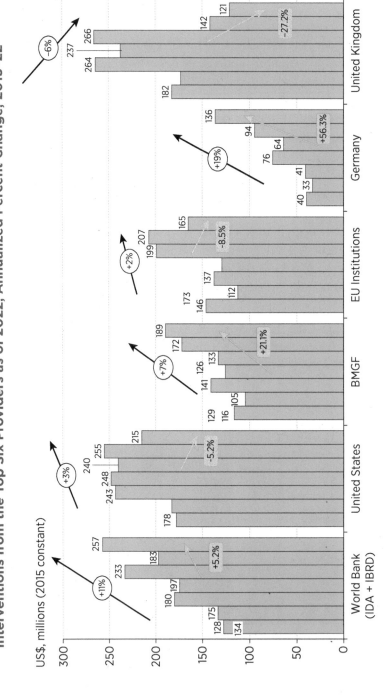

US$, millions (2015 constant)

Source: Andridge et al. 2024.

Note: BMGF = Bill & Melinda Gates Foundation; EU = European Union; IBRD = International Bank for Reconstruction and Development; IDA = International Development Association. OECD-CRS = Organisation for Economic Co-operation and Development Creditor Reporting System.

Figure 9.6 OECD-CRS Development Assistance Disbursements to Evidence-Based High-Impact Nutrition Interventions, by Funding Source, 2015–22

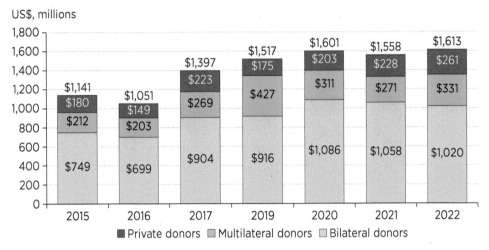

US$, millions

Source: Original figure for this publication, based on data extracted from the OECD-CRS, https://www.oecd-ilibrary.org/development/data/creditor -reporting-system_dev-cred-data-en, accessed May 16, 2024.
Note: Funding source groups are defined by OECD-CRS codes. See https:// web-archive.oecd.org/temp/2024-06-19/57753-dacandcrscodelists.htm for the list of funders in each category. Bilateral donors are traditional government donors; multilateral organizations include UN agencies, funds, and development banks (disbursements are mostly made up of International Development Association/International Bank for Reconstruction and Development); private donors include foundations that report to the OECD. OECD-CRS = Organisation for Economic Co-operation and Development Creditor Reporting System.

On the recipient side, LICs received a majority of the development assistance disbursements to evidence-based high-impact nutrition interventions, which steadily increased from 2016 and peaked in 2020. However, they declined by more than 10 percent between 2020 and 2022 (refer to figure 9.7).

Figure 9.7 OECD-CRS Development Assistance Disbursements to Evidence-Based High-Impact Nutrition Interventions, by Country Income Group, 2015–22

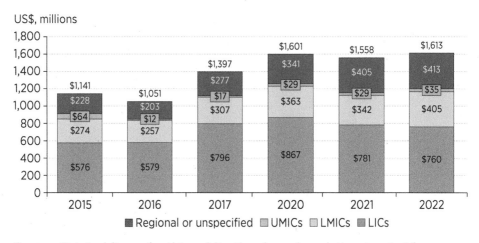

US$, millions

Source: Original figure for this publication, based on data extracted from the OECD-CRS, https://www.oecd-ilibrary.org/development/data/creditor -reporting-system_dev-cred-data-en, accessed May 16, 2024.
Note: LICs = low-income countries; LMICs = lower- and middle-income countries; OECD-CRS = Organisation for Economic Co-operation and Development Creditor Reporting System; regional or unspecified = the recipient is listed as a region or "bilateral, unspecified" recipient and therefore does not fit into an income group; UMICs = upper-middle-income countries.

It is noteworthy that much of the increase in development assistance disbursements to the set of evidence-based, high-impact nutrition interventions between 2018 and 2020 was for humanitarian assistance, which increased from $199 million in 2018 to $393 million in 2019, then flattened afterward (Andridge et al. 2024; refer to figure 9.4). Further disaggregated analyses reveal that across the four major nutrition targets of stunting, wasting, anemia, and breastfeeding, only the treatment of wasting received increased development assistance disbursements (refer to figure 9.8). These trends likely reflect post-COVID-19 humanitarian responses and have not continued thereafter. This confirms the 2020 modeled estimates that suggested likely impacts of the COVID-19 pandemic on development assistance flows toward nutrition (Osendarp et al. 2021). The study also forecast a slow recovery to prepandemic trends only by 2028, under a moderate scenario, without accounting for the potential impacts of the Ukraine conflict on development assistance financing (Osendarp et al. 2021). Such data are not available for nutrition-sensitive interventions.

Figure 9.8   Development Assistance Financing Disbursements to Priority Interventions, by World Health Assembly Target with Average Annual Change, 2015–22

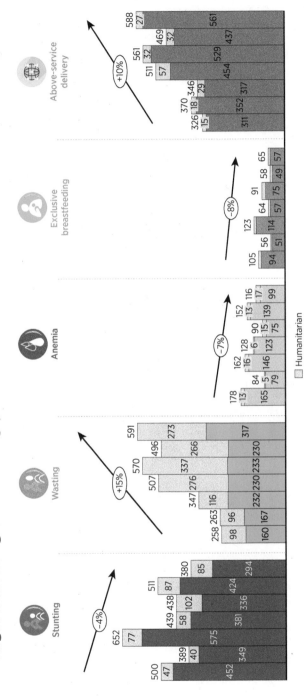

Source: Andridge et al. 2024.

Projected Domestic and Development Assistance Financing for Nutrition

Nutrition financing trends were projected for domestic and development assistance resources on the basis of annual rates of change in preceding years. Domestic nutrition expenditures as a share of domestic health expenditures increased from 2.6 percent to 3.3 percent between 2015 and 2025, which translates to annual increases of approximately 4.2 percent in that period. Applying this annual rate of increase, the model estimates that the 2025 baseline of $4.5 billion is projected to reach $6 billion by 2034. However, the projected trend of development assistance disbursements for nutrition shows only a 0.4 percent annual increase, which translates to less than a $0.1 billion increase per year from the 2025 baseline level of $1.9 billion (refer to figure 9.9). This projected trend is based on actual OECD-CRS development assistance disbursements for nutrition-specific interventions between 2015 and 2022.

Figure 9.9 Projected Domestic Expenditures for and Development Assistance Disbursements to Nutrition, 2025–34

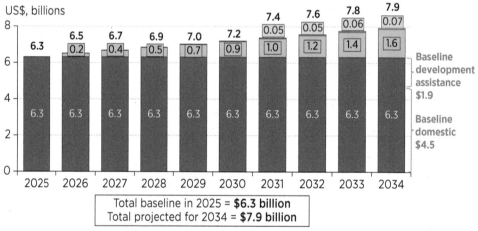

Total baseline in 2025 = **$6.3 billion**
Total projected for 2034 = **$7.9 billion**

■ Baseline (domestic + development assistance) ▢ Projected domestic
▢ Additional development assistance

Source: Original figure for this publication, based on data extracted from the Global Health Expenditure Database (World Health Organization), the Global Expected Health Spending database (Institute for Health Metrics and Evaluation), and the Organisation for Economic Co-operation and Development Creditor Reporting System, using the methodology described in annex 9A.

Overall, domestic expenditures for nutrition in the health sector are projected to increase between 2025 and 2034, driven by a multitude of factors, including global commitments made at the Tokyo N4G summit. It is also useful to note that data on domestic nutrition spending have become available for many more countries since 2016. This suggests that countries are starting to evaluate or track domestic nutrition spending, which will likely prompt more attention to nutrition in national budgeting processes.

However, the outlook for traditional donor aid is less encouraging, as a consequence, perhaps, of the Ukraine crisis, as well as the prolonged polycrises that have affected donor countries.

Nontraditional Sources of Nutrition Financing

The following sections highlight some potential opportunities to access nontraditional sources of financing from philanthropies, the private sector, innovative financing, and climate finance.

Philanthropies and Sovereign Wealth Funds

Philanthropic organizations have actively contributed financial resources to a wide range of nutrition activities across the world. However, levels and trends of philanthropic financing for nutrition were not analyzed in the past mainly because of the limited availability of data, except from a few large foundations, such as the BMGF and the Children's Investment Fund Foundation, which are included in the OECD-CRS. Recent data from 22 private foundations made available through the Stronger Foundations for Nutrition network reveal that a total of approximately $2 billion has been committed to nutrition activities (both nutrition specific and nutrition sensitive) for various time periods between 2014 and 2028.[3] Although approximately 8 percent of available grant data lack clarity on start and end years, rough estimates show $467 million, on average, per year.[4] Note that these figures are based on commitments, not disbursements.

Figure 9.10 breaks down these funds by intervention area. General maternal and child health and nutrition has the largest share (25.8 percent) because it includes activities not specifically assigned to other categories. The second-largest intervention area is micronutrient supplements (including multiple micronutrient supplements), at 15.6 percent, followed by nutritious and sustainable food systems, at 12.3 percent, which is anticipated to receive further increases in the coming 5 to 10 years through climate-related nutrition investments. Nutrition finance and capital and nutrition data and monitoring—which can be grouped together as institutional or system-strengthening investment—are ranked sixth and seventh. Although trends over time are not known, it is encouraging that some grantors also noted expected increases in other high-impact areas, such as micronutrient supplements, food fortification, and low birthweight and preterm births. These data are estimated to derive from approximately one-third of global nutrition philanthropies, by number, yet they are likely to represent closer to three-fourths of expected total philanthropic nutrition financing.

Figure 9.10   Philanthropic Financing for Nutrition, by Intervention Area, US$, Millions, 2014–28

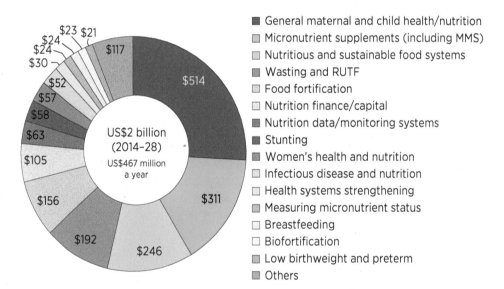

Source: Original figure for this publication, based on unpublished data from Stronger Foundations for Nutrition.
Note: MMS = multiple micronutrient supplements; RUTF = ready-to-use therapeutic food.

Sovereign wealth funds (SWFs) are also potential financing sources that have not, as yet, been tapped for nutrition. Globally, SWFs have grown more than 11-fold and, as of May 2024, hold assets of $11.9 trillion (SWF Academy 2024). Although SWFs are heterogeneous in their makeup and scope, and ambiguities still remain, the Sovereign Investment Laboratory offered the following detailed definition in 2015:

> (1) an investment fund rather than an operating company; (2) that is wholly owned by a sovereign government, but organized separately from the central bank or finance ministry to protect it from excessive political influence; (3) that makes international and domestic investments in a variety of risky assets; (4) that is charged with seeking a commercial return; and (5) which is a wealth fund rather than a pension fund—meaning that the fund is not financed with contributions from pensioners and does not have a stream of liabilities committed to individual citizens. (Bortolotti, Fotak, and Megginson 2015, 3001)

Traditionally, SWFs' primary role is to earn commercial returns through foreign investments. Yet, the financial and fiscal crises caused by the COVID-19 pandemic prompted SWFs to also be used as macrostabilization "rainy day funds" to stimulate domestic economies through measures such as industry bailouts or filling governments' domestic budget gaps (Megginson, Malik, and Zhou 2023). Arfaa et al. (2014) also note that multiple developing country governments had increased investments in their SWFs to fill persistent domestic infrastructure financing gaps. However, SWFs are not free from risks of being influenced by the political economy of the country, leading to challenges such as investments beyond the limits of macroeconomic or management capacity and political capture because SWFs are not subject to the market discipline required of development banks (Arfaa et al. 2014). At the same time, as large state-owned institutional investors, SWFs can play a unique and prime role in environmental, social, and governance (ESG) investments, which can be a significant source of financing for the food and nutrition agenda. SWFs' orientation toward ESG investments appears to be associated with their home countries' social norms regarding ESG (Megginson, Malik, and Zhou 2023).

Innovative Financing Opportunities

Several innovative financing opportunities have been identified in the development sector, ranging from gifts and donations to ESG financing, and are listed in box 9.1 (Shekar et al. 2023). However, the nutrition sector has yet to maximize these opportunities. Furthermore, the sector needs to focus on how donor or private sector financing can be designed to be more catalytic, as has been the case in other sectors, such as vaccine production and pricing and buy-downs for polio in key countries such as Nigeria and Pakistan.

Box 9.1

Existing Innovative Financing Opportunities

- *Gift and donation aggregation mechanisms.* There are mechanisms to aggregate voluntary donations, including in-kind contributions, from corporations or individuals to address specific social (or environmental) causes.

- *Pay-for-results mechanisms.* Funds are deployed only when predetermined outcomes are achieved and verified (as opposed to financing inputs).

- *Blended finance and impact investing.* Both of these instruments leverage development finance, philanthropic funds, and impact-driven capital to mobilize investment capital in vehicles, businesses, and projects for sustainable development.

- *Market guarantees and insurance instruments.* These instruments mitigate the risk (actual or perceived) that prevents capital flows.

- *Social bonds (capital markets).* Bonds or notes are issued in capital markets to finance businesses or projects for specific social (or environmental) impact, for which lenders receive principal and interest at maturity (unlike pay-for-results, where returns are tied to outcomes).

- *Strategic partnerships.* There are platforms designed to strategically structure partnerships for the purpose of mobilizing complementary resources.

Source: Adapted from Shekar et al. 2023.

Private Sector Sources

Food systems hold some of the most powerful opportunities to improve human and planetary health while increasing productivity—and the private sector plays a key role in this. Cognizant of this opportunity, the Food and Nutrition Security Global Challenge Program (FNS GCP) is designed to leverage these resources.

For food sector businesses, long-term reputational and financial risks are associated with poor health and malnutrition. These include social pressures and advocacy efforts to hold businesses accountable for their role in public health and global targets such as the Sustainable Development Goals (SDGs);

growing regulations, such as labeling, taxation, and marketing regulations (as highlighted in chapter 6); and increasing consumer demand for healthier and sustainably produced foods (Olayanju 2019). Reduced worker productivity in both the public and the private sectors as a consequence of poor nutrition is another key impetus for action. The corollary of these risks is the tremendous opportunity to drive financial success through the development and distribution of food products that respond to the global syndemic of malnutrition, as well as to maximize the market opportunity offered by the expanding demand for such foods. However, realistic and meaningful efforts at food systems transformation require managing serious conflicts of interest with so-called Big Food companies (Yates et al. 2021), and, currently, these efforts have been modest at best, despite investor pledges at the global level, such as the Tokyo N4G (Access to Nutrition Initiative 2021; Apampa et al. 2021),

A recent paper by Apampa et al. (2021) argues that the development finance community needs to collaborate with private financial institutions and investors to leverage limited public funding and increase investment. De-risking through smart blended finance is an effective development tool that will introduce new investors and demonstrate commercial viability of investments so blended finance can be phased out over time. Although the focus of the paper is agriculture, the same approach can also apply to nutrition.

In the agriculture and food space, several new initiatives have been launched to coordinate and catalyze new financing. These include, among others, the Good Food Finance Facility, convened by the EAT Foundation (GFFN n.d.), and Food Systems 2030 (World Bank n.d.) that provide advice and analytical products to underpin policy options, funds to pilot innovative approaches, and information to build support for change in different country contexts. It engages with the private sector by supporting the design, piloting, and de-risking of innovative public–private partnerships that advance development and climate goals. An innovative collaborative funding model is one mechanism that aims to go beyond existing blended finance solutions by bringing together a multitude of players and innovations to foster good food finance, optimizing investment cost and catalytic capital to de-risk innovative business model risk sharing, and reallocating public expenditures to reduce poverty and make nutritious food affordable and accessible in the context of "Food Finance Architecture: Financing a Healthy, Equitable, and Sustainable Food System" (World Bank 2021). Similar coordinated efforts have not yet materialized for nutrition, although the Multi-Donor Trust Fund for Scaling Up Nutrition hosted by the World Bank, has kick-started this effort and UNICEF's (n.d.) Child Nutrition Fund aims to catalyze coordinated action, albeit with a relatively narrow focus.

ESG Investing

Financial markets have witnessed burgeoning interest in ESG investing, which is based on the principle that companies that align their business practices, strategies, and governance with planetary and societal well-being are likely to yield financial success and shared value in the long term while also contributing to the global good. The value of global ESG assets tripled from 2012 to 2020 to $40.5 trillion—nearly half of the global financial assets under management (Baker 2020)—thereby representing a huge potential for social sector financing, including nutrition. However, although metrics and data systems for the environmental and governance components of ESG investing are more widely accepted and implemented, efforts in the social domain—especially as they pertain to health and nutrition—are still nascent (O'Hearn et al. 2022), despite ongoing efforts to strengthen these metrics and Nutrient Profiling Systems (Monteiro, Astrup, and Ludwig 2022).

ESG investing requires standardized, quantitative, and output-oriented metrics as well as an independent regulatory body to promote, oversee, and audit the findings of these metrics. However, when it comes to ESG investing and nutrition and health in the food sector (ESG–Nutrition), these minimum requirements are not currently being met, and there are significant limitations to the landscape of available ESG–Nutrition metrics. Major global ESG disclosure standards bodies have developed food sector–specific disclosure requirements to standardize business reporting on sustainability. In parallel, nonprofit groups such as the Access to Nutrition Initiative (https://accesstonutrition.org/) are developing comprehensive indices to track ESG performance and rank food sector businesses on key social and environmental sustainability issues (Food Foundation 2021; Global Reporting Initiative 2021; World Benchmarking Alliance 2021). However, although metrics aimed at quantifying the healthfulness of a business's product portfolio often single out specific nutrients of concern (for example, added sugar or calories) or broad product categories (for example, plant- versus animal-sourced foods), which are important considerations, they also need to evolve to consider healthfulness more holistically, to encompass equitable distribution of healthful foods and the relative affordability and accessibility of healthful products. Metrics for ESG investing in nutrition must therefore become nimbler to leverage substantive private sector resources for a healthier food system. Without this, "nutri-washing," similar to greenwashing in financial markets, becomes a concern.

Opportunities to Improve the Efficiency of Spending: More Nutrition for the Money

Effective and sustainable financing involves strategic deployment of public financial management (PFM) tools and processes. Opportunities exist in PFM reform processes in all nutrition-relevant sectors to improve allocative and spending efficiency, which can not only increase results but also create more fiscal space. Repurposing or reorienting existing sector financing for nutrition co-benefits is another opportunity that has yet to be fully leveraged.

Nutrition-Responsive Public Financial Management

Enhancing efficiency of nutrition spending requires nutrition-responsive PFM systems and tools that can facilitate PFM processes multisectorally. These processes include evidence-based budget allocation, tracking of nutrition expenditures across different sectors at different levels, analyzing expenditure data multisectorally, and making course corrections. By doing so, PFM systems can hold both implementers and financiers accountable to the financial resources and the results—all across relevant sectors.

Nutrition Public Expenditure Reviews

Nutrition Public Expenditure Reviews (NPERs) assess a country's nutrition budget allocations and expenditures and their links to nutrition outcomes. *A Guiding Framework for Nutrition Public Expenditure Reviews* (Wang et al. 2022) provides guidance on how to conduct a thorough assessment that goes beyond simply quantifying how much is allocated or spent on nutrition, to answer how well money is being spent across all relevant sectors—considering efficiency, effectiveness, and equity—to achieve nutrition outcomes. Several countries—such as Bangladesh, Bhutan, Indonesia, Nepal, Sri Lanka, Rwanda, and Tanzania—have conducted NPERs in recent years. They have found it critically important to have not only explicitly coded and adequately detailed nutrition budget data, ideally down to the activity level, but also mechanisms to conduct the assessments periodically to more meaningfully inform government budgeting processes.

Nutrition-Responsive Budgeting and PFM

On the basis of the lessons learned through NPERs and with a strong political will to invest in nutrition to build human capital, countries such as Indonesia, Pakistan, and Rwanda have undertaken nutrition-responsive PFM reform to allow tracking of nutrition expenditures across sectors through their financial management information systems. On the basis of those countries' experiences, the World Bank developed *Driving Nutrition Action through the Budget: A Guide to Nutrition Responsive Budgeting* (Piatti-Fünfkirchen et al. 2023), which proposes a five-step framework to help make budgets and PFM processes responsive to nutrition needs. The guide draws from literature related to budgeting on poverty, gender, and climate and recommends the following:

- Agreement on costed nutrition priorities between ministries of finance and sector ministries to guide budget allocations

- Preparation of a nutrition-responsive budget through a budget call circular and technical sector guidelines to explicitly recognize nutrition in the budget

- Obtainment of legislative approval of a dedicated nutrition budget statement

- Implementation of the budget by prioritizing timely budget release against the nutrition budget statement and execution reporting

- Course correction through collective nutrition financial and programmatic progress review so that priority interventions and costing are agreed on before the start of the new budget process (Piatti-Fünfkirchen et al. 2023).

Making nutrition financing visible across sectors is the first step toward better managing existing resources. Indonesia's budget tracking system helped to make nutrition spending visible to decision-makers for the first time, which led to a commitment announced at the Tokyo N4G summit in 2021 to maintain more than $2 billion worth of annual budget allocation to nutrition until 2024. In Rwanda, data generated from a similar system contributed to an increase in the nutrition budget allocation by over 20 percent between 2021 and 2022, although the growth of the total domestic resource envelope was much smaller.

Allocative Efficiency Analytics: Optima Nutrition

Chapter 7 lays out how the Optima Nutrition tool can be used to maximize impacts with limited budgets. Countries are being trained in the use of this tool, and many are already using it to improve their national plans.

Opportunities for Leveraging Existing Investments in Related Sectors for Nutrition

Nutrition is increasingly recognized as a multisectoral development agenda, yet existing investment strategies and financing plans of nutrition-contributing sectors, such as health, agriculture, social protection, and education, have not been fully calibrated to achieve nutrition objectives. For example, nutrition plays a critical role in attainment of Universal Health Coverage (UHC) objectives. Repurposing of agrifood public support policies, such as subsidies, to optimize economic and climate impacts has gained considerable political attention in the current crisis, whereas health and nutrition impacts of agrifood subsidies have only recently been included in ongoing repurposing efforts. Evidence-based advocacy can make the case for nutrition sensitivity and co-benefits across key sectors.

Including Nutrition in Universal Health Coverage Financing

Nutrition services are often not explicitly prioritized in UHC financing. Ensuring explicit inclusion of nutrition services in UHC packages offers a critical opportunity to leverage health finances to work toward nutrition outcomes that health systems ought to produce. Well-designed, targeted financing strategies and incentivization for primary health care delivery is of paramount importance to reaching vulnerable women and children with quality nutrition services when and where they need them. By optimizing the specific health financing levers of revenue raising, pooling, and purchasing, countries can do the following:

- Include and prioritize a costed and well-defined set of nutrition services in the UHC benefits package

- Increase domestic nutrition investment through innovative fiscal policies and strategic advocacy to save future health care costs

- Institute and implement strong accountability measures to deploy existing nutrition resources more effectively, efficiently, and equitably

- Align health financing arrangements with nutrition objectives to address underlying financing and service delivery challenges

- Strategically invest in strengthening health system components, such as program and financial data systems, to enable improved nutrition outcomes (Subandoro et al. 2022).

More specifically, optimizing health financing levers can address underlying service delivery and financing bottlenecks that contribute to low nutrition service coverage and quality by improving the following:

- Equity, by pooling prepaid resources to spread financial risk for nutrition services across population groups or contracting community-based providers who have the greatest access to the most vulnerable target users

- Efficiency, by incentivizing delivery of essential nutrition services in primary health care by using output-based payment methods such as capitation, fee-for-service, and results-based financing

- Transparency and accountability, by raising awareness among consumers, health workers, and community-based workers about nutrition service entitlements and monitoring the use of public funds for nutrition to ensure that they are managed appropriately.

Further work has been done to strengthen the understanding of how nutrition services can be incentivized in purchasing arrangements for primary health care to improve its quality, coverage, and efficiency (WHO 2021, 2022).

Nutrition-targeted health taxes can curb the consumption of unhealthy foods and simultaneously generate additional revenue, increasing fiscal space to pursue development priorities. Such tax revenue, however small in size, could be earmarked to health- and nutrition-promoting activities, for example in the case of Thailand (Ozer et al. 2020). Additional details are found in chapter 6.

Integrating Nutrition with Other Life-Saving Interventions

Many children continue to lack access to essential services, and often those at the highest risk of malnutrition are also those who are underimmunized. Evidence suggests that combining nutrition interventions with vaccination services can improve the success of both interventions, saving more lives and boosting vaccine demand (Davis, Rana, and Sarriot 2023). Tapping into financing opportunities for immunizations could therefore be mutually beneficial.

Gavi, the Vaccine Alliance, and the Eleanor Crook Foundation (ECF) have announced a modest US$2 million joint investment in the NutriVax Project, an integrated nutrition and immunization research partnership aiming to combine life-saving interventions that are typically delivered separately (ECF 2023). Despite the fact that immunization and nutrition services can both be delivered through community-based primary health care delivery systems such as outreach services, they are often financed and managed separately, which creates inefficiency. Lessons from this experience can inform future programming at scale.

As highlighted by Davis, Rana, and Sarriot (2023), there are two main types of integrated nutrition and immunization programming approaches, each with slightly different rationale and operational requirements:

- *Combined service provision.* This approach involves delivering both immunization and nutrition interventions at the same high-coverage health system touchpoint. These methods generate value through efficiency by codelivering compatible interventions to overlapping target populations. By delivering both services simultaneously, health systems can achieve cost savings or greater impact, reaching more children with the same combined budget. For families, the reduced time required to access health services can lead to higher overall utilization and lower dropout rates from multistep series. To enhance this approach, stakeholders should focus on bundling interventions with similar delivery modalities, human resource requirements, and logistical needs for efficient codelivery. The best-documented example is the integration of immunization with vitamin A supplementation.

- *Enhanced demand generation and case finding.* This approach uses a wider range of integrated methods, including joint demand generation, incentive approaches, and cross-referral, to increase program reach by leveraging the complementary strengths of immunization and nutrition programs. The advantage of this type of approach is that it does not require close matching of compatible services to integrate, thus offering more flexibility. Proven community-based integrated demand generation approaches should be deployed where appropriate. One such example is the care group approach, where social and behavior changes are encouraged through peer-to-peer knowledge sharing, primarily among mothers.

Integrating nutrition with other complementary life-saving interventions holds the potential to leverage health finances and make significant improvements in boosting coverage and quality of community-based delivery of life-saving interventions.

Repurposing Agrifood Public Support to Food Systems

As detailed in chapter 6, agrifood subsidies and public support add up to anywhere between $638 billion across 79 countries from 2016 to 2018 (Damania et al. 2023) and a post-COVID estimate by the OECD of $851 billion globally from 2020 to 2022 (OECD 2023). However, as highlighted in chapter 6, a large share of these subsidies is either regressive or focused on the wrong agricultural produce. Figure 6.2 demonstrates that sugar is among the most subsidized commodities globally, whereas fruits and vegetables receive the least amount of subsidies. The food, agriculture, climate, and health sectors are starting to work together to reorient subsidies channeled through food systems toward healthier diets, healthier people, healthier economies, and a healthier planet. Nutritional considerations are on the table in these discussions, but stronger political commitment and more investment through a nutrition lens are needed to ensure that when repurposed, these subsidies will improve nutrition rather than do harm.

Nutrition-Responsive Social Protection

The current prolonged polycrises have elevated the importance of social protection systems. Some countries are considering "cash-plus" assistance programs, where nutrition specificity is key to making such programs truly meaningful and maximizing the investment returns on human capital. The World Bank's new FNS GCP proposes to provide wraparound nutrition and health services along with adaptive safety net programs. Delivering some of the high-impact nutrition services (such as multiple micronutrient supplements and small-quantity lipid-based nutrient supplements, as well as breastfeeding advice) through these adaptive safety nets can significantly increase coverage of these key services, with modest additional costs, and achieve potential win–wins for both social protection and nutrition outcomes. In addition, social protection programs can scale up procurement of fortified foods through institutional food procurement.

Nutrition Investments through Climate Financing

Climate finance flows through various channels, offering recipient countries multiple avenues to access funding. These channels include multilateral funds, which—unlike contributor country-dominated governance structures—often provide developing country governments with more representation in decision-making. Several developed nations have also launched their own climate finance initiatives or are directing funds through their bilateral development assistance institutions. Additionally, numerous developing countries have established their own regional and national channels and funds, supported by international finance, domestic budget allocations, and contributions from the domestic private sector, each with distinct forms and functions (Watson and Schalatek 2023). Despite the significant impact of climate change on nutrition, highlighted in chapter 4, the scope of financing dedicated to related actions is currently extremely limited. Only less than 4.3 percent of climate financing is committed to the agrifood sector for both mitigation and adaptation activities, even though food systems are among the largest contributors to greenhouse gases (GHGs) and have a tremendous impact on food and nutrition security. This reflects a huge disconnect between GHG emissions and climate impacts and the financing currently mobilized from climate funds (Sutton, Lotsch, and Prasann 2024).

When looking for opportunities to leverage nutrition investments through climate adaptation funds, one potential avenue would be to channel resources to activities promoting nutrition with a human rights and gender lens. The Paris Agreement, negotiated in 2015, called for upholding human rights, including the right to health and the rights of vulnerable populations, as well as gender equality, women's empowerment, and intergenerational equity, as priorities to consider when taking action to address climate change. Because of this, some climate funds have incorporated environmental and social considerations into their policies and overarching action plans, providing targeted funding and support for capacity building to ensure implementation (Watson and Schalatek 2024) Food and nutrition security, for example, are central to individual dignity and foundational to the enjoyment of human rights, and gender equality and women's empowerment are high-priority areas in nutrition interventions. Therefore, aligning nutrition interventions with the principles outlined in the Paris Agreement is not only ethically imperative but also strategically beneficial to mobilize funding.

One example of a fund that has incorporated these principles into its operations is the Adaptation Fund. Programs funded by the Adaptation Fund primarily cover food security, agriculture, water management, and disaster risk reduction, thereby presenting numerous avenues to fund nutrition-sensitive yet climate-smart interventions (Adaptation Fund 2021). These focus areas are not uncommon: the Green Climate Fund and the emerging Enhanced Adaptation for Smallholder Agriculture Programme, among others, also have an explicit focus on intersectoral climate action, underscoring the potential for countries to unlock funding for activities that simultaneously benefit nutrition and climate outcomes.[5] Table 9.1 further outlines examples of multilateral funds that provide avenues for nutrition-sensitive climate adaptation initiatives.

Another opportunity to access climate financing is through mitigation efforts targeting the food system. Annual investments need to increase to $260 billion a year to put the world on track for net zero emissions by 2050, but mitigation finance for the agrifood sector has most recently, as of 2019–20, been estimated to equal only $14.4 billion. However, investments in low-emission agriculture and in reshaping food and land use practices can be highly profitable, because they have the potential to yield health, economic, and environmental benefits amounting to a 16-fold return of $4.3 trillion by 2030 (Sutton, Lotsch, and Prasann 2024).

Table 9.1 Examples of Multilateral Climate Adaptation Funds for Nutrition

Climate fund	Scope	Entry point for nutrition
Adaptation Fund	Supports initiatives aimed at assisting vulnerable communities in developing countries to adapt to climate change.	Strives to fund activities that are gender responsive and, wherever feasible, gender transformative, adopting an intersectional approach. Primarily covers food security, agriculture, water management, and disaster risk reduction.
Green Climate Fund	The world's largest climate fund; aims to bring forth transformative climate action in developing countries via country-owned partnerships and flexible financing solutions.	Among its eight result areas are an explicit focus on health, food, and water security; it recognizes improving nutrition as a desired co-benefit of its operations. Projects such as Akamatutu'anga To Tatou Ora'anga Meitaki in the Cook Islands enhance health and nutrition security, particularly for mothers and children.
Enhanced Adaptation for Smallholder Agriculture Programme	Launched in 2021; poised to become the largest initiative dedicated to supporting small-scale producers.	Initial priorities focus on the intersection of climate, conflict, and fragility in a few countries, but it is expected to expand its scope to include the intersection of climate, biodiversity, gender, and nutrition. Will also facilitate the implementation of new financial mechanisms to stimulate private sector investment in climate adaptation for small-scale agriculture, which a large part of the world depends on to maintain food security and nutrition.

Source: Original table for this publication.

Although climate mitigation financing can take many shapes, an important target is the industries responsible for a large share of GHG emissions. Agrifood industries could attract financing by implementing transition pathways to mitigate their climate and environmental impact, demonstrating their commitment to meeting sustainability goals. Stakeholders need to recognize these opportunities and encourage new investments, because limiting climate financing to traditionally "green" activities could hinder large GHG emitters from accessing essential capital for much-needed sustainable transitions. As highlighted in chapter 4, the Climate Bonds Initiative and Credit Suisse (2020) offer a framework for assessing credible and ambitious transitions, ensuring transparency and effectiveness. Private agrifood companies with a focus on nutrition should embrace these guidelines to establish strong transition plans and attract climate financing. Two major Brazilian agrifood companies have developed transition plans using the tools provided by Climate Bonds and can serve as the standard by which companies should be assessed. They offer recommendations on the core activities to be continued, those that should be reviewed, and areas in which further disclosure may be required. A recent report reviews sustainable debt instruments that can be accessed by those operating in the Brazilian agrifood sector to finance their transition to net zero (Climate Bonds Initiative 2023). Lessons from these examples can be helpful for private sector companies in the nutrition sector.

Finally, an important climate mitigation financing pathway for nutrition is through the reorientation of public investments toward breastfeeding. The economic value of this high-quality, locally sourced, and most sustainable first-food system is often overlooked and undervalued, in contrast with high GHG-emitting commercial milk formulas, for which expanding markets count toward gross domestic product growth. Financing breastfeeding protection, support, and promotion activities should be recognized not only as an investment for nutrition and health but also as a valuable carbon offset in global sustainable development plans. Integrating breastfeeding into a United Nations–backed carbon finance mechanism such as the Kyoto Protocol's Clean Development Mechanism would mean that investments in breastfeeding support could be financed by high-emission countries buying carbon credits, thereby reducing reliance on commercial milk formulas and supporting both human and planetary health (Smith et al. 2024).

The Way Forward

Overall, financing trends suggest that traditional financing sources from both development assistance and domestic sources continue to be constrained and are unlikely to meet financing needs, which will be in excess of $128 billion between 2025 and 2034 (approximately $13 billion annually). If the trajectory is unchanged, it leaves a financing gap of $120 billion between 2025 and 2034 (refer to figure 9.11). In 2017, it was suggested that the financing gap could be met if high-burden country governments would increase the share of their projected spending on health that is directed to nutrition from about 1.0 percent to 2.9 percent, and development assistance partners would boost nutrition support from an average of 1.0 percent of total development assistance resources to about 2.8 percent. Given the large financing gap that persists, despite a 4.2 percent increase in domestic financing, these recommendations for development assistance support stand as is.

Figure 9.11 Total Financing Needs and Gaps for Full Scale-Up of Nutrition Interventions, 2025–34

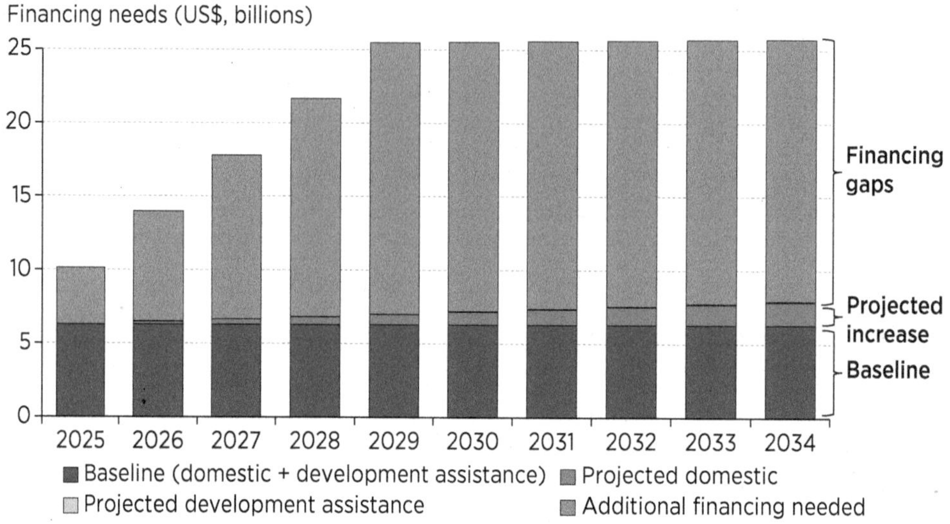

Financing needs (US$, billions)

Legend:
- Baseline (domestic + development assistance)
- Projected domestic
- Projected development assistance
- Additional financing needed

Financing gaps
Projected increase
Baseline

Source: Original figure for this publication, based on data extracted from Global Health Expenditure Database (World Health Organization), the Global Expected Health Spending database (Institute for Health Metrics and Evaluation), and the Organisation for Economic Co-operation and Development Creditor Reporting System, using the methodology described in annex 9A.

Note: The lower bars represent the costs of maintaining existing intervention coverage, and the top bars represent the annual additional financing requirements to increase the coverage of interventions to 90 percent over a five-year period (2025–29) and maintain coverage for an additional five years.

Given this scenario, it is imperative for the nutrition community to support country efforts to strengthen nutrition-responsive public financial management, step up to renew financial commitments at the Paris N4G summit, and at the same time explore new and innovative sources of financing to support countries to scale up high-impact nutrition actions. We need more money for nutrition, but we also need to deliver more nutrition for the money that is available by improving the efficiency of spending (refer to figure 9.12). There are untapped opportunities, such as leveraging UHC financing and adaptive safety net programs for nutrition, repurposing agrifood subsidies for healthier diets, and accessing climate funds. Nontraditional and innovative sources, including SWFs and private sector ESG investing, offer other new opportunities. Nutrition lags behind other sectors in catalyzing these sources, even though food systems hold some of the most powerful opportunities to improve human and planetary health while increasing productivity. And the private sector has a key role to play in this.

Figure 9.12 The Way Forward: More Money for Nutrition, More Nutrition for the Money

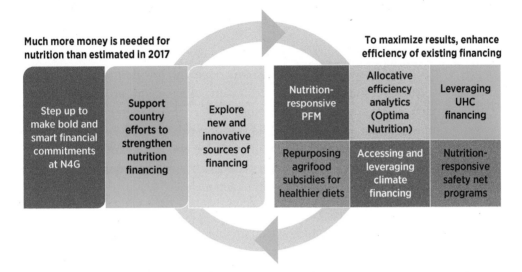

Much more money is needed for nutrition than estimated in 2017

To maximize results, enhance efficiency of existing financing

Source: Original figure for this publication
Note: N4G = Nutrition for Growth; PFM = public financial management; UHC = universal health coverage.

The World Bank's new FNS GCP is designed with a strong line of sight to private capital mobilization as well as innovative sources, recognizing that domestic resources and other development financing will not suffice to address the scale of global challenges.

In mobilizing private capital, the nutrition sector has much to learn from the climate movement, which has benefited from public capital investing in new technologies to the point at which renewable energy can now be generated more cheaply than fossil fuel energy. To catalyze significant ESG investing for food and nutrition security from the private sector, for example, the nutrition community needs to bring together metrics, advocacy, catalytic capital (leveraging the balance sheets of the development finance institutions and multilateral development bank communities), and strategic capital by incentivizing and encouraging companies and investors to invest in the food systems of tomorrow. With these four elements in place, private sector investment groups will pivot toward nutrition-positive investments, just as they did with climate investments and initiatives. The key here is to educate investors on the return potential of investing in nutrition, not just from an investment perspective but also for increasing labor productivity in the private sector (Shekar et al. 2023).

Areas for Further Work and Research

As the nutrition community congregates to generate new resources, this analysis also highlights the need for further work in the following five key domains:

- *Development assistance and domestic resources.* Ensure that development assistance resources are catalytic in converging actions across donors and national governments and that they balance the current focus on humanitarian aid to reduce child wasting with forward-looking preventive actions that will build resilience and reduce future needs for humanitarian financing. Support countries to enhance domestic resource allocations for preventive nutrition actions.

- *Innovative financing approaches.* Explore additional innovative financing sources, including climate finance, repurposing agrifood subsidies, and mobilizing private sector sources such as ESG investing. Further enhance mechanisms and tools to integrate preventive nutrition interventions and policies as well as fiscal policies, such as taxation and regulation of marketing of unhealthy foods and so forth, into national UHC plans and packages.

- *Empirical research.* Conduct additional empirical research on links between climate; gender; water, sanitation, and hygiene (WASH); and nutrition for which biological underpinnings are known but for which evidence on the size of their impact on nutrition outcomes is insufficient. Develop empirical estimates of the costs, opportunities, and challenges of implementing obesity reduction policies. Once estimates and costs are available, they could all be included in future iterations of impact models, such as Optima Nutrition.

- *Maximization of delivery platforms for scale-up.* Continue to explore how adaptive safety net programs can be designed to deliver high-impact nutrition interventions and how the synergies with the WASH, education, and agriculture sectors could be maximized. Identify setting-specific approaches that might influence the scale and effectiveness of interventions.

- *Technical and implementation support to countries to scale up.* Provide technical and implementation support to countries to scale up nutrition programming and policies across all relevant sectors; work with countries to understand how resources can be optimized, public financial management enhanced, and nutrition budgets better tracked in ways that align with their strategic plans and drive results.

The economic benefits associated with the investments in child and maternal nutrition alone far outweigh the costs of inaction, which run at about $41 trillion over 10 years. This is a combined estimate of the economic productivity losses up to $2.1 trillion a year due to undernutrition and micronutrient deficiencies (FAO 2013) and the latest estimate of $2 trillion as economic and social costs of overweight and obesity, which is predicted to reach $3 trillion a year by 2030 (Okunogbe et al. 2022). If we act together and fill the gaps, trillions of dollars' worth of human capital and economic productivity gains will be enjoyed by generations to come.

Notes

1. Those countries include Bangladesh, Bhutan, Ethiopia, Indonesia, Nepal, Rwanda, Sri Lanka, and Tanzania, among others.

2. The data were extracted from the OECD-CRS database to estimate total disbursements to the defined set of evidence-based, high-impact nutrition interventions by providers categorized under official development assistance, other official flows, and private development finance.

3. Calculation based on unpublished data provided by Stronger Foundations for Nutrition.

4. Calculation based on unpublished data provided by Stronger Foundations for Nutrition.

5. For more on The Green Climate Fund's initiatives on health, food, and water security, see Green Climate Fund (n.d.). For more on the IFAD's Enhanced Adaptation for Smallholder Agriculture Programme, see IFAD (n.d.).

References

Access to Nutrition Initiative. 2021. "N4G Investor Pledge." Utrecht: Access to Nutrition Foundation. https://accesstonutrition.org/app/uploads/2021/10/Investor-Pledge-Submitted-20211202-final.pdf.

Adaptation Fund. 2021. "About the Adaptation Fund." Washington, DC: Adaptation Fund. https://www.adaptation-fund.org/about/.

Andridge, Caroline, Abbe McCarter, Mary D'Alimonte, and Albertha Nyaku. 2024. *Tracking Aid for the WHA Nutrition Targets: Progress toward the Global Nutrition Goals between 2015 to 2022*. Washington, DC: Results for Development. https://r4d.org/resources/tracking-aid-wha-nutrition-targets-global-spending-roadmap-better-data/.

Apampa, Andrew, Chris Clubb, Bethany Emma Cosgrove, Gretel Gambarelli, Hans Loth, Richard Newman, Vanesa Rodriguez Osuna, et al. 2021. "Scaling Up Critical Finance for Sustainable Food Systems through Blended Finance." Discussion Paper, CGIAR Research Program on Climate Change, Agriculture and Food Security. Wageningen, the Netherlands. https://www.convergence .finance/resource/scaling-up-critical-finance-for-sustainable-food-systems -through-blended-finance/view.

Arfaa, Noora, Alan Harold Gelb, Havard Halland, Gregory Smith, and Silvana Tordo. 2014. "Sovereign Wealth Funds and Long-Term Development Finance: Risks and Opportunities." Policy Research Working Paper No. 6776, World Bank, Washington, DC.

Baker, S. 2020. "Global ESG-Data Driven Assets Hit \$40.5 trillion." *Pensions & Investments,* July 2, 2020. https://www.pionline.com/esg/global-esg-data-driven -assets-hit-405-trillion#:~:text=The%20value%20of%20global%20assets, to%20%2440.5%20trillion%20in%202020.

Bortolotti, Bernardo, Veljko Fotak, and William L. Megginson. 2015. "The Sovereign Wealth Fund Discount: Evidence from Public Equity Investments." *Review of Financial Studies* 28 (11): 2993–3035. https://doi.org/10.1093/rfs/hhv036.

Climate Bonds Initiative. 2023. "Investment Opportunities: Agrifood Sector in Brazil." London: Climate Bonds Initiative. https://www.climatebonds.net/files /reports/investment_opportunity_report_brazil_.pdf.

Climate Bonds Initiative and Credit Suisse. 2020. "Financing Credible Transitions: How to ensure the transition label has impact." London: Climate Bonds Initiative and Zurich: Credit Suisse. https://www.climatebonds.net/transition -finance/fin-credible-transitions.

Damania, Richard, Esteban Balseca, Charlotte de Fontaubert, Joshua Gill, Kichan Kim, Jun Rentschler, Jason Russ, and Esha Zaveri. 2023. *Detox Development: Repurposing Environmentally Harmful Subsidies—Overview.* Washington, DC: World Bank. https://hdl.handle.net/10986/39423.

Davis, Tom, Yashodhara Rana, and Eric Sarriot. 2023. *A Literature Review and Proposed Learning Agenda on Immunisation-Nutrition Integration.* San Marcos, TX: Gavi, the Vaccine Alliance, and Eleanor Crook Foundation.

ECF (Eleanor Crook Foundation). 2023. "Gavi, the Vaccine Alliance, and the Eleanor Crook Foundation Announce \$2 Million Investment in an Integrated Child Survival Project." Press release, June 14, 2023. https://www.prnewswire .com/news-releases/gavi-the-vaccine-alliance-and-the-eleanor-crook -foundation-announce-2-million-investment-in-an-integrated-child-survival -project-301851010.html.

FAO (Food and Agriculture Organization of the United Nations). 2013. "The State of Food and Agriculture, 2013." Working Paper 5511, FAO, Geneva.

Food Foundation. 2021. "Plating Up Progress." London: Food Foundation. https://foodfoundation.org.uk/plating-up-progress-home-page/.

France. 2024. "Décret no. 2024-124 du 21 février 2024 portant annulation de crédits." https://www.legifrance.gouv.fr/eli/decret/2024/2/21/ECOB2405177D/jo/texte.

GFFN (Good Food Finance Network). n.d. "Good Food Finance Facility." GFFN. https://goodfood.finance/workstreams/cip/.

Global Reporting Initiative. 2021. "GRI Standards by Language." Amsterdam: Global Reporting Initiative. https://www.globalreporting.org/standards/download-the-standards/.

Green Climate Fund. n.d. "Health, Food, and Water Security." Incheon, Republic of Korea: Green Climate Fund. https://www.greenclimate.fund/results/health-food-water-security.

IFAD (International Fund for Agricultural Development). n.d. "The Enhanced Adaptation for Smallholder Agriculture Programme (ASAP+)." Rome: IFAD. https://www.ifad.org/en/asap-enhanced.

IHME (Institute for Health Metrics and Evaluation). 2022. "Global Expected Health Spending 2016–2040." IHME, Seattle. Accessed May 31, 2024, https://ghdx.healthdata.org/record/ihme-data/global-expected-health-spending-2016-2040.

IHME (Institute for Health Metrics and Evaluation). 2023. "Global Expected Health Spending 2020–2050." https://ghdx.healthdata.org/record/ihme-data/global-expected-health-spending-2020-2050.

Megginson, William L., Asif I. Malik, and Xin Yue Zhou. 2023. "Sovereign Wealth Funds in the Post-Pandemic Era." *Journal of International Business Policy* 6: 253–75. https://doi.org/10.1057/s42214-023-00155-2.

Monteiro, Carlos A., Arne Astrup, and David S. Ludwig. 2022. "Does the Concept of 'Ultra-Processed Foods' Help Inform Dietary Guidelines, beyond Conventional Classification Systems? YES." *American Journal of Clinical Nutrition* 116 (6): 1476–81. https://doi.org/10.1093/ajcn/nqac122.

OECD (Organisation for Economic Co-operation and Development). 2023. *Agricultural Policy Monitoring and Evaluation 2023: Adapting Agriculture to Climate Change*. Paris: OECD Publishing. https://doi.org/10.1787/b14de474-en.

OECD (Organisation for Economic Co-operation and Development). 2024. "OECD Data Explorer" (database). Paris: OECD. Accessed May 16, 2024, https://stats.oecd.org/Index.aspx?DataSetCode=crs1.

O'Hearn, Meghan, Suzannah Gerber, Sylara M. Cruz, and Dariush Mozaffarian. 2022. "The Time Is Ripe for ESG+Nutrition: Evidence-Based Nutrition Metrics for Environmental, Social, and Governance (ESG) Investing." *European Journal of Clinical Nutrition* 76: 1047–52.

Okunogbe, Adeyemi, Rachel Nugent, Garrison Spencer, Jaynaide Powis, Johanna Ralston, and John Wilding. 2022. "Economic Impacts of Overweight and Obesity: Current and Future Estimates for 161 Countries." *BMJ Global Health* 7: e009773. https://doi.org/10.1136/bmjgh-2022-009773.

Olayanju, Julia B. 2019. "Top Trends Driving Change in the Food Industry." *Forbes*, February 16, 2019. https://www.forbes.com/sites/juliabolayanju/2019/02/16/top-trends-driving-change-in-the-food-industry/.

Osendarp, Saskia, Jonathan Kweku Akuoku, Robert E. Black, Derek Heady, Marie Ruel, Nick Scott, Meera Shekar, et al. 2021. "The COVID-19 Crisis Will Exacerbate Maternal and Child Undernutrition and Child Mortality in Low- and Middle-Income Countries." *Nature Food* 2 (7): 476–84.

Ozer, Ceren, Danielle Bloom, Adolfo Martinez Valle, Eduardo Banzon, Kate Madeville, Jeremias Paul, Evan Blecher, et al. 2020. "Health Earmarks and Health Taxes: What Do We Know?" World Bank Health, Nutrition and Population Knowledge Brief. World Bank, Washington, DC.

Piatti-Fünfkirchen, Moritz, Ali Winoto Subandoro, Timothy Williamson, and Kyoko Shibata Okamura. 2023. *Driving Nutrition Action through the Budget: A Guide to Nutrition Responsive Budgeting*. Washington, DC: World Bank. http://hdl.handle.net/10986/39856.

Shekar, Meera, Jakub Kakietek, Julia Dayton Eberwein, and Dylan Walters. 2017. *An Investment Framework for Nutrition: Reaching the Global Targets for Stunting, Anemia, Breastfeeding, and Wasting*. Washington, DC: World Bank. https://doi.org/10.1596/978-1-4648-1010-7.

Shekar, Meera, Meghan O'Hearn, Ellina Knudsen, Kenji Shibuya, Simon Bishop, Hélène van Berchem, Christopher Egerton-Warburton, et al. 2023. "Innovative Financing for Nutrition." *Nature Food* 4: 464–71.

Smith, Julie Patricia, Phillip Baker, Roger Mathisen, Aoife Long, Nigel Rollins, and Marilyn Waring. 2024. "A Proposal to Recognize Investment in Breastfeeding as a Carbon Offset." *Bulletin of the World Health Organization* 102 (5): 336–43. https://doi.org/10.2471/BLT.23.290210.

Subandoro, Ali Winoto, Kyoko S. Okamura, Michelle Mehta, Huihui Wang, Naina Ahluwalia, Elyssa Finkel, Andrea L. S. Bulungu, et al. 2022. "Positioning Nutrition with Universal Health Coverage: Optimizing Health Financing Levers." Health, Nutrition and Population Discussion Paper, World Bank, Washington, DC.

Sutton, William R., Alexander Lotsch, and Ashesh Prasann. 2024. *Recipe for a Livable Planet: Achieving Net Zero Emissions in the Agrifood System*. Agriculture and Food Series, Conference Edition. Washington, DC: World Bank.

SWF Academy. 2024. "Global SWF Data Platform." New York: SWF Academy. Accessed May 27, 2024, https://globalswf.com/.

UNICEF (United Nations Children's Fund). n.d. "The Child Nutrition Fund." New York: UNICEF. https://www.unicef.org/child-health-and-survival /the-child-nutrition-fund.

United Kingdom, Foreign, Commonwealth & Development Office. 2024. "Statistics on International Development: Final UK Aid Spend 2022." East Kilbride, UK, Foreign, Commonwealth & Development Office. https://www.gov.uk /government/statistics/statistics-on-international-development-final-uk-aid -spend-2022/statistics-on-international-development-final-uk-aid -spend-2022.

Wang, Huihui, Kyoko Shibata Okamura, Ali Winoto Subandoro, Yurie Tanimich Hoberg, Lubina Fatimah Quereshy, and Mamata Ghimire. 2022. *A Guiding Framework for Nutrition Public Expenditure Reviews*. International Development in Practice. Washington, DC: World Bank.

Watson, Charlene, and Liane Schalatek. 2023. "The Global Climate Finance Architecture." Climate Finance Fundamentals 2. Washington, DC: Climate Funds Update. https://climatefundsupdate.org/about-climate-finance /climate-finance-fundamentals/.

Watson, Charlene, and Liane Schalatek. 2024. "10 Things to Know about Climate Finance (2024)." Washington, DC: Climate Funds Update. https:// climatefundsupdate.org/about-climate-finance/10-things-to-know -about-climate-finance/.

WHO (World Health Organization). 2021. *Global Expenditure on Health: Public Spending on the Rise?* Geneva: World Health Organization.

WHO (World Health Organization). 2022. *Strategic Purchasing for Nutrition in Primary Health Care: Overview*. Geneva: World Health Organization.

World Bank. 2021. "Food Finance Architecture: Financing a Healthy, Equitable, and Sustainable Food System." Washington, DC: World Bank. http://documents .worldbank.org/curated/en/879401632342154766/Food-Finance-Architecture -Financing-a-Healthy-Equitable-and-Sustainable-Food-System.

World Bank. n.d. "Food Systems 2030: Overview." Washington, DC: World Bank. https://www.worldbank.org/en/programs/food-systems-2030/overview.

World Benchmarking Alliance. 2021. "Food and Agriculture Benchmark." London: World Benchmarking Alliance. https://www.worldbenchmarkingalliance.org /food-and-agriculture-benchmark/.

Yates, Joe, Stuart Gillespie, Natalie Savona, Megan Deeney, and Suneetha Kadiyala. 2021. "Trust and Responsibility in Food Systems Transformation. Engaging with Big Food: Marriage or Mirage?" *BMJ Global Health* 6 (11): e007350.

ECO-AUDIT
Environmental Benefits Statement

The World Bank Group is committed to reducing its environmental footprint. In support of this commitment, we leverage electronic publishing options and print-on-demand technology, which is located in regional hubs worldwide. Together, these initiatives enable print runs to be lowered and shipping distances decreased, resulting in reduced paper consumption, chemical use, greenhouse gas emissions, and waste.

We follow the recommended standards for paper use set by the Green Press Initiative. The majority of our books are printed on Forest Stewardship Council (FSC)–certified paper, with nearly all containing 50–100 percent recycled content. The recycled fiber in our book paper is either unbleached or bleached using totally chlorine-free (TCF), processed chlorine–free (PCF), or enhanced elemental chlorine–free (EECF) processes.

More information about the Bank's environmental philosophy can be found at http://www.worldbank.org/corporateresponsibility.

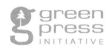